Go Dairy Free

The Guide and Cookbook for Milk Allergies, Lactose Intolerance, and Casein-Free Living

By Alisa Marie Fleming

Important Note from the Publisher

Copyright © 2008 by Alisa Fleming
Cover Designed by Andrea Schaaf
Cover Photography by Hannah Kaminsky

ISBN-10: 0-9791286-2-5
ISBN-13: 978-0-9791286-2-2

Printed in the United States
Published by Fleming Marrs, Inc
Henderson, Nevada

Table of Contents

My Story

Over the years, so many of you have been kind enough to email me with your dairy-free stories. You have even allowed me to post them on www.godairyfree.org, offering others a place for inspiration. I feel it only fair that I share my story with you, now …

At the age of 33, as I was in the midst of working on this guidebook, my father handed me a baby book he found while cleaning out some boxes. It was mine, but I had never seen it before. As it fell open in my hands, the first words I laid eyes upon were "4 months – Allergic to milk." I am not sure whether I was more amazed that it flipped right to that page, or that it took me decades to discover this fact for myself, the one that was so casually and plainly written in those memoirs.

My parents knew that I had a milk allergy as an infant, but the doctors assured them that such a thing is always quickly outgrown, not lasting past that first year … no testing required. In my childhood, it was never spoken of.

You might be wondering, how someone could live so long with a milk allergy and not know it. Fortunately, I hated almost all dairy; milk, cheese (yes, seriously), and cream ranked at the very bottom of my food-craving list. I naturally avoided most dairy on my own, instinctually … unless it was out of my control; I was a child after all.

Plus, there were symptoms, many symptoms during those uncontrollable times. Ear infections (including surgery), eczema, frequent and often violent illness, gastrointestinal symptoms, sudden bouts of weakness, and sporadic breathing difficulties … all written off as an unlucky childhood, though I missed more days of school than any of my classmates. In fact, during the final quarter of my senior year in high school, the vice-principal called me in to offer a kind word of warning that I was one missed school day away from not graduating, even though I liked school, was active in sports, and maintained good grades.

Yet, I still wasn't prepared for what lay ahead, in my twenties, when the doctors insisted that I must increase my dairy intake "for the sake of my bones." I reluctantly obliged, adding tolerable things like frozen yogurt and chocolate milk to my daily regime, and slowly working myself up to cheese. The next five years brought a continuous downward spiral in my health. During everyday activities, I would suddenly become severely ill, followed by weakness and pain, and if I tried to stand, I would lose consciousness. On a few unfortunate occasions, I had convulsions. My trips to the emergency room were becoming more frequent, until not a week passed without a visit. Yet, the doctors had no answers. There were blood tests, MRI's, EKG's, and heart monitors, but I was deemed "healthy." I was scared, and my husband could no longer hide his own fear.

It was only by luck that I stumbled across a western doctor who believed in alternative medicine and diet as treatment. In my first visit he sat with me for a full 90 minutes, asking all types of questions, from medical to psychological. At the end of the time, he said, "Have you tried cutting out milk?" I thought he was insane. That's it? I am having what feel like near death experiences, and that's all you've got?! I nearly walked out, but my husband said, "Why not? *We* should give it a try." Yes, that wonderful man went dairy-free with me.

Within three days, all of my symptoms ceased, and to this day, over five dairy-free years later, they have not returned. It felt like nothing short of a miracle. Of course, since I still wanted "real proof" (stubborn as I am) the doctor ordered a food allergy test. Sure enough, I was in fact allergic to milk, specifically casein (milk protein). Those test results could have brought on disappointment and stress, but I was elated. I had an answer and I felt better than I had in years.

I began researching the dairy-free diet like a madwoman. At that time, the data was actually quite difficult to find, but I wanted to know everything about how to live healthfully and actually enjoy a life free from dairy.

In all honesty, many external factors did make the transition difficult. My stint on a dairy-rich diet quickly created an ice cream addiction that I had to overcome. Plus, grocery shopping, dining out, and social gatherings with friends added some unexpected complications.

The good news is that it all became easy, very easy. My dairy cravings gradually melted away, and my diet is now rich with more delicious foods than I ever would have imagined. Just like riding a bicycle, living dairy-free has become very natural and virtually effortless. Yet, even after I felt my own life was well under control, I knew there was still some purpose for all of the information I had gathered. Thinking that perhaps a *few* others would find my data and recipes useful, I created www.godairyfree.org to be an online information resource for living without milk.

It seems I was right, but perhaps I did underestimate things just a bit. From July 2006 to June 2008 (I didn't have any website data prior to that time in 2006), www.godairyfree.org received half a million visitors and over 2.5 million hits, as people stuck around to read various pages. Each month, as the word gets out, the traffic continues to grow. It is so exciting to see how many other people this information is helping. Though I could have been content with working on the website, I knew that a more in-depth, offline resource could aid even more people ... and thus, this guidebook was born.

Since some of you might be wondering, no I don't bother with testing for my milk allergy these days. Even if I did someday, miraculously "outgrow" it, I would remain dairy-free. Both my husband and I are much healthier for it.

Best Wishes,
Alisa Marie Fleming

P.S. – Go Dairy Free the website (www.godairyfree.org) is updated every week (typically every day) with new product reviews, recipes, news articles, announcements, discounts ... really anything that I think might be useful for free-from dieters. Much of the content is written by yours truly, but I do have several wonderful, regular contributors, and I always welcome reviews, personal stories, recommendations, and recipes from you. Not to mention, I enjoy fielding your dairy-free questions. If you have anything to share, or you are looking for an answer, don't hesitate to email me at alisa@godairyfree.org.

A Great Big Thank You

What would any book be without a special thank you to all those who have helped and inspired? While I could begin with a long list, no one deserves my kind words more than my loving husband. To him I dedicate this book. Without a moment's hesitation, my cheese-loving hero abandoned all dairy in his diet for me. He has been my encouragement and inspiration (not to mention my web designer and tech support); if it weren't for him (and some of his nagging) this book never would have been written.

In terms of guidance, I must thank the vegan community as a whole. Following the 80/20 rule, vegans are a mere subsection of what would seem to be an enormous dairy-free community, yet they have contributed so many of the most helpful resources, recipes, and food products. Since the vegan diet has provided so much assistance to the much larger but less cohesive dairy-free community, I felt it only fair to make this guidebook as vegan-friendly as possible, without straying from the more expansive dairy-free theme. So to all you vegans who have honored me by purchasing this guidebook, thank you, and I hope you enjoy it!

Of course a special thank you goes out to my most devoted vegan contributor, Hannah. Her passion and kindness is a blessing ... and trust me, you will love the recipes she has created just for this book. I also want to thank Sarah, my most trusted recipe tester, editor, and mom to a milk allergic daughter, and Barb, a good friend who is a big help with the "little" details. While I would love to continue giving out heartfelt thanks to hundreds of people, it could get rather lengthy and boring, so I apologize if I miss anyone! I must thank my family for always being supportive, Dr. Cyrus Pourzan for thinking outside of the box, my wonderful friends from Lake Tahoe for never quite "getting" me, but always being there, and Rosey, my cat and muse.

In this industry I have come across so many wonderful people (hundreds if not thousands) who haven't hesitated to answer my many questions. Therefore, you can consider the resources section of this book to be one giant "thank you" chapter. It is filled with people, books, blogs, and websites that have brought me guidance and delight over the years. However, from this section I must highlight a special group, all ladies as it happens. These talented women were kind enough to share a favorite recipe (or three) or some words of wisdom, to give you a sampling of their work, whether it is a fabulous cookbook, website, or foodie blog:

Hannah Kaminsky, author of *My Sweet Vegan*
Sarah Hatfield of No Whey Mama
Barb Nicoletti, Go Dairy Free Reviewer
Celine Steen of Have Cake Will Travel
Susan Voisin of Fat Free Vegan
Karina Allrich of Karina's Kitchen
Melisser Elliott of The Urban Housewife
Gina Clowes of Allergy Moms
Nicole Smith of Allergic Child
Julie Hasson of Everyday Dish TV
Liz Stark of VeggieGirl
Ricki Heller of Diet, Dessert, and Dogs
Janet L. Doane of The Healing Feast
Jennifer McCann, author of *Vegan Lunch Box*
Dayna McIsaac of Vegan Visitor
Sloane Miller of Allergic Girl Resources
Sarena Shasteen of The Non-Dairy Queen
Amy of What Do I Eat Now?
Jill Robbins, author of *Allergen Free Baking*
Meghan Telpner of the National Post

Cynthia Mosher of VegFamily
jae steele (yes, lower case), author of *Get it Ripe*
Jo Stepaniak, author of numerous vegan cookbooks
Emily Hendrix, author of *Sophie-Safe Cooking*
Linda Coss, author of several food allergy books
Dreena Burton, author of several vegan cookbooks
Cybele Pascal, author of *The Whole Foods Allergy Cookbook*
Levana Kirschenbaum, author of *Levana Cooks Dairy-Free!*
Robin Robertson, author of several vegan cookbooks
Rachel Albert-Matesz, author of *The Ice Dream Cookbook*
Cathe Olson, author of *The Vegetarian Mother's Cookbook*
Beverly Lynn Bennett, author of several vegan cookbooks
Bryanna Clark Grogan, author of several vegan cookbooks

Section 1

Understanding Dairy & Dairy-Free From a Health Perspective

CHAPTER 1:
WHAT IS DAIRY?

As you venture into the world of non-dairy, you will likely be confronted with a barrage of news and information on cow milk and various other types of milk on the market. Arming yourself with enough information to understand dairy and its alternatives will allow you to feel confident in your choices. That said ...

With respect to the American diet, dairy most often refers to cow milk and its derivatives. Typical dairy foods produced from cow milk include cheese, butter, yogurt, and cream. However, cow milk has many purposes in our food supply well beyond these obvious applications. The proteins, fat, and sugar within cow milk are commonly extracted for use in processed foods to add flavor, structure, or other enhancements. Additional mammal milks, which are less common in western societies, may also fall under the dairy header. I will address several of these later in this chapter.

Individuals who follow a general non-dairy diet may opt to restrict only whole dairy foods, such as milk, cheese, and cream. Those who follow a strict dairy-free diet would also cut out processed foods that are manufactured with milk ingredients of any kind (proteins, sugars, etc.). The rare few who have severe milk allergies or intolerances may need to scrutinize products down to the manufacturing processes. Even trace amounts of milk (parts per million) may elicit a reaction in the highly sensitive. For these individuals, cross-contamination of milk in production must be ruled out prior to consumption of any packaged foods.

Though frequently found in the dairy section, eggs are not technically a dairy food. Due to the nutritional make-up of eggs, it would make more sense to classify them with meat rather than milk. Aside from those who follow a vegan diet or who have an egg allergy or intolerance, eggs are suitable for dairy-free dieters. Nonetheless, to accommodate those who follow a vegan diet, or who have multiple food allergies, I have written this guide to accommodate both dairy and egg-free diets. A few of the recipes do contain or suggest eggs for a superior product, but in those cases a tested egg-free option or alternate recipe is offered. See the food allergy index on p277 for specifics.

To the best of my knowledge any food or recipe referred to within this guide is made without any milk ingredients. However, you should always check ingredient labels prior to consumption, and if necessary, check the manufacturing processes for cross-contamination concerns. Ingredients, products, and processes are subject to change by the manufacturer at any time. Yes, you will catch me repeating this phrase on many occasions.

What Makes Milk So Special?

As it comes from cows, milk has many nutrients. After all, its natural purpose is for the development of calves, just as breast milk is intended for the development of human babies. Interestingly, humans are the only mammals that consume milk past infancy, let alone milk from another species. Nonetheless, since milk has become such a staple in the American diet, it is important to understand what nutrients we have come to rely on it for, and how to ensure a milk-free diet provides adequate nutrition.

Let's start with a little Milk 101. Cow milk can be broken down into seven major components:

Water

Cow milk boasts approximately 88% water. Basic as it may seem, if you have been consuming one or more glasses of cow milk in a day, be sure to replace it with a liquid that is equally hydrating. Of course, plain old water will do the trick.

As an interesting side note, it takes up to 2000 gallons of water (for the day to day functions of a dairy cow) to produce just one gallon of cow milk. That excess water could surely provide a great deal of hydration, since your water needs will undoubtedly be quite a bit less than the dairy cow's.

Protein

Cow milk contains roughly 3 to 4% protein, of which about 80% is casein and 20% is whey. Unfortunately, both casein and whey are top allergen sources. For non-meat eaters, several beans, nuts, and even grains (quinoa is a personal favorite) can serve as excellent sources of protein. I will also address protein-rich foods and protein powders beginning on p58; many wonderful options have emerged which are dairy-free and often soy-free.

Fat

Naturally, the fat content of cow milk can range from 3% to 6%. In the United States, whole milk must contain at least 3.25% milk fat, while caps of 2%, 1%, and 0.5% milk fat are regulated for reduced fat, low-fat, and skim varieties, respectively.

This doesn't sound too bad, but the fat content is actually much higher than we perceive. These percentages are by weight, not calories. This means that the 88% water is not only diluting the milk itself, but also the percentage of fat. Whole milk derives 50% of its calories from fat, 2% milk gets 35% of its calories from fat; 1% milk weighs in with 23% of its calories from fat; and skim milk is the lone lightweight with 5% of calories from fat. Keep in mind; the fat in milk is mostly saturated (not the heart-healthy kind). Too little consumption of saturated fat is rarely a problem in our society.

However, I have received countless emails from moms who are concerned about weight gain in their little ones. During growth and even times of illness, receiving adequate amounts of fat can be a crucial issue. Since North Americans and Europeans tend to rely heavily on milk products for dietary fat, alternative fatty food options may be required. I go into more detail on this topic beginning on p57, and you can read more about the various oils in the butter alternatives chapter on p111.

Carbohydrate

When it comes to fiber and complex carbohydrates, milk is not a top contender. It contains sugar, lactose to be specific. Approximately 5% of milk is sugar, and not the fun, sweet kind either. In fact, a glass of milk contains half the sugar found in a serving of soda pop! Lactose is also a significant source of suffering for up to 70% of the world's population. More on this topic later, but for now, getting enough sugar and carbs probably isn't high on your concern list.

Water-Soluble Vitamins

Natural, raw milk contains a fair amount of C and B vitamins. However, during pasteurization most of the Vitamin C is weakened or destroyed, and about 38% of the B vitamins suffer a similar fate. Better sources of these vitamins can be found in a diet full of fresh fruits, vegetables, and grains, with the exception of vitamin B12. Vitamin B12 is primarily found in animal-based foods, such as meat, fish, and dairy, but there are a few alternative sources. Nutritional yeast (a popular cheesy addition to dairy-free recipes) contains a generous supply of B vitamins, including B12, and many breakfast cereals and milk substitutes are fortified with B12. Nonetheless, vegans or those who seldom consume meat or fish may need to consider supplementation of vitamin B12.

Fat-Soluble Vitamins

Cow milk contains the fat-soluble vitamins A, D, E, and a very small amount of K. However, these vitamins are removed with the fat in the production of reduced fat, low-fat, and nonfat milks.

To counteract one of these deficiencies, dairy farmers are required to fortify low-fat and nonfat milks with at least 2,000 IU of vitamin A per quart. There is just one BIG problem with this. A moderate to high intake of Vitamin A (specifically retinol, rather than plant carotenes) has now been linked to an increased risk for hip fracture. Scientists speculate that the Vitamin A used to fortify most milk may actually interfere with the activity of Vitamin D, a crucial bone-building nutrient. Better sources of Vitamin A, in the form of beta-carotenes, are incredibly abundant in greens (spinach, kale, etc.), carrots, red bell peppers, and sweet potatoes.

As for Vitamin D, dairy farmers may choose to fortify with vitamin D (it is not required), but if they do, then it must be at least 400 IU per quart. These days, most milk alternative manufacturers also fortify their products with Vitamin D. Plus Vitamin D can be absorbed via 15 minutes of sunshine per day (or even just a few times per week). If you live in a gloomy place, it may be wise to take a Vitamin D supplement. If you are a vegan living in a gloomy place, a multivitamin may be warranted.

Minerals

The primary minerals in milk are phosphorous and calcium. The body needs to maintain a perfect balance of phosphorous and calcium; when too much of one is present, it depletes the other. High blood phosphate levels are the top concern in westernized diets, which are rich in dietary phosphorous in the form of carbonated beverages and processed foods. Too much phosphorus can reduce the body's ability to utilize Vitamin D (convert it into its active form), reduce blood calcium levels, and eventually lead to poor bone mineral content. As you might expect, this could have a negative effect on the growth and development of little ones, and could promote osteoporosis later in life.

Since westernized diets tend to rely on milk for the bulk of calcium intake, the calcium/phosphorus balance can be further upset when dairy-free consumers substitute milk with carbonated beverages, which happens all too often. Carbonated beverages are typically high in phosphoric acid, yet void of calcium.

Luckily, some wise food and beverage choices can ensure that your mineral intake is adequate for healthy bones while maintaining a milk-free diet. For starters, skip the soda. Enjoy some good old H2O as a beverage substitute for milk, and consume a balanced diet that includes healthy, dairy-free sources of calcium. An entire chapter is dedicated to the discussion of calcium later in this book (beginning on p38.), which includes a chart of milk-free foods that can help you reach your calcium quota.

So what does make milk so special? It certainly isn't the proteins, saturated fat, sugar, phosphorous, or Vitamin A. Milk is touted almost exclusively for its calcium, B Vitamins, fortified Vitamin D, and water. A well balanced diet and some occasional sunshine will supply the dairy-free individual with each of these essential nutrients. Plus, the various non-dairy milks on the market are frequently fortified with calcium, vitamin D, and B vitamins. If in doubt take a multivitamin, even milk drinkers do!

Organic Milk is it worth it?

Organic milk is still cow milk. It contains all of the same proteins (i.e. casein), fats (i.e. saturated), sugars (i.e. lactose), and cholesterol that may be problematic for allergies, intolerances, special diets, and/or general health. However, for those who can and do consume even small amounts of dairy, organic milk products appear to be well worth the extra cost.

Milk repeatedly makes the top ten lists for foods you should buy organic, and for good reason. Beyond dangerous pesticides, U.S. Organic Milk is also produced without the use of added antibiotics and hormones. Are hormones and antibiotics in the foods supply a true concern, or has the issue been stretched a bit too far by organic farmers and anti-milk campaigners? I was curious to know, so I pooled together some unbiased facts as evidenced by regulations and scientific studies.

Whether you would like to include some dairy products in your diet, or you could use another reason to go dairy-free, the following offers some important information on hormones and antibiotics in the dairy industry that you may find interesting:

Why Dairy Farmers Use Synthetic Hormones....
~ Bovine Growth Hormone, or BGH, is a naturally occurring hormone in cows that stimulates the production of another hormone, IGF-1 (insulin-like growth factor-1). IGF-1 in turn initiates the production of milk.
~ The FDA approved the use of rBGH, a synthetic version of BGH, in 1993. The injection of rBGH into cows has become standard practice on many dairy farms, as it has the ability to unnaturally increase a cow's output of milk by up to 20% (according to the rBGH manufacturer). Higher production per cow means a better bottom line for the dairy farmer.

The Effects of Synthetic Hormone Use on Humans....
~ Cows treated with rBGH produce greater levels of IGF-1. In fact, numerous studies have confirmed that cows treated with rBGH produce milk with 2 to 10 times the levels of IGF-1 found in untreated cow milk.
~ The IGF-1 found in cows is a bio-identical hormone to the IGF-1 produced by humans.
~ Dairy supporters argue that the IGF-1 in milk is not absorbed into the body; however, the consumption of cow milk has been scientifically shown to increase the serum level of IGF-1 in humans by 10%. In contradiction of their prior claims, the Dairy Council has even utilized a study confirming this increase in IGF-1 as a supporting document for bone health.
~ Higher levels of IGF-1 in humans have been linked to a significantly increased risk of prostate, colon, lung and breast cancer.

Other Consequences of Hormone Use....
~ Cows treated with rBGH were found to have a 25% increased risk of acquiring an udder infection (mastitis). Other major side effects (as noted by the manufacturer of rBGH) include infertility, lameness, cystic ovaries, uterine disorders, digestive disorders, lacerations, and calluses of the knee.

Cue the Antibiotics...
~ An increase in infections results in an increase of antibiotic use, both legal and illegal.
~ Antibiotic residues in milk may cause allergic reactions in sensitive individuals, and may be an important factor in the growth of antibiotic resistant bacteria.
~ Testing for antibiotics is limited in its effectiveness. Mandatory screenings by milk processors are only for a few select antibiotics (while dozens of types are in use). Additional testing is randomized and on more of an "audit" level.
~ Even for those batches that pass inspection, low levels of antibiotic residues are typically permitted. The effects of these low levels, in addition to the potential antibiotic levels of untested milk, are largely unknown, but greatly feared.
~ In 2001, 6.7 million pounds of milk were dumped in Minnesota alone due to the detection of antibiotic residue. This was only from the 10% of loads randomly inspected on a quarterly review. You might either be shocked by the idea of how much "tainted" milk may have gone untested and continued on into our milk supply, or by the incredible amount of waste. Waste, which may have potentially negated the "increased production" from the use of rBGH. And so the cycle continues.

Though hotly contested by the United States, the European Union has maintained a ban on the use of rBGH since 1985. They have deemed rBGH as unsafe for public health and from a veterinary perspective. In 1999, Codex Alimentarius (the United Nations' food safety organization), ruled in favor of the European moratorium on hormone treated milk products. Australia, New Zealand, and Canada have upheld a similar ban on the use of hormones in the dairy industry. So why on earth did the FDA approve rBGH, and why are dairy farmers in the United States, Mexico, and South Africa still routinely administering it? We as consumers are still waiting for an answer.

Those who do consume conventional dairy products should use caution; dairy farmers within the United States are not currently required to disclose the use of rBGH on their labeling. In fact, some states have attempted to block manufacturers from disclosing on the package if they do not use rBGH.

Beyond synthetic hormones, it is still unclear how the growth hormones that naturally occur in the milk of untreated cows affect humans in the long run. Some may opt to follow a dairy-free diet for this very reason. However, for those who can and choose to consume some milk products, reach for organic or at the very least those products specified as rBGH free. Be aware though, that these dairy products are still subject to pasteurization and homogenization ...

What is Pasteurization & Homogenization?

What is Pasteurization?
According to the U.S. Centers for Disease Control (CDC), pasteurization is "the process of heating milk or other liquids to destroy microorganisms that can cause disease or spoilage." During pasteurization, raw milk is heated to 145ºF for 30 minutes, 163ºF for 15 seconds (Flash Pasteurization), or 285ºF for a second or two (Ultra High Temperature (UHT) Pasteurization). It is estimated that pasteurization kills 95 to 99% of pathogenic bacteria in milk. What about the other 1 to 4%? I digress.

On the typical dairy farm, unpasteurized milk can be a source of tuberculosis, diphtheria, salmonellas, typhoid fever, undulant fever, Q fever, and listeria. Pasteurization is also a handy way to increase the shelf life of refrigerated milk. The FDA requires that all packaged or bottled milk shipped interstate be pasteurized.

What Could Be Wrong With Pasteurization?
This is quite a controversial question. A few of the typical responses are:

~   It allows otherwise "unfit" milk to be given to the general public.
~   It strips away many of the essential vitamins.
~   It destroys "beneficial" bacteria, leaving behind small amounts of dangerous bacteria and germs, which are now free to multiply.
~   Its introduction can be directly correlated with a sudden increase in the incidence of heart disease.
~   It alters the nutrients in milk, creating more "allergies."

Although few studies are readily available regarding pasteurization and disease, it is well proven that pasteurization destroys and alters many beneficial nutrients. Plus, dairy farmers who pasteurize are blessed with more relaxed regulations on their sanitary practices and the quality of milk they use, as it is assumed that the pasteurization will take care of things.

What is Homogenization?
Homogenization is really just "pretty packaging." Natural milk separates, leaving skim milk on the bottom and a thick layer of cream on top. This cream can be easily skimmed off, similar to the layer of coconut cream that

forms atop an unshaken can of coconut milk. However, the westernized palate looked down on this type of presentation, so the food industry responded with process of homogenization to give milk that consistent, creamy look. Homogenized milk has been forced through ultrafine mesh at high pressure to break up the milk fat globules and disperse them evenly throughout the milk, thereby creating a uniform product. Wait a minute; milk is actually a processed food? Sad, but true, the milk as we see it in the refrigerated section is a far cry from natural or raw milk.

While it does in fact look better, it doesn't take a heart surgeon to point out (although a good one will) that whole foods are a much better choice than processed foods. Processing destroys healthy vitamins and minerals and actually alters the state of many nutrients in a way that is not fully understood. Homogenization showed up on the scene around the same time as pasteurization. Therefore, many physicians believe it may also be linked to the increased incidence of high cholesterol and heart disease.

Homogenized milk has also been accused of harboring more casein and whey proteins. This could be a potential factor in the substantial rise in milk allergies over the past few decades.

Is Raw Milk a Good Alternative?
Many dairy-based health enthusiasts promote the consumption of raw milk over commercial brands. Like organic milk, raw milk is expected to be free of hormones and antibiotics. However, dairy farmers of raw milk take "natural" one step further. Unlike organic and conventional cow milk, raw milk is not homogenized or pasteurized.

Some proponents of raw milk do feel that it is a safe solution for the prevention of milk allergies and heart disease. Since raw milk is in fact cow milk, many more studies would need to be conducted before these bold claims could be validated. It still harbors a good amount of lactose and allergenic proteins, and it may not be suitable for those who forgo milk for social or religious reasons. Plus, raw milk can be very difficult to find, expensive to purchase, and the jury is still out on if it is truly "fit" for human consumption. The U.S. Department of Health and Human Services still expresses concern that contaminated raw milk may be a source of harmful bacteria and illness.

When I last checked, raw milk was available to purchase for human consumption on farms in 28 states. Each state has varying levels of restrictions. Raw milk may be purchased in retail stores within California, Connecticut, Maine, New Mexico, Arizona, Washington, and South Carolina. All 50 states permit the sale of raw milk cheeses that are aged for at least 60 days.

What is Acidophilus Milk?

Acidophilus milk has the same nutritional make-up as the milk from which it is made, most often cow milk. It differs in that the bacterium Lactobacillus acidophilus, a common probiotic (aka "good bacteria"), has been added directly to the milk to theoretically aid in digestion.

Traditionally, the bacterium was added to the milk, which was then fermented to create acidophilus cultured milk. This process did lower the lactose level in the milk, but it also increased the acidity of the milk, consequently resulting in a sour flavor that was unappealing to most taste buds.

To combat the flavor issues, a new process was developed to grow the bacterial culture first and then add it to the milk, skipping the acid forming fermentation altogether. The result was the product we see most commonly on store shelves today, Sweet Acidophilus Milk (SAM). Unfortunately, this "sweet" version retains the same lactose level as regular milk.

SAM proponents argue that the acidophilus aids in digestion regardless of the production process. However, a study reported in the American Journal of Nutrition showed that although SAM does contain lactase-rich organisms, it does not enhance lactose digestion.

If you are lactose intolerant, and very interested in finding a cow milk substitute, then it may be worth your while to seek out traditionally fermented acidophilus milk, but sweet acidophilus milk will likely yield no benefits. None of these options will be suitable for those who are milk allergic or who are cutting milk for other health, social, or religious reasons.

What is Kefir?

Kefir is another interesting option for lactose intolerant individuals. It is an obscure substitute for milk that likens itself to a drinkable yogurt. In fact, kefir's benefits are very similar to yogurt.

Kefir contains a high level of probiotics (that "good bacteria" again), which aides in digestion. Like yogurt (but unlike SAM), kefir is a cultured or fermented product, and studies have shown that it typically produces little to no digestive symptoms when ingested by lactose intolerant individuals. Kefir is not a cure for lactose intolerance, nor is it lactose-free, but rather a tolerant food for some who may crave a little mammal milk. Use caution though, as neither yogurt nor kefir is a safe haven for all lactose intolerant individuals.

Originally, kefir was made from camel milk. Today, you are more likely to find commercially available kefir that is made from the milk of sheep, goats, or cows, though soy versions of kefir have emerged. Both kefir and regular yogurt are considered good sources of calcium, potassium, and protein, and both can provide a helpful dose of probiotics, though studies show that kefir contains a wider array of these digestion-boosting bacteria than yogurt.

Store-bought kefir, aside from the soy-based versions, is not believed to be a good choice for those who are seeking a milk alternative for reasons other than lactose intolerance. While you can make homemade kefir using other liquids, such as coconut water, almond milk, and even lemonade, it is very difficult to find dairy-free kefir starter powder or granules. They do best when cultured on dairy milk, and likewise when stored in milk for reuse. I have been told that any traces of dairy from the starter granules are eliminated during the fermentation process, but it is up to the individual on whether this is a worthwhile and "safe" option. If you are interested in experimenting with kefir, see the Body Ecology website (www.bodyecology.com).

What is Lactose-Free Milk?

There are no major secrets to lactose-free milk. It is simply milk with all of its original properties, minus the lactose. So how do they do it? Rather than simply pasteurizing the raw milk, the dairy-farmers ultra-pasteurize it. They basically turn up the heat. They then add lactase to the milk, a natural enzyme that converts lactose into glucose and galactose. Since lactose intolerant individuals are short on their own internal lactase supplies, the dairies are in essence pre-digesting the lactose in milk for them.

Lactose-free milk is another product that should only be considered by the lactose intolerant. It won't be suitable for those with milk protein allergies or for those who forgo dairy for religious, social, or other health reasons.

What is A2 Milk?

There are three types of casein proteins in milk: alpha, kappa and beta-caseins. A2 milk addresses the latter of the three, beta-caseins. There are two major types of beta-caseins, and they are affectionately referred to as A1 and A2. Cow milk (and other mammal milks) can differ in their proportions of A1 and A2 beta-caseins, but milk designated as "a2 milk™" has been tested to ensure that it contains a higher proportion of A2 than regular milk.

Why is this important? There have been claims circulating that a2 milk™ might be less allergenic for those who have an allergy to the casein proteins in standard A1 cow's milk. This theory is compared to the fact that goat milk, which has a higher ratio of A2 beta-casein, is tolerated by some milk allergic individuals. Unfortunately, this concept has not been formally tested, to date, and even the company who owns the trademark to a2 milk™, A2 Corporation (yes, that is their real name), says that these claims are unwarranted. According to the A2 Corporation's website (www.a2corporation.com), both regular cow milk and a2 milk™ contain the casein proteins indicated in milk allergies, and they are unaware of any reason why a2 milk™ would cause a reduction in allergic reactions.

Also, in contrast to the aforementioned milk products, a2 milk™ has shown no benefits for those with lactose intolerance. It differs only in its protein make-up, and still contains comparable levels of lactose to standard cow milk. At the time of writing, the distribution of a2 milk™ was limited to New Zealand, Australia and select locations in the United States.

Are Other Mammal Milks the Same as Cow Milk?

Over the past few years, many claims have emerged about the hypoallergenic nature of various mammal milks. While these "better than cow milk" statements may sound ludicrous ... at least they did to me ... research has shown that a few might actually hold a grain (or should I say drop?) of truth. Scientists have found that the allergenic nature of certain animal food proteins could lie in how related they are to their equivalent human protein.

In theory, all proteins have the potential to become allergenic, but a study out of the Institute of Food Research in Norwich and the Medical University of Vienna found that the ability of a particular animal food protein to trigger a food allergy might correlate with its "evolutionary distance" from a human equivalent.

The researchers sought to define how closely an animal protein must resemble its human counterpart to lose its allergenic potential. In general, proteins that were more than 62% identical to a human equivalent were rarely allergenic, while those that fell below the 54% marker had a much higher ability to become allergenic. The more distant proteins may hinder the ability of the human immune system to discriminate between foreign and self-proteins, resulting in immune responses that are otherwise known as allergy symptoms.

This study does shed light on why cow and goat milks, which both fall under the 54% identical mark, are fairly prevalent food allergens; while mare (horse) milk is up to 66% identical to human milk proteins, and can often be tolerated by the milk allergic. The researchers are very hopeful that their extensive findings will bring them closer to a vaccine for food allergies.

Since a bit more can be said about the mammal milks currently on the market, I will continue ...

Goat Milk

Goat milk is slightly closer in composition to human milk than cow milk is, with proteins that may be easier to digest. It is estimated that 20 to 40% of milk allergic individuals do not react to goat milk. However, milk allergic individuals should obtain an allergy test prior to trialing, as most people who are allergic to cow milk have similar reactions to goat milk. Plus, a rare few are in fact more allergic to goat milk.

Nonetheless, there are some additional benefits of goat milk, which are worth noting. Unlike cow milk, goat milk does not contain agglutinin, a substance that clusters fat globules together and makes them more difficult to digest. Goat milk is also higher in calcium, vitamin B-6, potassium, and niacin than cow milk. However, it is significantly lower in vitamin B-12 and folic acid. These vitamins would need to be compensated for in other portions of one's diet or through supplementation.

The lactose levels in goat milk versus cow milk are very similar (4.1% and 4.7% respectively), so lactose intolerant individuals might experience little to no relief from making the switch.

Sheep Milk

Sheep milk is considered by many to be highly nutritious and richer in vitamins (A, B, and E specifically), calcium, phosphorus, potassium, and magnesium than cow milk. It has also been noted that the fat globules in sheep milk are smaller than the fat globules in cow milk, making sheep milk more easily digested. Nonetheless, sheep milk is much higher in both fat and protein than either goat or cow milk. For this reason, it would rarely be a good option for the milk allergic or other dairy-free dieters.

The commercial sheep dairy industry is concentrated in Europe and in countries surrounding the Mediterranean Sea. Sheep milk has yet to hit the mainstream in North America, though it is sometimes found in the form of cheese.

Camel Milk

Camel milk has not yet hit North America, but it is all the rage in the Middle East. Traditionally, it has been a staple of the Bedouins throughout the Middle East. More recently, camel milk, camel milk ice cream, and camel milk cheese (with the nickname 'camelbert') have hit the scene, and it may be only a matter of time before these products head west.

In a study of eight children with severe food allergies who did not benefit from conventional treatment, camel milk appeared to emerge victorious. According to the study, all eight children reacted well to the milk and recovered fully from their cow milk allergies. In fact, after following a camel milk diet, many saw an increase in their ability to digest other foods.

The success of the camel milk is suspected to be due to the difference in proteins between camel milk and cow milk. Camel milk is free of the specific beta-casein protein and beta-lacto-globulin protein (whey) that are known instigators of milk allergies. In addition, the immunoglobulins in camel milk are similar to those in mothers' milk, which reduce children's allergic reactions and strengthen their future response to foods.

Beyond allergies, camel milk is being touted for numerous medicinal benefits. Nonetheless, structured clinical trials will need to take place before any health claims or camel milk deliveries will be made to North America.

Mare Milk

As previously mentioned the affinity of mare milk to human milk has sparked some curiosity in the scientific and milk allergy communities. While this type of mammal milk may sound like a very new concept in English speaking countries, it is old school throughout other parts of the world. It just happens to be enjoying a revival in continental Europe, including Belgium, France, the Netherlands, and Norway. Mare milk is also fairly common in central Asia, but it is typically served in a fermented form, similar to kefir, called kumis or airag.

In addition to its possibilities for milk allergies, some believe that mare milk contains curative properties for digestive problems. This theory is still quite anecdotal. In fact, in my search to discover the lactose levels of mare milk, I read that it is much higher in lactose than cow milk and much lower in lactose than cow milk within the same article!

As you can imagine, milking a horse could pose many more challenges than a cow, so mare milk is still quite scarce and expensive. However, if the food allergy studies continue to prove fruitful for mare milk, then we might eventually see its availability on a grander scale to consumers.

Donkey Milk?
Yes, donkey milk. At present, you will only run across this when traveling, perhaps in France, Belgium, or Ecuador. However, speculators say that it may be on its way to North America, so I will briefly address it.

Donkey milk is being touted as the closest to human milk (I will politely refrain from commentary on this one), low in fat, high in vitamins and minerals, and low in allergenic proteins. But, until there is further scientific evidence of its composition and benefits, donkey milk won't be on the most recommended list for non-dairy dieters. Due to the very low milking output of donkeys, the price would likely deter any consideration, regardless.

Other Mammal Milk
Beyond those noted above, buffalo, yak, water buffalo, reindeer, zebra, and even moose have been known to provide milk used by humans for dairy products. Plus, wallaby milk is being studied for its potential anti-Candida effects. While each may vary in composition, they are all mammal milks containing water, fat, lactose, whey protein, and casein in higher amounts than is found in human milk. Like cow milk, these various milks may elicit allergic reactions, upset lactose intolerance, and may not be suitable for those who forgo dairy for social, political, religious, or other health reasons. Research on each would be required before any opposing claims could be made.

Keep in mind that all mammal milks still possess the lactose, proteins, fat, and hormones that do in fact make them milk. To date, the only mammal milk that seems to be inarguably healthy for human consumption in most cases (see galactosemia on p29 and lactose intolerance on p24) is human breast milk. If you are interested in exploring other mammal milks, consult a physician first.

CHAPTER 2:
WHY WE LIVE DAIRY-FREE

Just ten years ago the concept of living without milk was viewed as radical and impossible by most. Today, the non-dairy industry is thriving as individuals from all walks of life focus on healthier diets. In 2006, the Vegetarian Resource group conducted a dietary poll that estimated over 22.8 million Americans were following a non-dairy lifestyle, up from the estimates of 10 million dairy-free consumers in their 2000 poll.

The reasons for following this "free-from" lifestyle are as diverse as the people themselves. This chapter focuses on the most common motives for living sans dairy, and some facts you may just find useful.

Milk Allergies

Dairy milk contains over 25 different molecules that have the potential to elicit an allergic reaction. No wonder milk is ranked as one of the top eight food allergy offenders! In fact, many doctors, scientists, and health specialists recommend going dairy-free as an initial test when a food allergy is suspected.

What is a Milk Allergy?
Although they are often muddled together in conversation, milk allergies and lactose intolerance are quite different. A food allergy is identified as an abnormal and heightened response of the immune system to certain components (most notably proteins) within the offending food. On the contrary, a food intolerance is indicated when symptoms develop after eating a food that your body can't cope with effectively, but it does not involve an immune response. I will address lactose intolerance further beginning on p24, but for now, more on allergies …

Our immune systems are designed to detect and launch an attack on harmful invaders, such as viruses. However, when things go awry, the immune system may identify a perfectly harmless substance, like a peanut, as a threat. The food allergy reactions we see are actually the immune system attempting to attack the "invader." Ironically, by trying to protect us, our immune system can in turn cause harm with these false alarms.

In milk, the two leading allergy offenders are the proteins known as casein and whey. Casein is the curd that forms when milk is left to sour. Whey is the watery part that is left after the curd is removed.

Some scientists believe that there is only one type of "true food allergy" while others report studies on two, three, and even four variations of food allergies. For simplicity sake I will just note the two most commonly sited allergy categories: immediate hypersensitivity reaction and delayed hypersensitivity reaction. In immediate hypersensitivity situations, symptoms may begin to appear within minutes of ingesting the offending food. Like the way your friend's Aunt Martha blows up like a balloon the second she takes a bite of a chocolate bar laced with peanuts.

Delayed hypersensitivity reactions have received little attention until recently, so not too much is known about them as of yet. It is believed that these types of reactions elicit a different response from the immune system than the immediate hypersensitivity. With delayed hypersensitivity, symptoms have an onset time of 6 to 24 hours after eating an offending food, tend to reach their peak at about 48 hours, and gradually subside over 3 to

4 days. For both immediate and delayed reactions, symptoms may be very mild, and even go unnoticed (i.e. rash or eczema), or they may be quite severe (i.e. Aunt Martha).

How Common are Milk Allergies?
It was previously thought that milk allergies occurred only in infants, and that the problem subsided prior to adulthood. Unfortunately, for many of us this just isn't so. While prior estimates had stated that roughly 80% of milk allergies are outgrown by the age of 6, a newer study out of the Johns Hopkins University School of Medicine in Baltimore, Maryland claims that these numbers are far too optimistic.

They estimated that the prevalence of milk allergies in the general population is 2 to 3%, or roughly 6 to 9 million Americans, including infants, children, and adults. According to their findings, the rates of milk allergy resolution were found to be 19% by the age of 4, 42% by the age of 8, 64% by the age of 12, and 79% by the age of 16. However, it is also possible for adults to develop a milk allergy with no childhood history of allergies.

To complicate things further, symptoms associated with milk allergy have the potential to morph over time. One study followed a group of milk allergic children and found that at the beginning of the study most of the children had primarily gastrointestinal symptoms (vomiting, diarrhea), but by the end of the study, many had switched over to respiratory symptoms such as wheezing.

What are the Symptoms of Milk Allergies?
Similar to other food allergies, the majority of milk allergy symptoms can be lumped into four "reaction" categories:

Skin
- ~ Itchy Red Rash
- ~ Eczema
- ~ Hives
- ~ "Shiners" Or Black Eyes
- ~ Aphthous Ulcers (Canker Sores)
- ~ Swelling of Lips, Mouth, Tongue, Face, Or Throat

Digestive
- ~ Abdominal Pain
- ~ Abdominal Cramps
- ~ Abdominal Bloating
- ~ Diarrhea
- ~ Gas / Flatulence
- ~ Nausea
- ~ Vomiting

Respiratory
- ~ Runny Nose / Congestion
- ~ Sneezing
- ~ Watery Eyes
- ~ Itchy Eyes
- ~ Coughing
- ~ Wheezing
- ~ Shortness of Breath
- ~ Recurrent "Colds"
- ~ Recurrent Ear Infections
- ~ Sinusitis

Behavioral
Current research has uncovered this fourth category of symptoms, which may clear up some issues for "psychological" sufferers. Many doctors now believe that food allergies could be a direct cause of:
- ~ Fatigue
- ~ Migraine Headaches
- ~ Hyperactivity (ADHD)
- ~ Irritability
- ~ Night Waking
- ~ Anxiety
- ~ Sore Muscles and Joints

As noted above, these symptoms may be mild or life threatening; they could appear immediately or over a period of several days; and they may vary in response to mild, moderate, or large quantities of milk intake.

For an unlucky few, anaphylaxis is a reality. Anaphylaxis is a systemic allergic reaction that may involve multiple areas of the body, including the skin, cardiovascular system, respiratory tract, and gastrointestinal tract. Symptoms are sudden, and may come on immediately or up to four hours after coming in contact with the allergen (in this case milk). Anaphylactic reactions can be mild. However, some cases are potentially fatal, and therefore require urgent medical attention. If you are concerned that you or a loved one may be at risk for anaphylactic reactions, a doctor should be consulted immediately.

How do I know if I Have a Milk Allergy?
There are three primary methods utilized by doctors for the diagnosis of food allergies: skin tests, blood tests, and elimination-challenge tests.

<u>Skin Tests</u>
The skin-prick test has been around for decades, and it is typically administered by an allergist referred by your doctor. This test involves placing a drop of the suspect food on a person's arm or back and pricking the skin, thereby allowing a tiny amount of the suspect allergen to enter the skin. If a red spot flares up, then an allergic reaction is indicated. The results are almost immediate, as reactions should occur within about 15 minutes.

Anti-allergy medications, such as over-the-counter antihistamines, may need to be discontinued 2 to 3 days before the skin prick test, as they can interfere with the results. Cold medications, some antidepressants, beta-blockers, and other medications may also promote inaccuracy.

In some parts of the world (currently France, the Middle East, Mexico, New Zealand, and Australia), a newer skin-patch test known as Diallertest® Milk is also available. Slightly less intimidating than a skin-prick test, it is boasted for its ease of use and non-invasive nature, but it is essentially the same type of test.

Skin testing is useful only in the diagnosis of IgE mediated food allergies, or those allergies in which your immune system produces IgE antibodies to attack a specific food. IgE antibodies are associated with immediate hypersensitivity reactions, those occurring within minutes of consuming a suspect food, and may include cases of hives, anaphylaxis, and eczema. However, many gastrointestinal allergic reactions do not involve IgE antibodies.

Some doctors like the ability to test for many allergies at once and the overall reliability of skin tests, but others question the level of accuracy since false positive tests are fairly common. Skin-prick tests are ill advised for those who may have a life-threatening reaction to milk or other food allergens being tested, as they may be dangerous. Blood tests are the preferred method where life-threatening reactions are a concern.

<u>Blood Tests</u>
The relative newcomers on the food allergy diagnosis scene are blood tests, but they are quickly gaining in popularity. I will address three of the more popular types of food allergy blood tests, which are now available in most developed countries.

The RAST (RadioAllergoSorbent Test), otherwise known as the CAP-RAST or ImmunoCap test, involves sending a small blood sample to a medical laboratory to be analyzed for reactivity to a set of food allergens. The results of the RAST are usually received within one week. Similar to skin-prick tests, the RAST measures only IgE antibodies to detect allergies to specific foods.

Though not perfect (this test is also known to produce false positives with some regularity), many doctors prefer this test for its relatively high level of accuracy. Since it is quite accurate when IgE levels are high, the RAST is often useful as a first test to determine if an elimination-challenge test (discussion coming up!) will be safe. This strategy is frequently used when testing to see if a child has outgrown a severe food allergy. The RAST is also useful for patients who have eczema or other skin problems that may complicate reading the results of a skin-prick test. Plus, this blood test is not affected by the presence of medications.

However, some medical professionals argue that nearly 60% of milk reactions in young children are delayed, and therefore unlikely to be detected with the skin-prick test or RAST. In turn, they may request the ELISA / ACT (Enzyme-Linked Immunosorbent Assay). The ELISA is a food sensitivity test that typically measures both the IgE and IgG antibodies that your immune system allegedly produces in response to specific foods. IgG antibodies are said to be associated with delayed food reactions and sensitivities. The IgG theory tends to be supported more by naturopathic medicine than by traditional allergists and immunologists, because there is a great deal of controversy about whether or not IgG-mediated food allergy reactions actually exist. It isn't uncommon to find "anti-food" IgG antibodies circulating in the blood of people who have no signs or history of adverse reactions to the suspect foods. Nonetheless, some doctors feel that this test offers a good starting point for resolving underlying health issues.

Like the RAST, the ELISA is a simple blood test, and the results are often available within one to three weeks, depending upon the laboratory used. The patient receives a detailed printout that may include several hundred foods and potential allergens, and any level of reactivity to these substances is indicated. Though the ELISA is available from several home-testing companies, it is best to undergo the test under the supervision of your doctor to ensure the results are interpreted properly. Many of the labs give dietary recommendations based on the results, which is realistically out of their jurisdiction.

A third, and even more controversial, food allergy blood test is the ALCAT Test (sometimes referred to as a leucocytotoxic or NuTron test). Like proponents of the ELISA, ALCAT supporters argue that the RAST misses the boat entirely by only detecting IgE mediated reactions. However, ALCAT supporters also feel that the ELISA cuts out a big piece of the pie by relying on just two immune pathways, serum levels of IgG and IgE. Rather than looking for a particular immune response (such as IgE or IgG antibodies), the ALCAT measures the reactivity of leukocytes, white blood cells in the immune system that are responsible for defending the body against foreign materials.

As the theory goes, when you consume a food that your body is sensitive to, your immune system will, in some way, attack it as if it is "foreign." But your immune system has several ways in which to attack an invader, so by looking at just one or two types of immune responses (again, those IgE or IgG antibodies) it could be possible to miss several food sensitivities. The ALCAT goes to the source, the white blood cells, to detect which foods they are labeling as invaders, regardless of the type of attack that is launched.

Like the RAST and the ELISA, the ALCAT test can cover hundreds of commonly consumed foods. It too is available as a home-test kit, but it is best to perform the test under the supervision of a health practitioner. Test results can be obtained within a week. Though it is a medical test, the ALCAT receives the most support from alternative health practitioners and is not as readily accepted by the medical community, as it is believed to produce many false positives.

Elimination-Challenge Test
With an elimination test, suspicious foods are temporarily removed from the patient's regular diet. Depending on the doctor used, the recommended period of elimination may be anywhere from one week to one month, or possibly longer. Then, under the direct supervision of a physician (this is crucial), the suspect foods are slowly reintroduced one at a time to see whether symptoms are reproduced.

It is important to note that reactions may be heightened following a period of elimination. If a significant change in symptoms is noted during the period of elimination, then your doctor may opt to skip the challenge phase altogether, and recommend a continued elimination of the suspect food. A detailed journal of diet and symptoms should be kept for one to two weeks prior to the elimination diet, during the period of elimination, and throughout the reintroduction/challenge phase.

This type of allergy testing may take a longer period of time for diagnosis. However, many consider it to be the gold standard for determining food allergies and sensitivities. An elimination diet can easily identify a negative effect to a food, whether it is an allergy, intolerance, or a pure mystery, regardless of what the individual test results say. Doctors and patients are often pleased with this method as it is simple, free, highly effective, and tailored to the individual.

A free, downloadable journal is offered at www.godairyfree.org to help log your diet and track symptoms. This journal offers 14 days of detail that you can access to download and/or print at any time.

Other Allergy Tests
In addition to the ALCAT, you may come across a few other "alternative" tests when venturing into complimentary medicine. These could include the Vega test, kinesiology, or hair analysis, among others. These may also carry a high rate of false readings, so it is important to consult a physician before undergoing any type of allergy testing.

Can Milk Allergies Be Treated?
As with most allergies, avoiding the offending substance is the most recommended form of treatment. Though there are many medical concepts circulating, a universal cure or vaccine for food allergies has not yet been confirmed. But … that isn't to say scientists aren't working on it …

For years, a procedure known commonly as "desensitization" has been used as a treatment against environmental allergies. It involves subjecting the patient (under strict medical supervision) to minute amounts of their known allergen in gradually increasing quantities over time, with a goal to "desensitize" them to the allergen. Though not always successful, desensitization does work for many individuals, lessening the severity of their symptoms and in some cases acting as a virtual "cure" of the allergy.

Because the subjects in food allergy cases may risk life-threatening reactions to even trace amounts of the offending food, desensitization (otherwise known as specific oral tolerance induction) has been difficult to test in this arena. However, in February 2008, a study was reported in the Journal of Allergy and Clinical Immunology that successfully demonstrated the potential of desensitization against food allergies.

The small study, led by Dr. Egidio Barbi from 'Burlo Garofolo' University of Trieste, carefully administered a desensitization program to 30 children with severe allergic reactions to cow milk proteins. After one year, 11 (36%) of the children had become completely tolerant, 16 (54%) could tolerate limited amounts of milk (5 to 150 mL / 0.1 to 5.0 oz), and 3 (10%) were not able to complete the program due to persistent respiratory or abdominal complaints.

As I write, desensitization for food allergies is still in the investigation phase, however, more scientific programs are popping up to study this possible treatment.

Lactose Intolerance

If you are not lactose intolerant yourself, odds are you know someone who is. According to the National Institute of Diabetes and Digestive and Kidney Diseases (NIDDK), 30 to 50 million people in the United States alone are lactose intolerant. Look around, that is up to 1 in every 6 people you see.

What is Lactose Intolerance?
Otherwise known as "milk sugar," lactose is the primary carbohydrate in milk products. During the digestion process, lactose is broken down into glucose and galactose for proper absorption. This step occurs in the small intestine with the assistance of an enzyme known as lactase. Many people have or develop a shortage of lactase, and therefore are unable to properly digest some or all of the lactose they consume. The unabsorbed lactose passes into the colon where the party ensues. This lactase deficiency and any resulting gastrointestinal symptoms are what we typically refer to as lactose intolerance.

Could it Just Be Maldigestion?
The true prevalence of lactose intolerance has been put into question by the dairy industry. I know - big surprise. The National Dairy Council suggests that most people are not actually lactose intolerant, but rather they are suffering from lactose "maldigestion."

If you want to get technical about it, they may be correct. Within the very sparse literature I was able to uncover on the term lactose "maldigestion" or "malabsorption" (pretty much the Dairy Council website and a study in Sicily) it stated "Lactose maldigestion occurs when digestion of lactose is reduced as a result of low activity of the enzyme lactase..." In other words, maldigestion is a reduction in the ability to digest lactose while intolerance is the complete inability to digest lactose.

As confirmed by its very definition, both maldigestion and intolerance "can cause uncomfortable gastrointestinal symptoms and overall poor health." Since you may experience some very strange looks if you told people you were a lactose maldigester, and both an intolerance and maldigestion can cause discomfort following milk consumption, I think they may be splitting hairs with the terminology. For the purpose of this book, we will keep it simple by just using the expression lactose intolerance.

Who is Most Likely to Be Lactose Intolerant?
Lactose intolerance rates are much higher among adults than children and are known to be significantly increased in certain nationalities. According to the NIDDK's 1994 study, the incidence of lactose intolerance in the United States was reported as follows:

~   90% of Asian American Adults
~   70% of African American Adults
~   74% of Native American Adults

~   53% of Mexican American Adults
~   15% of Caucasian Adults

Internationally, it has been estimated that 70% of the world's population is lactase deficient and at risk for the symptoms of lactose intolerance. Men and women are affected equally, although some women may temporarily regain the ability to digest lactose during pregnancy.

What are the Symptoms of Lactose Intolerance?
Lactose intolerance symptoms may vary from person to person. They can range from mildly uncomfortable to quite severe. The most notable byproducts of lactose intolerance are:

~   Abdominal Pain
~   Abdominal Cramps
~   Intestinal Bloating

~   Gas / Flatulence
~   Diarrhea
~   Nausea

These symptoms typically emerge about 30 minutes to 2 hours after ingesting lactose-laden foods.

How Does Lactose Intolerance Develop?
For most, lactose intolerance is developed through the progression into adulthood; for some it is acquired as a result of an acute illness; but for a very few lactose/lactase issues may be present from birth.

Primary Lactose Intolerance stems from a natural and gradual decrease in lactase activity after weaning. This is the most common cause of lactose intolerance. Due to the progression, symptoms may develop as early as 5 years old, and often worsen with age. Some may have a complete loss of lactase activity, but many will retain 10 to 30% of their initial level of the enzyme activity (those maldigesters again). This may allow for digestion of very low levels of lactose.

Secondary Lactose Intolerance may occur during episodes of acute illness. This can happen at any age, and following full recovery it is possible for the damage to be reversed. A few potential causes of secondary lactose intolerance are irritable bowel syndrome, acute gastroenteritis, celiac disease, cancer, and chemotherapy. The lactose intolerance may subside once the underlying condition has resolved, though for many it persists.

Congenital Lactose Intolerance is a very, very rare metabolic disorder in which a baby is born with lactose intolerance. Congenital lactose intolerance must be passed through the generations via autosomal recessive inheritance. In other words, both the mother and father must possess and pass on the defective form of the gene in order for their child to be affected. Infants with congenital lactose intolerance are actually intolerant of the lactose in their mothers' breast milk and will typically present with symptoms (diarrhea, vomiting, dehydration, and failure to thrive) within a few days following birth. This condition seems to be most common in Finland.

How is Lactose Intolerance Diagnosed?
Lactose intolerance is typically diagnosed through one of three commonly utilized tests: the lactose tolerance test, the hydrogen breath test, and the stool acidity test. Each of these tests is performed on an outpatient basis at a hospital, clinic, or in a doctor's office.

The Lactose Tolerance Test
This test begins with a 24-hour fasting period. At the end of this fasting, the patient's blood is drawn, and the glucose level is tested. The patient then receives a lactose-rich beverage, and for the next 2 to 3 hours blood samples are taken to check their glucose level. Normally, when lactose reaches the digestive system, the lactase enzyme breaks it down into glucose and galactose. The liver then changes the galactose into more glucose, which in turn enters the bloodstream and raises the patient's blood glucose level. If lactose is incompletely broken down then the blood glucose level does not rise as it should, and a diagnosis of lactose intolerance may be confirmed.

The Hydrogen Breath Test
Very little hydrogen is detectable in the breath of someone who has a normal healthy gut. However, in lactose intolerant individuals bacteria ferments undigested lactose in the colon and hydrogen is produced.

In the hydrogen breath test, the patient drinks a lactose-rich beverage, and their breath is analyzed at regular intervals. Increased levels of hydrogen in the breath indicate improper digestion of lactose and may confirm a diagnosis of lactose intolerance. Prior to the hydrogen breath test, certain foods, medications, and cigarettes should be avoided, as they may interfere with the accuracy of the results.

The lactose tolerance and hydrogen breath tests are not given to infants and very young children who are suspected of having lactose intolerance. The large lactose load administered in these two tests may be dangerous for very young individuals, since they are more prone to the dehydration that can result from lactose-induced diarrhea.

The Stool Acidity Test
Undigested lactose fermented by bacteria in the colon also creates lactic acid, which can be detected in a stool sample. This third test is suitable for infants and young children and may be an easy option to help identify the presence of lactose intolerance.

Some pediatricians may simply recommend that a baby or young child be switched to a lactose-free diet as a trial to see if the symptoms subside. Likewise, many doctors feel that this short-term "elimination" diet may be a good testing option for adults who believe they are suffering with lactose intolerance. A doctor should be consulted to see if any of the above tests, including an elimination diet, would be appropriate.

What are the Treatment Options for Lactose Intolerance?
Unfortunately, scientists have not yet discovered a way to boost the body's ability to produce lactase, so the best treatment is dietary avoidance of lactose-laden foods. As mentioned, many people are not completely intolerant, and will be able to digest limited quantities of lactose. However, there are a few things to keep in mind.

Naturally low lactose dairy foods can include butter, hard cheeses, and yogurt. Yet most doctors would be hesitant to recommend cheese and butter for daily consumption or as major sources of calcium. They are rich in animal-based saturated fats, proven instigators of heart disease. Plain yogurt, specifically with live yogurt cultures (aka probiotics), may be well tolerated. However, the yogurt we Americans love is typically loaded with fruit, flavors, and sweeteners (sometimes in the form of milk solids / lactose), combating the power of these digestion-boosting bacteria.

Unlike milk allergies, primary lactose intolerance (the most common type) is rarely, if ever, outgrown. In fact, lactase production typically decreases with age. It is not uncommon for individuals to experience a worsening of lactose intolerant symptoms, or for those with a previous record of good digestion to suddenly begin experiencing symptoms of lactose intolerance. In other words, that hunk of cheese may be okay today, but it might spell disaster tomorrow. It really is a system of trial and sometimes unpleasant error for lactose intolerant individuals who choose to consume dairy.

For those who must have that ice cream sundae, lactase enzymes are available over the counter. However, these are not 100% effective, and dosage can be quite the balancing act. Lactase enzymes only function well in very acidic environments (aka the human gut), but too much acid can denature them. For this reason, it is best not to take them on an empty stomach. Yet, the enzymes will not be effective if they don't reach the small intestine before the problematic food arrives. They must be taken prior to, or at the time of, each bout of dairy intake. There is also the risk that the enzymes will not provide enough lactase to digest the lactose being consumed, allowing the symptoms to ensue regardless.

Some people have such severe lactose intolerance that a strict dairy-free diet is the only way to go, but I have received numerous stories from *moderately* lactose intolerant people who have simply chosen to go dairy-free. In general, they found that complete avoidance broke their cheesy cravings, that the experimentation was more of a hassle than it was worth, and while they were able to "tolerate" some milk products, they actually felt better when they didn't bother to consume any.

How Much Lactose is in Dairy?
Like milk protein, lactose is a water-soluble molecule that is not found in the fat portion of milk. Therefore, curdling processes and fat percentages can have a big impact on the prevalence of lactose. Unlike weight loss dieters, low-fat and fat free products can be the nemesis of lactose intolerant individuals. Plus, lower fat dairy foods often have milk solids or other dairy derivatives added back in to enhance sweetness, which may consequently increase the lactose content.

Surprisingly, finding lactose percentages in dairy foods is no easy feat. I turned to the lactose intolerance guru, Steve Carper, for some guidance in this area. Steve runs the websites Planet Lactose and the Lactose Intolerance Clearinghouse (www.stevecarper.com), and has written THE book on the subject of lactose intolerance, *Milk is Not for Every Body*. Because processes can vary among dairies and manufacturers, and so many new types of dairy products are continuously coming online, reported lactose levels can vary. The following is just intended to give you a general idea. Also, as Steve mentions, lactose levels below 2% are considered low-lactose, and may be well tolerated by many lactose intolerant people in reasonable quantities.

Human Breast Milk – 9.0% - While milk protein-allergic infants are able to thrive on mom's breast milk, lactose intolerant infants simply cannot digest lactose, regardless of the source. Human milk contains nearly double the lactose of other mammal milks.

Cow Milk - 3.7 to 5.7% - This range does apply to whole, low-fat, nonfat / skim milk, and buttermilk, but in general lowering the fat will cause a slight bump up in lactose levels. It should also be noted that the lactose levels for other mammal milks, including goat, sheep, buffalo, and yak, are similar to cow milk, varying only by fractions of a percentage.

Lactose Reduced Milk – 0.0 to 1.6% - Not all lactose-reduced milk is completely lactose-free, but it can usually be considered a low lactose beverage.

Cream - 2.8 to 4.3% - Like beverage milk, the fat in cream matters when it comes to lactose. Whipping cream will fall around the 3.0% mark, while light cream will be closer to 4.0%, and half and half will weigh in at over 4%. Sour cream also fits comfortably into this range with roughly 3.0 to 4.0% lactose.

"Cultured" Products - 1.9 to 6.0% - This range is wide due to the variability among commercial yogurt. Sweet Acidophilus Milk (SAM) and part-skim kefir have lactose levels around 4.0%.

Concentrated Milk - 9.7 to 16.3% - Sweetened condensed milk and evaporated milk (whole and skim) possess more lactose than regular cow milk, with sweetened condensed milk being the highest offender.

Ice Cream - 3.1 to 8.4% - This includes ice cream and ice milks, but sherbet is often a low lactose food with less than 2% lactose.

Butter and Margarine – 0.0 to 1.0% - In a perfect world, butter would be lactose-free, but this rarely happens. However, both butter and margarine are considered low-lactose foods, when consumed in reasonable quantities of course!

Dry Milk Powders – 36.0 to 55.0% - This concentrated form of milk is very high in lactose and best avoided by any lactose intolerant individuals. Dry milk powders include nonfat and buttermilk versions (which are on the high end of the scale) and whole milk powder.

Whey, Dry – 52.0 to 80.0% - Whey is very high in lactose, whether it is sweet, sour, or reduced lactose. The only exceptions are whey protein concentrate (ranges from 10 to 55%), whey protein isolate (only around 0.5%), and liquid whey (4.5 to 5.0%).

Cheese – 0.0 to 5.1% - Cheese is tricky, as the lactose percentages don't just vary by the type of cheese, but also by how the cheese is manufactured. Hard and soft ripened cheeses that are produced via traditional methods are often better tolerated than milk, as the fermentation processes and higher fat content contribute to lower lactose levels. Plus, the traditional aging of cheese (over 2 years) reduces the lactose content to near zero. However, modern processes used in the production of most cheeses today rarely assist in lactose reduction, and typically involve minimal aging. Swiss cheese, for example, could easily range from zero lactose up to 3.4% lactose, depending on how it was manufactured. Cheeses that are moderately high in lactose with some regularity are lower fat soft cheeses, including ricotta, feta, and cottage cheese. Also, highly processed cheeses (American processed, Velveeta®, etc.) are often very high in lactose and best avoided by the lactose intolerant.

Galactosemia

Galactosemia is a very rare metabolic disorder that affects how the body processes galactose, one of the simple sugars created when lactose is broken down in the digestive system. Not to be confused with lactose intolerance, galactosemia is a much more dangerous disorder. While someone with galactosemia may have no problem in digesting lactose, they have a shortage or absence of the liver enzyme GALT, which is needed to break down galactose. As a result, galactose accumulates in the body, where it may damage the liver, central nervous system, eyes, kidneys, and other body systems.

The classical form of galactosemia presents itself quite soon after birth, with symptoms of vomiting, diarrhea, jaundice and failure to thrive. Diagnosis is usually made during the first week of life with a heel prick blood test as a part of standard newborn screening. Since galactose is a lactose byproduct, babies with the more severe forms of galactosemia will not be able to consume any lactose-containing foods, including their own mother's milk.

Treatment requires the strict lifetime exclusion of lactose / galactose from the diet. This includes milk products, but it can also include processed foods, some fruits and vegetables, meats, and some children's medicines. Even with a prompt diagnosis and treatment, galactosemic children are known to have long-term complications.

As mentioned, galactosemia is very rare, with the classical form affecting 1 in 30,000 to 60,000 newborns. For more information on galactosemia, visit the Parents of Galactosemic Children website, at www.galactosemia.org.

The Vegan Diet

While vegetarians typically shun meat and fish, strict vegans consume a diet that is free of all animal products. This includes (or should I say excludes) meat, fish, eggs, dairy, and often honey. This eating style was once associated almost exclusively with socially aware individuals. However, with each passing year thousands of people are realizing the benefits of this plant-based diet (rich in vegetables, grains, fruits, nuts and seeds), and switching to it for health reasons.

The vegan diet has been touted time and time again for its incredible health benefits in the areas of heart disease, cancer prevention, weight loss, fibromyalgia, rheumatoid arthritis, etc., etc., etc. In fact, according to a recent study from George Washington University and the University of Toronto, the vegan diet beat out the American Diabetes Association (ADA) diet in the treatment of diabetes! Not only was the vegan diet much more effective in shedding pounds and reversing type 2 diabetes symptoms, but the researchers also noted that it seemed easier to follow. Unlike the ADA diet, the vegan diet was simple and straightforward with no calories to count, portion sizes to measure, or carbohydrates to limit.

Vegan websites and cookbooks are fantastic tools for all dairy-free dieters, omnivorous or not, since the primary difference between typical vegan and vegetarian diets is the dairy. For those who do consume meat and/or fish, it is easy to use vegan recipes as the base for meals, adding in your protein of choice. As a dairy-free dieter I owe a great deal of thanks to the vegan community for bringing so many wonderful recipes and foods to the mainstream. It is fairly safe to say that vegan is "the new vegetarian."

Autism

Public awareness of autism has increased exponentially since the U.S. Centers for Disease Control (CDC) released a report announcing the prevalence of autism. In 2003 and 2004, two national health organizations interviewed the parents of approximately 98,000 school-aged children, combined. The results estimated that nearly 1 in every 175 children is living with autism. In a follow-up study in 2007, the CDC revised these numbers upwards, to close to 1 in 150 children. This equates to roughly 350,000 autistic school-aged children in the U.S. alone. To most people, this news came as quite a shock. However, for the hundreds of thousands of parents with autistic children it is a mere affirmation that this condition deserves far more attention than it has been receiving.

Autism is a brain disorder that typically makes its presence known in early childhood. It affects several crucial areas of development including social interaction, communication, behavior, creativity, and imagination. Autism was formally identified around the mid-1900s, but it has persisted as a misunderstood and often mislabeled condition.

For decades, the parents of autistic children have been experimenting with various medical and alternative treatments. Although a cure has yet to surface, their network of trial and error has yielded some surprising and positive results.

In 2005, The Autism Research Institute published their findings from an ongoing study, focused on the usefulness of different treatment interventions. Overall, they questioned nearly 23,700 parents of autistic children. The parents were asked to rate the therapies they had trialed according to effectiveness. The treatment options fell into three major categories: drugs; biomedical non-drug therapies, such as vitamin supplements; and special diets. Much to the dismay of major drug companies, the results swung largely in favor of alternative therapies and diet.

Approximately 50 different drugs were reported as tested. On average, 30% of the cases showed an improvement of symptoms, however, 31% actually got worse while on one or more of the drugs. Biomedical non-drug therapies faired far better. 45% of the cases reported a decline in symptoms with only 5% exhibiting an increase. Yet amazingly, special diets rated as the most successful treatment category overall. Among the autistic children who were put on a special diet, 50% of the cases exhibited signs of improvement, while only 2% experienced a rise in symptoms.

The simple removal of dairy products was the special diet option trialed most, with over 5,500 parental reports. On par with the special diet category results, 49% of those who chose a dairy-free treatment option found it to improve their child's symptoms, while only 2% found it to worsen symptoms. Of those who were willing to take it a step further to a gluten-free / casein-free diet, a resounding 65% saw an improvement in symptoms. Gluten is a protein found in wheat and other flours.

Gradually, the gluten-free / casein-free diet is becoming a mainstream recommendation for the treatment of autism. Other alternative treatments are beginning to receive similar recognition, particularly in the areas of reducing chemical exposure (in food, water, and the environment) and detoxification. Although numerous research studies do support the hypothesis that alternative therapies and special diets can dramatically aide in the severity of autism, the reason behind their success is still somewhat elusive. For this reason, experts recommend that parents consult a gastroenterologist before their autistic child undergoes a dietary modification.

ADHD

Attention Deficit Hyperactivity Disorder (ADHD) is frequently coupled in studies with autism, as these two developmental disorders seem to share many similarities in terms of symptoms. This has prompted scientists to consider the two together when researching their root cause and potential treatments.

Consequently, a study out of Norway found that, like autism, a casein-free diet might improve mental health in children with ADHD. This ten year study, led by Dr. Karl Ludvig Reichelt, placed 23 children diagnosed with hyperactive disorders on milk-free and/or gluten-free diets. Reichelt believes that people with this type of disorder lack an enzyme that breaks down proteins like casein. As a consequence, the inability to efficiently digest these proteins inhibits optimal brain function. By reducing the intake of these aggravators, he felt that hyperactivity could be brought under control. Based on his research results, this may very well be true.

Twenty-two of the Norwegian children who were taken off milk products and other casein-containing foods exhibited almost immediate improvement in their mental health and overall behavior, longer attention spans, and increased learning capabilities. However, the symptoms returned as soon as the milk-based foods were reintroduced into their diets. Most of the children involved in this study had been taking behavioral medications, such as Ritalin, prior to changing their diets. However, after following a casein-free diet, they were soon taken off the medicines.

Long-term follow-up with these children has found their disorders to be manageable, with the virtual disappearance of past behavioral challenges. Beyond autism and now ADHD, this protein/digestive disorder has also been linked to schizophrenia.

Weight Loss

In 2007, the dairy industry lost some serious promotional footing when the People's Committee for Responsible Medicine (PCRM) petitioned the Federal Trade Commission (FTC) to shut down their infamous milk / weight loss campaigns. According to Dan Kinburn, PCRM's general counsel, "Milk and cheese are more likely to pack on pounds than help people slim down." It seems the FTC believed that Mr. Kinburn might be right. From my personal experience, I agree with him whole-heartedly.

When my husband opted to go dairy-free he dropped over ten pounds in two months (all from his waist) without changing any other aspect of his diet or lifestyle. It was then that I began to think about the true purpose of milk. Calves are roughly 50 to 100 lbs at birth, but they mature within a year to weigh around 500 lbs (continuing on to their full weight of around 1500 lbs, give or take a few hundred) primarily with the assistance of their mother's milk … the stuff that we pump and consume by the gallon. Milk is used as a shortcut for growth in our own species, but what happens when we are done growing and still consuming milk with all of its natural (and sometimes synthetic) hormones, fats, and proteins?

Every month I receive emails from Go Dairy Free readers who proclaim how good they feel and how much weight they have lost since they cut out dairy. For most, it wasn't their original intent. They changed their diet for a milk allergy, intolerance, veganism, or other health or social reason, but to their great surprise a side benefit emerged … unwanted pounds melted away. This is all the proof I needed to form my own opinion on the dairy and weight loss topic, but you might be interested in a few more facts …

The Cheese Generation: Where Would You Like That Extra <u>32.5 Lbs</u>?
On the surface, it looks as though our society has taken on healthier eating habits in recent decades. Coffee jitters have been traded in for antioxidant rich tea; red meat has taken a back seat to lean proteins such as fish and poultry; egg consumption has been cut in an effort to lower cholesterol levels; superfood sales are soaring; and cartons of low-fat/nonfat milk have been crowding out the whole milk on grocery store shelves. But … underneath it all … our fat, sugar, and overall calorie consumption has increased dramatically.

Some may point to alcohol and butter consumption, which are both on the rise. Yet, they are mere slugs compared to the growing popularity of the number one fat offender: cheese. According to the United States Department of Agriculture (USDA) Economic Research Service, the average American's appetite for cheese grew from 7.7 lbs per year in the 1950's to 32.5 lbs per year in 2006. That is a 420% increase! Not to mention, imagine the damage that 32.5 lbs of cheese (approximately 53,400 calories and 4300 grams of fat) could do.

How does one eat this much cheese? Are consumers literally sitting around eating big wedges? Maybe some, but in this day and age approximately two-thirds of cheese consumption is in the form of commercially manufactured and prepared foods, such as frozen pizzas, sauces, instant pasta meals, bagel spreads, and packaged snack foods. The good news is those who choose a non-dairy lifestyle can dramatically decrease their intake of saturated fats and hydrogenated oils by dumping the cheese along with the additional processed food ingredients and chemicals that accompany it.

What about Low-Fat Options Like Plain Old Milk?
Beyond the fat and calories, there may be a bit more to the weight and dairy issue. Several studies have linked milk consumption specifically (whether low-fat, skim, or whole) to weight gain and diseases such as diabetes and heart disease. Here are two examples that you may find interesting:

Dairy Effects on Diabetes, Obesity, and Heart Disease in Women - The British Women's Heart and Health Study examined 4,286 British women ranging in age from 60 to 79 for links to the Metabolic Syndrome. The Metabolic Syndrome was defined as those women who had Type 2 Diabetes or Pre-Diabetes (insulin resistance or high fasting glucose) and at least two of the following: obesity, hypertension, and lipid disorders (i.e. high triglycerides or low HDL). Those women who *avoided* milk were about half as likely to have the Metabolic Syndrome when compared to milk drinkers. The non-milk drinkers benefited from lower insulin resistance levels, lower triglyceride levels, lower BMI's (Body Mass Index) and higher levels of that healthy HDL cholesterol.

Children & Milk Consumption: Are They Growing Up or Out? - A large study led by Catherine S. Berkey of Harvard Medical School and Brigham & Women's Hospital in Boston, followed the diets and weight of 12,829 United States children. The children were diversified across all 50 states, and ranged in age from 9 to 14 years when the study began in 1996. Data was collected from the children through 1999, and the results were a bit of a surprise. Those children consuming more than 3 servings of milk per day were approximately 35% more likely to become overweight than those children who drank just 1 or 2 glasses of milk per day, even though most of the children were drinking low-fat milk. This association still held after the researchers took into consideration physical activity, other dietary factors, and growth. This study has emerged at a time when obesity among children is at an all time high, the rate has more than tripled since 1980.

The bottom line … overall dairy consumption in the U.S. has been rising steadily over the years, mostly in the areas of low-fat milk, yogurt, and cheese. The average waistline of Americans has also been expanding, along with reports of heart disease, cancer, and various other ailments that are directly linked to extra pounds. Coincidence?

General Health & Disease Prevention

A growing number of nutrition-oriented doctors are recommending dairy-free diets to encourage better overall health and disease prevention. From their perspective, every calorie we consume takes on an internal function. Unfortunately, for many individuals, the proteins, sugar, and fat found in milk products can act in a very counterproductive role. The consumption of dairy may cause, aggravate, inflame, or even masquerade as a serious medical condition. The following covers a few of the more common health concerns that may prompt a dairy-free diet.

Ovarian Cancer: The Milk Connection

It is no secret that some rather large studies have identified dairy consumption as one of the strongest links to ovarian cancer. But the real kicker is that a significant increase in ovarian cancer risk was shown in women who consumed higher levels of low-fat and nonfat milk. Prior research had already suggested that a high consumption of whole milk, yogurt, and cheese may increase the risk of ovarian cancer, but now the fat free varieties are out too? Perhaps.

One U.S. study of over 80,000 women showed that those who consumed just one or more servings of skim or low-fat milk daily had a 32% higher risk of developing any ovarian cancer and a 69% higher risk of serous ovarian cancer when compared to women who consumed 3 or less servings per month. Another study from Sweden of over 60,000 women confirmed these results. Their researchers found that women who consumed more than 4 servings per day of dairy products had twice the risk of serous ovarian cancer as women who consumed fewer than 2 servings of dairy products per day. To further their evidence against milk in particular, women who drank as little as 2 or more glasses of cow milk per day were twice as likely to develop ovarian cancer as women who consumed little to no milk.

For once, added fat and hormones may not be to blame. The main theory circulating indicates galactose as the true culprit. As mentioned previously, galactose is one of the two main components produced when lactose is broken down in our digestive systems. Many researchers believe that high levels of galactose over-stimulate, overload, or damage the ovaries, thus leading to ovarian cancer.

Prostate Cancer: Research Studies Vote 'Soy Yes, Dairy No'

Controversy abounds on this topic; however, numerous studies have shown a solid connection between dairy consumption and the risk of prostate cancer. Prior theories circled around the increase in IGF-1 (insulin growth hormone) seen in milk drinkers. High levels of IGF-1 have been directly linked to various hormonal cancers. Although this theory may still hold some validity, research has uncovered a potential cause that has further heated the debate on dairy and prostate cancer, calcium.

A study led by the Harvard School of Public Health in 2001 observed over 20,000 men, and concluded that men who consumed more than 600mg of daily calcium from dairy products had a 32% higher risk of prostate cancer than men who consumed less than 150mg of daily calcium from dairy products. The results of this study came as quite a shock for a couple of reasons. First, the researchers noted that the men who consumed the most dairy per day tended to be, by definition, healthier. On average, they smoked less, exercised more frequently, and were more likely to pop a multivitamin than their non-dairy counterparts. Second, it presented an odd twist on convention, since the USDA has recommended a minimum of 1200mg of daily calcium for men over 50, and 1000mg for men aged 19 to 50.

A cohort study published in mid-2005 by the American Journal of Clinical Nutrition showed that men with the highest dietary intake of dairy foods were 2.2 times more likely to develop prostate cancer than men with the lowest dietary intake of dairy foods. This dramatic increase in prostate cancer risk held true for men with the highest dietary calcium intake over those with the lowest.

A report in April 2008 detailed the work of researchers at the National Cancer Center in Tokyo who followed over 43,000 Japanese men aged 45 to 74 for an average of 7.5 years. They found the prostate cancer risk was increased by more than 50% in those whose intake of dairy products was in the highest quartile, compared to those in the lowest quartile.

The Tokyo study was quickly followed by a June 2008 report in the British Journal of Cancer. The investigators utilized the European Prospective Investigation into Cancer and Nutrition database of 145,250 participants to study the relationship between diet, lifestyle, environmental factors and cancer. In this group, 2,722 men had been diagnosed with prostate cancer at the time of follow-up. While there was no association between meat, fish, or eggs and the risk of prostate cancer, there was a strong correlation with dairy protein and dairy calcium intake. Dairy products and yoghurt showed an increased risk in prostate cancer, as did calcium intake from dairy foods (but not calcium intake from non-dairy foods).

Luckily, the news on prostate cancer isn't all that bad. Several other nutrients, vitamins, and minerals have been given a gold star for their potential to reduce the risk of prostate cancer. Fructose (fruit), selenium (seafood, mushrooms, grains), vitamin D (sunshine), vitamin E (nuts, seeds, & greens), lycopene (tomatoes), soy...did I just mention soy in a discussion of men's health? Oh yes, it seems that a prospective study in the U.S. indicated a 70% reduction in the risk of prostate cancer among men who consumed more than one serving of soymilk per day.

Acne: Is Traditional Pizza Back on the Blacklist?
While the acne-milk link is frequently dismissed as an old wives' tale, there have been several medical studies demonstrating the validity of this association. The most notable of which, was a portion of the landmark Nurses Health Study involving 47,355 women in 1998. The good news is, this enormous body of research did not find a link between chocolate and acne. However, it did find one between women who had suffered with acne and those who had consumed a lot of milk.

The researchers hypothesized that the hormones in milk, not the fat, were the true acne instigators. It has been estimated that 75 to 90% of milk and milk products on our shelves comes from pregnant cows. This milk contains progesterone and other hormones that are known precursors to DHT, the primary acne-producing hormone in humans. These hormones are carried primarily in the butterfat, and are known to make frequent appearances in milk, cheese, and butter.

In addition to the hormones above, there are about 60 growth hormones and growth factors present in dairy products. One of these, insulin-like growth factor (IGF-I), is likely partially responsible for acne during the teen years. Back in the 1960's, Dr. Jerome K. Fisher conducted a clinical study on the cause and effect relationship of milk and acne for a presentation to the American Dermatological Association. His research looked at more than 1000 teenage acne patients over a 10-year period. He concluded that the severity of their acne was directly correlated to their milk consumption. Along with the hormones in milk, Dr. Fisher hypothesized that milk sugar (lactose) and butterfat might be acne triggers. His paper was never published but is now available on line at www.acnemilk.com.

Most dermatologists recognize the crucial role that diet plays in skin conditions, and many cite milk products as the top food culprit in acne. Dairy elimination may not be the solution for everyone, but something so simple to get rid of acne may be worth a shot. It should be tested with patience though. A dietary change may prevent new plugging, but it could take a few months for the already established acne to "cool."

Personal stories from several acne sufferers who have trialed non-dairy diets are available on www.godairyfree.org.

Headaches: Migraines Retreat with Diet Modifications

The research is clear, food intolerance, allergies, and hypersensitivities are frequently key triggers of headaches and migraines. Although each migraine sufferer may react to a different food or group of foods, there are a few which seem to pop up as frequent offenders: dairy (including milk, cheeses, and yogurt), wheat, eggs, soy, corn, citrus, chocolate, coffee, beef, yeast, red wine, and processed foods with additives and preservatives.

In the pursuit to identify these top instigators, scientists and physicians often enlist the oligoantigenic diet. This is a hypoallergenic "elimination" diet, consisting of a selection of foods that are presumably well tolerated. During their studies, patients are told to eat only the "safe" foods outlined on their version of the oligonantigenic diet in an effort to eliminate any symptoms. Once the symptoms have gone into remission, the "high risk" foods are re-introduced into the diet one at a time to assess their potential trigger effect on symptoms. This type of diet should be undertaken with the assistance of a physician, in order to ensure adequate nutritional intake. In each of the 3 case studies listed below, some form of an oligoantigenic diet was used:

~ 60 migraine patients followed an elimination diet after a 5-day withdrawal from their normal diet. Upon reintroduction, specific foods elicited migraine reactions in a significant percentage of patients: wheat (78%), oranges (65%), eggs (45%), tea and coffee (40% each), chocolate and milk (37% each), beef (35%), and corn, cane sugar, and yeast (33% each). When an average of ten common trigger foods was avoided, there was a dramatic decline in the number of headaches per month and 85% of patients actually became headache-free! As science would have it, an added benefit was welcomed by the 25% of these patients who also had hypertension – their blood pressure returned to normal levels.
~ In a clinical trial, 93% of 88 children who suffered frequent and severe migraines recovered on oligoantigenic diets. Most of the patients responded to several foods, which suggested the probability of an allergic rather than a metabolic cause. An added bonus... abdominal pain, behavior disorder, fits, asthma, and eczema also improved in several of these patients.
~ A research study trialed an oligoantigenic diet on 63 children with epilepsy, 45 of which also suffered from migraines, hyperkinetic behavior, or both. The 18 children who had epilepsy alone saw no improvement on the oligoantigenic diet. However, of the 45 children with additional symptoms, 25 ceased to have seizures and 11 had fewer seizures while on this diet. Migraines, abdominal pain, and hyperkinetic behavior halted in the 25 children who stopped having seizures, and also in some of those who did not stop having seizures. Reintroduction of foods one by one confirmed that the seizures, migraines, hyperkinetic activity, and abdominal pain these children were experiencing related to 42 different "trigger" foods.

Why do so many people suffer from migraines and other headaches when they consume these foods? The medical community is getting closer to an answer. Researchers in Germany have discovered a genetic mutation responsible for the "faulty wiring" and the subsequent pain. Although clinical scientists have known for a while that migraines are hereditary, the exact "defect" being passed on was previously unknown.

IBS: Tummy Troubles

Irritable Bowel Syndrome (otherwise known as IBS) is a common, yet vague disorder of the gastrointestinal (GI) tract. IBS is characterized by recurrent abdominal pain and bloating, accompanied by diarrhea, constipation, or an alternating combination of both. These symptoms tend to be chronic, but may come and go over a period of several months or years. Research estimates that 10 to 20% of adults within the United States suffer from IBS, placing it at the top of the list for the most common functional GI disorders.

Dairy is a potential offender for many IBS sufferers, and it may attack from various angles:

Lactose Intolerance - Lactose intolerance has the ability to mimic or aggravate IBS symptoms. The International Foundation for Functional Gastrointestinal Disorders (IFFGD) references two studies on lactose intolerance / malabsorption in which patients diagnosed with IBS were given a hydrogen breath test to clinically identify lactose intolerance. The first study estimated that almost 25% of IBS patients had evidence of lactose malabsorption. The second study was performed on IBS patients who had no noticeable symptoms related directly to the ingestion of milk. Lactose malabsorption was identified in 68% of these patients. Symptoms improved on a lactose-limited diet.

High Fat Content - Eating foods that are too high in fat is a well-known trigger of IBS symptoms. The majority of dairy foods consumed have a high fat content, including cheese, ice cream, and other whole milk products.

Milk Protein - For the allergic, or just the hypersensitive, whey and casein may cause severe digestive problems. Food hypersensitivities among the general population have been estimated at about 5%, but the prevalence may increase to 65% in IBS patients. Diet exclusion studies are now underway. If proof positive, then even skim milk products may serve as aggravators to IBS sufferers.

Crohn's Disease: Increased Risk of Lactose Intolerance
Inflammatory Bowel Disease (IBD) is the name given to a group of disorders, which cause the intestines to become inflamed. Although less common than Irritable Bowel Syndrome, it is estimated that more than a half a million adults in the United States suffer from IBD each year. General symptoms tend to "flare-up" periodically, and may include abdominal cramping, abdominal pain, diarrhea, weight loss, and bleeding from the intestines. The two most well known types of IBD are Crohn's Disease and Ulcerative colitis. Diagnosis by a physician is essential for IBD.

The cause of IBD is still quite a mystery; however, many individuals find some symptom relief through dietary modifications. In particular, research has shown a significant increase in the prevalence of lactose malabsorption among patients with Crohn's Disease. For this reason many doctors recommend a lactose-limited diet to individuals with Crohn's Disease.

High Cholesterol: Real-Life Experiences
I debated including a section on cholesterol in this guide, as studies in relation to dairy consumption (versus dairy-free living) and cholesterol, pro or con, were sparse ... very sparse. Yet, the purpose of this guide is to help people, so if just one other person discovers the cure for their own high cholesterol based on my personal experiences, then I feel it is a story worth sharing.

In my early twenties, I had my first cholesterol test. Though I was slight of build and athletic, my total cholesterol was high - bordering on very high - at 240. This included 200 LDL ("bad cholesterol") and 40 HDL ("good cholesterol"). If you are not familiar with cholesterol numbers, let's just say this is not a good ratio for anyone, let alone someone so young. Yet it wasn't too much of a shock, since high cholesterol runs in my family, with all of my immediate family on cholesterol medication. My doctor made dietary recommendations (more oats, low fat, etc.) and sent me on my way with a warning that I would need to start medication soon. Of course, my diet was already in line with a "good cholesterol diet" so I was stumped. For the next five years every test came back with the exact same numbers, but I refused to start on the medication. I just knew there had to be a natural answer ... but I never would have guessed that it would be a dairy-free diet.

My annual cholesterol test came up just 3 months after I leapt into the dairy-free diet with both feet. To everyone's shock, my cholesterol had dumped 100 points! This is not an exaggeration; I had not changed anything else in my diet, exercise habits, or lifestyle, but I was down to 100 LDL and 40 HDL. Since that time, my total cholesterol has not only continued at this "healthy" level, but the ratio has also improved. The "good cholesterol" numbers have continued to rise to just under 60 while the "bad cholesterol" numbers have fallen to just over 80.

I had my father trial the dairy-free diet before one of his annual cholesterol checks, and he also saw a surprise downward leap in his numbers. This is obviously a hereditary link, yet it doesn't seem like such a bizarre concept that others might not see the same benefits. Over the years, I have received two other personal stories from readers who gave up all dairy, only to discover a side benefit in their cholesterol.

Feeling Good: The Most Important Reason of Them All
It seems like we always need a medical explanation or a profound external reason of sorts to keep from feeling silly about following a special diet. When I was in a funk, an alternative doctor recommended that I cut out sugar and wheat-based foods for a little while. I wasn't diagnosed with celiac disease or gluten intolerance, but I thought, "Why not give it a try?" Within a week, my energy perked up dramatically. I simply felt better.

When asthma, allergies, or general malaise have someone down, holistic practitioners often recommend avoiding dairy products. If they begin feeling better, it doesn't necessarily mean that they have a milk allergy or lactose intolerance. Perhaps dairy just doesn't work for them, as is true for so many people. It is hard to argue a diet that optimizes your general well being.

CHAPTER 3:
STRONG BONES, CALCIUM & BEYOND

What if I told you that citrus may be better for your bone health than milk? What if I even suggested that milk might not be a good option for fighting osteoporosis? Would you think I was insane? If so, I wouldn't blame you. Ten years ago, I would have balked at the very notion that any food could be more powerful at battling brittle bones than the almighty glass of milk.

More often than not, the media has led us to believe that dairy is the superior, and perhaps the only suitable choice for building and maintaining strong bones. Yet in recent years this notion has been put to the test, and shown by many studies to be alarmingly false. According to the enormous 12-year Harvard study of 77,761 female nurses, as published in the American Journal of Public Health (1997, volume 87):

> "...women consuming greater amounts of calcium from dairy foods had significantly increased risks of hip fractures, while no increase in fracture risk was observed for the same levels of calcium from nondairy sources."

Yes, you read that correctly, dairy products could actually be a *cause* of hip fractures from osteoporosis. This landmark study has risen more than a few eyebrows in the medical community, and although it was a giant study in its own right, it certainly does not stand-alone.

In a review of 34 published studies in 16 different countries, researchers at Yale University discovered that the countries with the highest rates of osteoporosis, including the United States, England, Sweden, and Finland, were coincidentally the highest consumers of dairy products. As further proof, countries with historically low rates of osteoporosis and hip fracture, such as China, are seeing a proportionate increase in the incidence of osteoporosis with the adoption of Westernized dietary habits.

How is this possible? According to the USDA, isn't milk one of our major food groups? The answer is not completely clear, but there are a couple of sound theories circulating in the scientific community. For starters, high dairy intake provides a good dose of animal protein, which in turn is rich in sulfur-containing amino acids. The body buffers the effects of these amino acids by releasing calcium from the bones, and excreting it from the body. In addition, animal-based foods, particularly milk, contain very high levels of phosphorous, which may interfere with calcium absorption.

The tides are turning on the osteoporosis front. Many renowned researchers are changing their healthy bone vote from milk to plant-based foods, such as vegetables, fruits, and nuts.

Surprising Secrets to Strong Bones

Don't get me wrong, calcium is very important. After all, when combined with phosphorous it composes approximately 80 to 90% of the mineral content of our bones. Yet, over the years, study after study has revealed that maintaining strong bones isn't as much about our intake of calcium as it is about how well we absorb it, and at what level we are able to keep it in our bones. The suggestions below include baseline tips for building and keeping strong bones, followed by some potential bone "superfoods" that I hope you will find as interesting as I did …

Exercise

Exercise is recognized throughout the medical community as essential for keeping calcium in its place. Use it or lose it really is the name of the game; active people tend to absorb and keep calcium in their bones, while sedentary people lose it. Our bones may be thought of as hard and inflexible, but in reality they are constantly being remodeled with new bone cells replacing old ones. The impact of weight bearing exercise assists in the bone building cycle. This may include the obvious strength training, but for those of you who loathe the weight room, baseball, basketball, soccer, tennis, aerobics, dancing, running, jumping, and walking are all considered weight bearing activities. However, "easy on the joints" sports, such as swimming are not.

Keep a Balanced Diet

Magnesium, potassium, iron, zinc, copper, sodium, vitamin D, vitamin K, and antioxidant vitamins (such as C & E) each play a vital role in calcium absorption and/or retention. Enjoying a healthy, varied diet rich in these essential nutrients is definitely an insurance policy worth taking out. Eat a wide selection of fruits, vegetables (including loads of those leafy greens and cruciferous types), beans, nuts, seeds, and whole grains. Keep in mind that it is better to obtain vitamins and minerals via your diet rather than supplements, whenever possible. Plus, when consumed as food there is far less risk for toxicity of a particular nutrient. For extensive information on these nutrients, and the foods you can find them in, visit The World's Healthiest Foods at www.whfoods.com. It is one of my favorite personal resources.

Absorb Some Vitamin D

In 2003, researchers at the Channing Laboratory out of Harvard Medical School found Vitamin D to be the true "healthy bone hero," reducing the risk for hip fracture by 37%. This massive 18-year prospective analysis followed over 72,000 postmenopausal women. Oddly enough, they found that neither a high-calcium diet nor milk was associated with a reduced risk for hip fracture.

Aside from mushrooms, fortified foods, and a small handful of other sources, it can be difficult to obtain enough Vitamin D via our diets. Luckily, the best source of Vitamin D is right above our heads; approximately 15 minutes of sunlight on the skin per day is typically enough to meet Vitamin D needs. If you obtain little to no sun exposure, then you may want to consider a multi-vitamin that contains Vitamin D.

Drink Alcohol in Moderation

Alcohol is believed to weaken your bones by reducing the body's ability to build new bone and replace normal losses. Of course, water is best, but if you must indulge, make sure you have no more than 1 or 2 servings of beer, wine, or liquor per day.

Cut the Caffeine

Several studies have shown a strong link between high caffeine intake and accelerated bone loss. If you still require that quick jolt, try to limit it to one or two cups a day of caffeinated beverages.

Hide the Saltshaker

While some sodium is necessary, removing that little saltshaker from the table may be a wise move. Limiting sodium to 1 to 2 grams (1000 to 2000 mg) per day will encourage calcium retention. Sodium hides in processed foods, so stick to whole and natural foods whenever possible.

Don't Smoke

Just in case you needed one more reason to quit the habit, there is a strong link between smoking and a higher risk of fracture and calcium loss.

Understand Medical Conditions

Steroid medications, such as prednisone, and hormone imbalances have been indicated as potential causes of bone loss and fractures. These risk factors should be discussed with a doctor.

Potential "Super-Bone" Foods

In recent years, scientists have uncovered numerous unsuspecting foods that are showing a good deal of promise in the fight against osteoporosis ...

Citrus - Superstars may soon be trading in their milk moustaches for pitchers of freshly squeezed orange juice. A 2006 study out of Texas A&M University cited citrus as a potential key to osteoporosis prevention. In the controlled study, they fed an abundance of orange and grapefruit juice to a group of lab rats. The results showed a surprising improvement in bone density. The researchers believe this success was due to the high concentration of antioxidants in the juice, but more research is on the way.

Dried Plums - My grandmother will be thrilled to know that her daily dose of prunes may be working double time. A study out of Oklahoma State University indicated that post-menopausal women who consume moderate quantities of prunes (just 12 a day) present increased rates of markers of bone formation. If the beneficial results continue, dried plums may have the potential to produce clinically significant increases in bone mass. Furthers studies are currently underway at the Florida State University College of Human Sciences. While these studies have focused on the primary risk group for osteoporosis, it seems the opposite sex need not feel left out of the prune frenzy. Scientists at the University of Oklahoma believe dried plums may also help prevent skeletal deterioration in men.

Tea - A 2007 study published in the American Journal of Clinical Nutrition, reported some potentially good news for tea drinkers. Australian researchers surveyed elderly women between the ages of 70 and 85 who were participating in a larger 5-year study on osteoporosis, about their green and black tea consumption. Bone density measurements were taken at the beginning and the end of the five-year study, and the tea drinkers exhibited a higher bone mineral density in their hips and less bone loss than women who didn't drink tea. Interestingly enough, they found no correlation between the number of cups consumed per day and bone density. The researchers took this as further confirmation on prior studies that have suggested a positive link between tea and osteoporosis prevention. Though they are not yet sure of the mechanism at work, the previous studies suggest that phytochemicals in tea, such as flavonoids, may be responsible for the protective effect against bone loss due to their estrogen-like properties.

How Much Calcium Do I Really Need?

The jury is still out on this one. The "official" recommendations for calcium were most recently set in 1998 by the Institute of Medicine at the National Academy of Sciences. They issued new Adequate Intake (AI) levels for calcium, which are as follows:

0 - 6 months	210 mg
6 - 12 months	270 mg
1 - 3 years	500 mg
4 - 8 years	800 mg
9 - 18 years	1300 mg
19 - 50 years	1000 mg
51+ years	1200 mg

Postmenopausal women not taking hormone replacement therapy	1500 mg
Pregnant and lactating women (younger than 18 years)	1300 mg
Pregnant and lactating women (older than 18 years)	1000 mg

However, many professionals in the medical and scientific community question these high calcium recommendations. They are more concerned with nutrient balance and preventing calcium loss. In countries such as Japan, India, and Peru, the average daily calcium intake is as low as 300 mg per day (less than one third of the U.S. recommendation for adults age 19 to 50), yet their incidence of bone fracture is quite low in comparison to the United States.

In another interesting comparison, the average daily calcium intake for African-Americans is more than 1000 mg, while it is only 196 mg for black South Africans. Oddly enough, the hip fracture rate for African-Americans is 9 times greater than the hip fracture rate for black South Africans.

Some speculate that the lower rates of fracture may be due in part to an increased level of Vitamin D, a new "healthy bone hero." It seems that excess calcium has a tendency to suppress circulating vitamin D. Others feel it may be a mix of cultural and dietary habits.

Calcium is essential for bone health, but what levels of calcium intake are optimal, is still in a heated debate. While the verdict is out, you may wish to reference the information below healthy dietary calcium options and consider supplementation for extra insurance.

Calcium-Rich Foods

Calcium is naturally abundant in a wide variety of foods, including most vegetables, fruits, and nuts. In fact, many green vegetables such as broccoli, bok choy, and kale have calcium absorption rates of 50 to 70%, much higher than the 32% calcium absorption rate found in milk. For your quick and easy reference, the following calcium charts list an abundance of healthy, dairy-free food options.

Dairy-Free / Gluten-Free / Vegan Calcium Chart
(*Calcium Content Shown in Milligrams*)

SOY FOODS
Serving Size: 1 Cup

Soy Beans, cooked	261
Soy Flour, defatted	241
Soymilk	93
Soymilk, calcium-fortified	368*
Tempeh	184*
Tofu, Firm, set w/ calcium	516*
Tofu, Medium Firm, set w/ calcium	260*

NUTS & SEEDS
Serving Size: 1 Ounce (unless noted)

Almonds, roasted	80
Almond Butter (1 Tablespoon)	43
Brazil Nuts	45
Hazelnuts	32
Pistachios	31
Sesame Seeds, hulled (1 Tablespoon)	37
Tahini (1 Tablespoon)	64

SALAD GREENS
Serving Size: 1 Cup, Raw (unless noted)

Borage	83
Chicory Greens	180
Collard Greens, boiled	226
Dandelion Greens	103
Kale, boiled	94
Lambsquarters, boiled	464
Lettuce, Looseleaf	38
Mustard Greens	58
Mustard Greens, boiled	104
Mustard Greens, frozen	152
Parsley	78
Turnip Greens	105
Turnip Greens, boiled	198
Watercress	40

GRAINS
Serving Size: 1 Cup

Amaranth, cooked	276
Amaranth Flour	300
Carob Flour	359
Corn Tortillas (2)	100*
Oats (not always gluten-free)	84
Quinoa, cooked	31

FRUIT & JUICE
Serving Size: 1 Medium (unless noted)

Blackberries (1 cup)	46
Figs, dried (1 cup)	241
Kiwi	46
Orange	56
Orange Juice, calcium-fortified	300*
Papaya	72
Raisins, Golden (2/3 cup)	52

BEANS
Serving Size: 1 Cup Cooked

Baked Beans	128*
Black Turtle Beans	103
Great Northern Beans	121
Mung Beans	56
Navy Beans	128
Refried Beans	88*
White Beans	161
Winged Beans	244
Yellow Beans	110

SPICES
Serving Size: 1 Tablespoon, Dried or Ground

Basil	85
Cinnamon	74
Cloves	39
Dill Seed	91
Mustard Seed	58
Oregano	48
Rosemary	38
Thyme	76

OTHER VEGETABLES
Serving Size: 1 Cup, Cooked (unless noted)

Acorn Squash	90
Artichoke (1 medium)	54
Asparagus	36
Bok Choy	158
Broccoli	72
Brussels Sprouts	56
Burdock Root	61
Butternut Squash	84
Cabbage, Green	50
Cabbage, Red	56
Carrots	48
Cassava, raw	33
Cauliflower	34
Celery, raw	44
Chinese Broccoli	88
French Beans / Haricot Verts	111
Green Beans	58
Kelp, raw	144
Kohlrabi	40
Okra	100
Peas, edible pod	62
Pumpkin, canned	64
Radishes, raw, sliced	29
Rutabaga, cubed	82
Seaweed, Agar, dried (1 Tablespoon)	50
Seaweed, Hijiki, dried (1 Tablespoon)	80
Squash, Summer	49
Sweet Potato, cubed	76
Turnips, cubed	51

MOLASSES / SWEETENER
Serving Size: 1 Tablespoon

Maple Syrup	21
Molasses, Blackstrap	172
Molasses, Light	33
Molasses, Medium	58

Dairy-Free / Gluten-Free / Non-Vegan Calcium Chart
(*Calcium Content Shown in Milligrams*)

SEAFOOD Serving Size: 3 Ounces (unless noted)	
Anchovies, canned (5)	45
Blue Crab, canned	86
Clams, canned	78
Ocean Perch Atlantic, cooked	116
Oyster, dried (3 medium)	45
Pink Salmon, canned w/ bones	181
Rainbow Trout, cooked	73
Sardines, canned	317
Shrimp, small dried (1 ounce)	167

A Few Notes on These Calcium Charts:
~ Most fruits, vegetables, seeds, and nuts contain some amount of calcium, but the above selections are limited to class leaders.
~ Spinach, rhubarb, beet greens, and Swiss chard are all very high in calcium. However, due to their very low absorption rates (approximately 5%), they have been excluded from the list.
~ With the exception of mung beans, the dried beans do have a fairly low absorption rate (approximately 17%), so only those with over 100mg of calcium have been included.
~ These numbers are intended for use as general information only. Actual calcium levels may vary.
~ For comparison, 1 cup of 2% cow milk has 297 mg of calcium.
~ Items with an asterisk (*) may vary quite a bit in calcium content based upon manufacturing processes.

Homemade Broth / Stock
One more calcium-rich food worth mentioning is homemade broth that is prepared using beef or chicken bones. Since results can vary significantly, there is no hard and fast calculation for how much calcium is in a batch of homemade broth, but in general, calcium from the bones makes its way into the soup as it cooks. To facilitate this, you should add some vinegar (1 Tablespoon for every 8 cups of water should suffice) to the cooking water, as it helps to extract calcium from the soup bones.

It's in the Water
Depending on where you live, you may be getting quite a bit of calcium via your tap water. England, the prairies of Canada, some parts of Australia, and most of the United States (with the exceptions of New England, the South Atlantic-Gulf, the Pacific Northwest, and Hawaii) have tap water that is quite high in minerals such as calcium, otherwise known as "hard water." It is important to know if you are already obtaining quite a bit of calcium from your drinking and cooking water, as too much calcium, as with any mineral, can have its drawbacks.

How to Become Calcium Fortified

Still concerned? Have no fear … the food manufacturers are listening. They have been stocking grocery store shelves with calcium-fortified versions of your old favorites. So much so that doctors are now waiving the red flag for calcium toxicity! These days you may find a good dose of calcium hiding in popular brands of frozen waffles, energy bars, soy yogurts, "healthy" pastries, granola, cereal, beverages, crackers, or other snack foods.

If you choose to reach for calcium-fortified foods, stick to the healthier options. An 8-ounce glass of calcium-fortified orange juice or milk substitute (soy, almond, rice, etc.) can supply you with the equivalent 300 mg of calcium found in an 8 ounce glass of skim milk. As an added bonus, orange juice is fortified with calcium citrate, the most usable source of calcium.

Use caution if choosing ready made hot and cold breakfast cereals as a calcium source. These are not a good option for the gluten-sensitive, and may be too high in calcium. One name brand cereal was fortifying each serving with 1000mg of calcium, which many doctors consider excessive.

Choosing the Best Calcium Supplement

Although a well-balanced diet is the best way to consume vitamins and minerals, some people prefer to take out an "insurance policy" or two in the form of supplements. One thing is for sure; there is no shortage of calcium supplements on the market. Here are some helpful consumer hints to narrow down your selections:

Types of Calcium Supplements
It is often best to ignore the sales pitches and consumer hype when purchasing calcium supplements. The least expensive and most basic brands of calcium carbonate or calcium citrate will typically do the trick:

Calcium Carbonate is the most inexpensive and readily available option. It contains the highest level of elemental calcium (40%); so fewer pills may be required in order to reach your desired daily intake. However, a big pill typically accompanies this big amount of calcium. A chewable or liquid version may be preferred for those who find the tablets too large to swallow. Calcium carbonate should be taken with meals or with an acidic beverage such as orange juice. It is alkaline-based and requires extra stomach acid for maximum absorption. For some, intestinal distress in the form of gas or constipation is a possibility. If this happens to you, try upping your dietary fiber intake, and drink more water. If that doesn't help, switch to calcium citrate.

Calcium Citrate usually costs just a bit more than calcium carbonate, and is not quite as easy to find, but overall it is an excellent option. Calcium citrate has less elemental calcium (21%), but it is better absorbed than calcium carbonate. It is acidic based, and may be taken at any time in the day, even on an empty stomach. If you are taking acid blockers for indigestion, acid reflux or other intestinal conditions, calcium citrate may be your best option from an absorption point of view.

Calcium Phosphate is rarely recommended. Although some types of calcium phosphate contain high levels of elemental calcium, the average diet already contains too much phosphorous from processed foods.

Calcium Lactate and Calcium Gluconate supplements are usually well absorbed, but they have a very low rate of elemental calcium (13% and 9% respectively). Calcium lactate is derived from lactic acid, but it should not be a problem for milk allergies or lactose intolerance.

Coral and Chelated Calcium options are frequently overpriced and over-hyped supplements. They supply no known advantages over any of the calcium compounds noted above. It is best to avoid supplements that contain dolomite, bone meal, or oyster shell. These products may be contaminated with lead, mercury, and/or arsenic.

What is Elemental Calcium?
Several different calcium compounds are utilized in supplements, such as calcium carbonate, calcium phosphate and calcium citrate. The elemental calcium represents the actual amount or percentage of calcium in the compound. It is important that you read the labels of calcium supplements to verify the amount of elemental calcium available. On the nutrition/supplement facts label a % of daily value is listed. This is based upon a

1000mg recommended daily value for calcium, so a supplement with a 25% daily value for calcium has 250mg of elemental calcium. Also, be sure to note the serving size, or the number of tablets, pills, etc. you must take in order to obtain that level of elemental calcium.

Isn't this Stuff Regulated?

Although the FDA does not currently regulate calcium supplements, you can check the label for the initials USP. This is a guarantee that the product meets with the U.S. Pharmacopeia's voluntary standards for quality, purity (lead content), and tablet disintegration.

Since the USP system is completely voluntary, it does omit some top brands. Sign up with Consumer Lab (www.consumerlab.com) for a broader selection of reputable vitamins and minerals. They test, and report on, various brands and types of supplements, utilizing the same basic markers as the USP (quality, purity, and disintegration / absorption).

Absorption Insurance

In reality, the body will easily absorb most brands of calcium products. However, if in doubt check for the USP symbol, select an approved product from Consumer Lab, or try a simple at-home test on a sample tablet. Place it into a glass of warm water or clear vinegar. Stir occasionally. If the tablet dissolves within 30 minutes, then the supplement will most likely dissolve in your stomach as well. Chewable and liquid calcium supplements are a good alternative to ensure proper absorption. As a general rule of thumb, calcium from diet or supplements is best absorbed when consumed throughout the day, in increments of less than 500mg.

Other Bone Builders to Consider

Adding to the confusion, calcium supplements can be found in varying combinations, often paired with other vitamins and minerals. Two of the most common calcium buddies you will find are magnesium and vitamin D ... and for good reason. Approximately half of the magnesium in our bodies is located in our bones, making it another important piece in the bone health puzzle. Vitamin D is essential for promoting calcium absorption in the gut and maintaining adequate concentrations of calcium in the blood. It is also required for bone growth and remodeling.

Many doctors argue that most healthy individuals do not need magnesium supplements. Magnesium is abundant in leafy greens, nuts, peas, beans, and whole grains, so in theory, those who consume a varied, well-balanced, whole food oriented diet should be well covered. However, other medical professionals argue that magnesium is deficient in most modern diets due to high fat consumption, the tendency to cook vegetables, depleted minerals in the soil, and excessive use of medications that can block the absorption of magnesium. Hence the popularity of calcium-magnesium supplements. Calcium and magnesium are quite synergistic, so if you do choose to supplement with magnesium, a combo of calcium and magnesium may simplify things. Those who believe they may have a magnesium deficiency due to illness should consult a physician.

On a different note, most doctors seem to agree that sunscreen, age, and increasing indoor activities are depleting the levels of Vitamin D we as humans are producing. This is prompting both the east and west sides of the medical community to unite in the recommendation of Vitamin D supplementation. You may opt to take calcium supplements that contain Vitamin D, which is great, but not an absolute must. Although Vitamin D enhances calcium absorption, it is taken in and stored in a unique way and at a different rate than calcium. Therefore, it can be taken separately from calcium, and still prove effective.

Will a Multivitamin Cover my Calcium Needs?

The multivitamin has become a convenient, one-stop vitamin & mineral insurance policy for today's hectic lifestyles. Not all multivitamins are created equal though. Multivitamins possess numerous vitamins and minerals; therefore quality is at greater risk. Be sure to select a USP or Consumer Lab verified product.

Precautions

Always check with your doctor or pharmacist before adding calcium or any other vitamins or supplements into the mix. This is particularly important if you are already taking any prescription or over-the-counter medications. Calcium has been shown to interfere with the absorption of iron supplements, Synthroid for hypothyroidism, bisphosphonate medication for osteoporosis (i.e. Fosamax or Didrocal), and certain antibiotics such as Tetracycline. A window of 2 hours or more between the medication and calcium supplementation is often recommended to prevent an interaction.

Also, if you choose to supplement, be careful not to go overboard. As sited by the National Institute of Health, the "Tolerable Upper Limit" of calcium for children and adults ages 1 year and older is 2500 mg per day (diet and supplements combined). It was not possible to establish an Upper Limit for infants under the age of 1 year.

CHAPTER 4:
INFANT & CHILDHOOD MILK ALLERGIES

If a food allergy or intolerance is suspected in an infant, then they should be under close pediatrician supervision. The following is merely baseline information for parents and parents to be. Always consult a physician before making any changes to a child's diet.

Recognizing Infant Milk Allergies

More than 100,000 babies suffer from a milk allergy each year. This condition causes digestive, respiratory and/or skin problems, but it is often very difficult to recognize, since infants are unable to put their discomfort into words. The following is a list of symptoms that may signal a potential milk allergy:

~ *Diarrhea* - Diarrhea is a common occurrence in babies, but if it is persists several times a day for more than a week, it could signal a milk allergy.
~ *Vomiting* - Babies often spit up bits of food, but a doctor should examine vomiting beyond the typical mealtime regurgitation. Reflux symptoms, such as excessive spit-up and difficulty swallowing can also be milk allergy symptoms.
~ *Skin Rashes* - There are many causes of red rashes and eczema, but it may signal an underlying milk allergy.
~ *Extreme Fussiness* - Every baby cries, but crying continuously and inconsolably for long periods of time is abnormal. When there is no apparent reason, this is usually called colic. Sometimes this extreme fussiness is actually caused by the gastrointestinal pain resulting from an allergy to the proteins found in milk.
~ *Respiratory Problems* - Colds are common for infants, but wheezing, struggling to breathe and developing excess mucus in the nose and throat is not. In some instances, these respiratory problems could be the baby's reaction to the proteins found in milk.
~ *Failure to Thrive* - Babies with milk allergies often suffer from a lack of proper nutrition characterized by dehydration, loss of appetite, low weight gain, and lack of energy.
~ *Recurrent Ear Infections* - It has been estimated that up to 79% of children with recurrent ear infections get them because of allergies. Signs of an ear infection may include a runny or stuffy nose, cough, fever, and/or irritability.

A few little known facts are important to understand when dealing with a food allergic child:

~ *Food Allergy Symptoms Vary in Severity*. Some children may experience dramatic respiratory symptoms, while others may develop a simple rash.
~ *Food Allergy Symptoms May Be Delayed*. An infant may experience allergic symptoms immediately upon feeding. However, the majority of allergic reactions are delayed, occurring a few hours to several days after consuming milk products. This can make diagnosis very difficult. Delayed reactions may include loose stools (possibly containing blood), vomiting, gagging, refusing food, irritability or colic, and skin rashes. Rapid-onset reactions come on suddenly with symptoms that can include irritability, vomiting, wheezing, swelling, hives, itchy bumps on the skin, and bloody diarrhea. In rare cases, a potentially life-threatening allergic reaction called anaphylaxis can occur and affect the baby's skin, stomach, breathing, and blood pressure.

~ *There Could Be Multiple Allergens.* If your child is allergic to milk, they have a greater chance of being allergic to other foods as well. If a milk allergy has been confirmed, but symptoms persist upon removal, consider having your child tested for other food allergies.

~ *Withdrawal May Be Difficult.* As noted in the next chapter, addiction is common with foods allergies. Just as a smoker craves the nicotine that causes negative reactions within their system, your child may actually crave the food they are allergic to once it is removed. If your child is allergic to milk, then their cravings should subside after a certain period of elimination, but it may take some time for the addiction cycle to be broken.

~ *Food Allergies Should Not Interfere with a Child's Growth.* Few foods are absolutely essential for growth. A child who is allergic to one food can certainly get the same nutrition in many other foods.

~ *Allergy Symptoms Can Change with Age.* Many children do "outgrow" milk allergies. However, when a food allergy or some level of sensitivity persists it is very possible for the symptoms to alter over time. A skin rash may morph into wheezing later in life.

Feeding Options

When a milk allergy or intolerance is considered, it is essential to consult with a physician for feeding recommendations and to monitor your child's condition. The following is a list of the options that may be useful to know about when speaking with your pediatrician.

Breastfeeding
The primary benefit of breast milk is nutrition. Human milk contains just the right amount of fatty acids, lactose, water, and amino acids for human digestion, brain development, and growth. It also contains at least 100 beneficial ingredients not found in formula.

Breastfed babies tend to have fewer illnesses because human milk transfers a mother's antibodies for disease to the infant. About 80% of the cells in breast milk are macrophages, cells that kill bacteria, fungi and viruses. Breastfed babies are protected, in varying degrees, from a number of illnesses, including pneumonia, botulism, bronchitis, staphylococcal infections, influenza, ear infections, and German measles. Mothers also produce antibodies to whatever disease is present in their environment, making their milk custom-designed to fight the diseases their babies are also exposed to. Furthermore, a breastfed baby's digestive tract contains large amounts of Lactobacillus bifidus, beneficial bacteria that prevent the growth of harmful organisms.

Babies are not allergic to their mother's milk, although they may have a reaction to something their mother eats. Babies with allergies or sensitivities may react adversely towards proteins within these foods, as they find their way into the breast milk. In cases of milk-allergic infants, nursing mothers would most likely be advised to follow a dairy-free diet. A lactose-free diet would not be sufficient since it is the proteins in milk, not the lactose, which instigates allergic reactions.

In rare conditions, such as congenital lactose intolerance (p25) or galactosemia (p29), an infant may be intolerant of their mother's milk. In these instances, a special formula and a strict lactose-free diet for the infant would be prescribed immediately. Unfortunately, it wouldn't matter if the nursing mother followed a lactose-free diet herself, as the infant would react to the lactose naturally occurring in her own breast milk.

Infant Formulas
Formulas available in the United States are approved by the Food and Drug Administration (FDA) and have been created through a very specialized process that cannot be duplicated at home. Regular, commercially available soymilk, goat milk, rice milk, and almond milk are not considered to be safe alternatives for infant formula. Here are a few types of infant formula to discuss with your pediatrician:

Soy Protein-Based Formula – Soy formulas are readily available, however, many doctors have differing opinions as to whether these are the best option. Some babies who are allergic to cow milk also have a sensitivity or allergy to soy. Do not confuse soy formula with soymilk; soymilk is not suitable for infants.

Hydrolyzed Formula – Hydrolyzed formulas are made from cow milk, but the proteins have been broken down or "pre-digested" to be less allergenic. Partially hydrolyzed formulas are of little benefit against milk allergies. Extensively hydrolyzed formulas may provide allergy symptom relief, and are frequently recommended by doctors as a first trial.

Amino Acid-Based Formula - Not all infants with cow milk allergies respond to hydrolyzed formulas. For these babies, amino acid-based formula is often the next option. It contains protein in its simplest form (amino acids are the building blocks of proteins). Though it is derived from cow milk, amino acid based formulas have a high rate of success among dairy allergic infants. However, this type of formula is extremely expensive, and not always covered by health insurance. The most well known brand of amino acid based formula is Neocate® (www.neocate.com, (800) 365-7354 – U.S., (877) 636-2283 - Canada).

Lactose-Free Formula – In rare instances, babies may be born with congenital lactose intolerance (p26). In this case, a lactose-free formula may be essential. Also, secondary lactase deficiency (p26) often occurs in babies suffering from acute diarrhea. In this case, a pediatrician may recommend the temporary use of a soy or lactose-free formula.

Once you switch your baby to another formula, the milk allergy symptoms should go away in 2 to 4 weeks if the new formula is successful.

Toddler Time
After their first year, your pediatrician may have some other options to recommend for your milk allergic child:

Milk Introduction – Even in children who have been milk allergic, doctors may recommend the gradual introduction of cow milk after one year of age. Some may have outgrown their allergy by this time, while others may not. Reintroduction of cow milk should always be done under the strict supervision of a doctor. It is up to the parents and their pediatrician to decide the diet that their child should follow.

Toddler Formulas - Otherwise known as "Nutritional Drinks," many on the market are dairy based, but options have emerged for rice, oat, and soy based nutritional drinks for children from the age of 13 months to 5 years. These drink mixes may be mixed into water or non-dairy "milks" for a tasty toddler beverage with essential vitamins and minerals.

Childhood and Beyond
Many children must live with a milk allergy throughout their growing years and into adulthood. Parents with a milk allergic child, or who opt to promote a dairy-free lifestyle in the home, may sometimes feel restricted in their selections. A few good recommendations I have found include:

~ *Follow Vegan Family Recommendations.* Though the information is limited for raising a child in a dairy-free household, vegan resources are abundant. If your family is most definitely omnivorous, it is simple to add meat, eggs, or fish to most vegan main dishes.
~ *Don't Ignore Healthy Fats.* Many parents are concerned that their children may not be getting adequate fat for growth and weight gain in the early years. Soymilk contains the most fat of the obvious dairy alternatives, which is similar to that of 2% milk. However, regular coconut milk (which can be used for pudding, soup, ice cream, etc.), avocados, and the wide array of nut butters are rich in plant-based fats. See p56 for more information on gaining weight.

~ *Keep Snacking Simple.* It is easier to prevent allergic reactions if the foods consumed contain few ingredients or are whole in nature. Try carrot sticks, celery, whole fruit (bananas, apples, pears, berries, melon, etc.), dried fruit, chunky applesauce, nuts, trail mix, olives, or popcorn. See the "Snacks & Apps" recipe chapter (p169) for more recipes and ideas.

~ *Get Them Involved.* Special diets can involve more made-from-scratch foods. Let children help in baking cookies, preparing snacks, and reading recipes. Not only will it be an excellent bonding experience, but it will also help them to better understand and cope with their diet in the future. Plus, you will have better odds in getting your little ones to eat some broccoli if they were the ones to stir those steamed florets into the pasta salad!

~ *Ask for Help.* Dealing with food allergies is no time to be shy. Ask questions, make requests, and help inform. When you come across people or companies that are resistant or unhelpful, then it is a red flag that this may not be the best option anyway. However, you may be surprised by how many "safe" foods you discover, and what companies and restaurants are more than accommodating.

~ *Join Forces.* Seek out or start a food allergy or dairy-free support group in your local area or virtually. Food allergy moms around the world have united via local groups and international Internet groups. These groups can offer everything from real world discussions on food allergies in school to recipe exchanges.

Infant Food Allergy Prevention

The "Official" Guidelines ...

In 2006, the American College of Allergy, Asthma and Immunology (ACAAI) released their recommendations for reducing allergy risk in infants. According to the ACAAI, whenever possible, new moms should breastfeed exclusively for six months to help protect their babies against developing food allergies. During this time, solid foods of all types should be avoided.

In the statement issued by the ACAAI, they also put forth suggestions for the introduction of top allergens. For infants who may show evidence of an increased risk for food allergies:

~ Cow milk and other dairy products should be avoided for the first year of life
~ Eggs should be avoided until at least age two
~ Peanuts, tree nuts, fish, and other seafood should be avoided until at least age three

These are the most common allergen triggers, but there are other foods that may pose a risk if introduced too early. Therefore the ACAAI contributed the following supplemental recommendations for "staple foods":

~ After 6 months of breastfeeding exclusively, solid foods such as fruits, vegetables, meats, soy, and cereal should be introduced "individually and gradually" to lessen allergy risk and to help identify any potential allergens.
~ Mixed foods containing a variety of potentially allergenic foods should be avoided until the baby's tolerance to each ingredient is known.
~ Beef, vegetables, and fruits should initially be given in the form of prepared baby foods that are cooked and homogenized. According to the studies they reviewed these "processed foods" may be less likely to cause allergies than the fresh varieties.

Wheat and cereals should be introduced gradually, though there are no specific guidelines for their introduction after 6 months of age. The ACAAI felt that the clinical evidence did not support wheat as a highly allergenic food for infants.

... Put into Question

But, according to two pieces of research released in 2008, many widely practiced methods for food allergy prevention in children may be ineffective. Former theory involved strict diets for both mom and baby, plus this strategic introduction of foods as mentioned above. However, the American Academy of Pediatrics (AAP) and a team of German Researchers have indicated that these strategies may simply be overkill.

Thousands of moms-to-be concerned that their newborns may be at risk for food allergies have proactively changed their own diets to avoid major allergens while pregnant and nursing. But, Dr. Frank Greer, author of a report on the topic and chairman of the AAP, stated that it probably does not matter what pregnant and lactating women eat in terms of prevention. Further, his report showed no evidence that mothers should hold out on the introduction of foods such as eggs, fish or peanut butter in the name of allergy prevention.

The AAP maintained their recommendation that atopic disease (eczema, asthma, and food allergies) may be delayed or prevented in high-risk infants if they are breastfed exclusively for at least 4 months or given infant formula without cow milk protein (casein). Along this line, they still recommend that parents delay the introduction of solid foods for 4 to 6 months in the name of allergy prevention.

Yet, even this guideline may not be well proven. A team of German researchers said that there is no evidence to support this recommendation. In fact, they found the delayed introduction of solids for the prescribed time did not lower a child's risk for nasal allergies, asthma, or food allergies. In fact, food sensitization was actually more frequent in children who were introduced to solids later rather than sooner. The one possible exception they observed was eczema. They did find that children given a more diverse diet before 4 months of age were more likely to develop eczema later in life. Of course, Dr. Joachim Heinrich, the senior researcher for the German study warns that parents should not ignore the advice to delay solid foods, as infants may not be developed enough to properly chew and swallow foods.

Regardless of the controversy on age, many doctors do recommend introducing one food at a time to high-risk infants, in order to help identify specific allergens. Only this new food would be added for roughly 4 to 5 days. With any food introduced, a record is kept noting any type of allergic reaction such as hives, rash, behavior change, or immediate coughing, and a physician is contacted immediately in the event of a severe reaction. Since each child differs in his or her needs and risk factors, you should speak with your pediatrician to decide what method of food introduction is best for your baby.

CHAPTER 5:
OTHER DAIRY-FREE CONCERNS

What about soy? Is a little dairy okay? How will I live without cheese? What if I need to gain weight? This chapter addresses these popular dairy-free FAQ's to help alleviate some additional concerns.

Battling with Dairy Food Addiction

Whenever I mention to someone that I do not eat dairy (never even suggesting that they should follow suit), they often interrupt to profess their extreme passion for cheese and proclaim that they could never give it up! You may think this is an exaggeration, but in a study that placed 59 overweight post-menopausal women on a strict vegan diet, the food most missed was not milk, chicken, bacon, or even ice cream, it was cheese. For those of you with this obsession for curdled milk or any other dairy-rich food, I have a few suggestions. Feel free to pick and choose which ones you think will suit your needs best:

Keep an Eye on the Prize
Odds are you are venturing dairy-free territory with a purpose. It could be for weight loss, food allergies, social reasons, or general health. Every time cravings strike, make a conscious effort to remind yourself of that goal. Will dairy cause distress to the little one you are nursing? Will it cause your own allergies to flare? Will it threaten to derail your dieting efforts? Will it promote embarrassing GI troubles? Will it sap your energy or up your risk for certain diseases of concern? Does it conflict with your animal rights beliefs? Enough of these reminders will keep you motivated on your path and may even help those once sought-after foods seem rather unappealing.

Look for Replacements Before Taking the Plunge …
Although there are no identical substitutes to dairy, there are many alternatives on the market that are pretty good. Delicious non-dairy "milks" and "ice creams" made from soy, rice, coconut, hempseed, and/or nuts seem to be all the rage. Admittedly, cheese is the toughest dairy product to find a good substitute for, but the options are growing and improving each year. Test a few brands out to find one or two that will suffice, or trial a homemade "cheese" recipe (p120) for a flavor boost.

… Or Break the Spell
Opposing the above recommendation, you may need to cut ties completely from dairy and alternatives to rid yourself of cravings. For some people, teasing the taste buds with cheese alternatives that aren't quite "there" can actually up their desire for the real thing. Rather than seeking out cheese subs, get cozy with recipes that are naturally cheese-free.

Create a Menu
All too often I read about people attempting a diet, only to find themselves eating apples and energy bars all day. A little forethought goes a long ways in transitioning to a free-from diet. If you have the time, plan that transition. Your dairy-free needs could be urgent, as you or a loved one may be very sick from a newly discovered food allergy. On the contrary, the symptoms may be mild to moderate ones that you have lived with for quite some time or you may be making the switch for personal reasons. If the latter is true, then you may

have some leeway in switching to a dairy-free diet; consider keeping your diet as is for a few days, using that time to plan out two weeks worth of menus while stocking your pantry and freezer.

As an example, my husband and I decided to trial the vegan diet for our health. I was a bit nervous about what we would eat, so I spent a lazy Sunday afternoon gathering recipe ideas before we took the plunge. With a prepared refrigerator and several meal ideas ready to go, it turned out to be a piece of cake and my very omnivorous husband actually loved every entrée. Plus, the planned meals and snacks bought me some time to become comfortable with vegan cooking. I had no trouble in coming up with food ideas, even after my original menus had been exhausted.

Choose Your Method Wisely
Sometimes weaning yourself off is easier, but other times quitting cold turkey is the only effective method. For myself, going back to a dairy-free diet happened overnight, and it worked very effectively for me. My vicious ice cream cravings stopped within three days, as did the food allergy symptoms I was experiencing. Yet, sugar withdrawal has been a gradual process. I tried to toss all of the sweet stuff, but even after a completely sugar-free month I was still wrestling with jumbo cookie cravings. With sugar I have found that gradually changing my diet is helping me to retrain my taste buds.

Keep an Eye Out for Saboteurs
You might switch to cheese-less pizza and change to a tofu-ricotta lasagna, but if the premade pizza crust or bottled pasta sauce you are using has some sneaky cheese or milk in it, then your cravings may continue. For many people, even small amounts of an offending food can often keep those cravings going in full force.

Don't Allow Yourself to Get Over-Hungry
When following a free-from diet it is all too easy to find yourself in a ravenous state, simply because you couldn't think of anything to eat. Make sure you always have a good supply of snacks on hand to keep hunger at bay while you are trying to figure out your next meal move. Otherwise you might be more likely to succumb to those dairy cravings.

Turn Your Attention Away From Food
Exercise can deter your attention from food, and it can actually change what foods you desire. After a good workout, the last thing I crave is heavy foods, such as cheese. Refreshing salads and fruit smoothies make the menu instead.

Make Your House a Dairy-Free Zone
It can be hard to cut out cheese, milk, or any other foods when temptation beckons from the other side of the refrigerator door. The support of your family, including sharing your special diet at home, makes the journey much easier. If they are reluctant, remind them that it will help you significantly ... and they can always sneak away for a slice of cheese pizza.

Check Your Addiction Level
If you are absolutely sure that giving up cheese or other dairy products would be the biggest torture you could imagine, then you may actually have a "food addiction." No, I am not joking. Food addiction has been a heavily researched issue. Strong and consistent cravings for a particular food are not considered healthy, and are often compared to the behavior of drug addiction, but on a much smaller scale of course.

Addictions to caffeine, sugar, and chocolate have been shown in studies, and now theories are circulating about milk and grain addictions. When casein, the primary protein in milk, is broken down in our digestive system it produces casomorphins, otherwise known as opioid peptides. This part is well proven. The controversy comes with respect to what happens next. Some believe that the opiate effect is neutralized, while others state that these peptides can pass to the brain and various other organs to elicit an opiate effect. Scientists believe that mother's milk (cows are also mothers when they are producing milk) possesses this opiate effect in order to heighten the mother-baby bond, calming the baby, and often resulting in them falling off to sleep following feeding. Cheese contains a high concentration of casein, and therefore is under scrutiny for this opioid related "food addiction."

Many people who have felt this strong "addiction" to certain milk products find that they actually have an allergy or a general heightened reaction to casein. Removal of the milk products for a certain length of time (varies by individual) usually eliminates the cravings altogether along with the symptoms or side effects (migraines, stomach pain, etc.). For some people it may just be a couple of weeks before the cravings and symptoms subside, but for others it may take a few months.

Am I suggesting that all cheese lovers are addicts who must give up milk? By all means no. If you feel it is impossible to take a short break from any particular food, it is time to do a reality check. This is particularly true if you have symptoms that could be the result of food sensitivities or a vitamin or mineral deficiency.

Milk Allergies & the Rotation Diet

If you do not experience severe allergic reactions to milk, some amount of dairy flexibility may be well tolerated in your diet if you wish. In this type of situation, doctors often recommend trialing a rotation diet.

Sometimes strict rotation diets are essential for people who have multiple food allergies, but they have been adapted in many ways to suit individual needs. The basic concept involves a 4-day rotation cycle with three days on followed by one day off. In other words, keep your diet dairy-free for three days, and the fourth day can be more relaxed. It is believed that this cycle allows your body to fully process a food, preventing a build up of the offender in your body, and thus minimizing any negative reactions. Many people rotate foods regularly for basic health, and to keep their diet varied.

Utilizing a dairy rotation diet can be quite simple if you keep your kitchen dairy-free. By following a dairy-free diet at home (where it is assumed you do most of your eating and lunch prep), you may not need to be as concerned about accidental milk ingredients slipping into your meal when eating away from home. It also allows you to schedule your "on" dairy days with more efficiency.

A rotation diet will not work for lactose intolerant individuals (lactase does not replenish, even on "off" days), but it may allow for better planning with those lactase enzymes.

Is Soy a Good Option?

Soy foods are growing in popularity throughout North America, particularly due to the rise in awareness of lactose intolerance, allergies, and chronic disease prevention. In fact, according to the United Soybean Board's 2006 annual report, 82% of Americans now view soy foods as healthy (up from 67% in 1998). However, concerns remain among the other 18% due to conflicting reports in the media.

I could write an entire book on the controversies of consuming soy, in fact, a few have already been written. It is safe to say that I am fairly objective on the topic, as I do agree with both sides of the soy equation to some extent. The following includes some of the facts that have helped me to address the issue of soy in my own diet.

Scientific interest in soy emerged from observational studies of geographically based populations. Researchers noted that groups who consumed a lot of soy, particularly those in eastern Asia, experienced a significantly lower incidence of breast cancer, prostate cancer, age-related brain diseases, and cardiovascular disease, in addition to fewer bone fractures. The topic became more interesting, as the researchers followed the health of Asians who immigrated to areas such as the United States. Those who altered their diets toward westernized foods experienced an upward change in disease rates. This indicated a strong tie to environmental and lifestyle influences, rather than ancestry.

Opponents to soy claim that the amount of soy consumed by Asians has been exaggerated. For the most part, this is true, yet the typical Asian diet is still significantly higher in soy than the Standard American Diet (SAD). A 2003 report from the UN Food and Agriculture Organization, estimated the per-capita consumption of soy protein per day to be almost nine times higher in Japan than in most European and North American countries. Beyond the statistics, a sociable chat with a current or former resident of Japan, China, or most other East Asia countries will confirm that soy foods have been an integral part of their diet for generations.

Though many medical professionals view it as a very nutritious product, soymilk is relatively new throughout the world. It is now consumed in Asia, but it is not typically considered a traditional food. Traditional soy foods primarily include tofu and fermented soy products, such as miso and tempeh. It should be noted that the various methods of preparing soy (i.e. fermentation) for consumption have a dramatic effect on the health properties of the food. In other words, specific reports on health benefits and/or detriments should probably not be blanketed across 'soy' as a whole. The portion of the bean which is utilized, and the method by which it is prepared will have a dramatic effect on its composition and digestibility.

Much of the positive research to date has focused on dietary soy in the form of whole foods such as tofu. The findings of concern tend to focus on animal and human intervention studies that used soy concentrates or isolated isoflavones (plant compounds or phytoestrogens), rather than soy as a whole food. This implies that these isolated chemicals, which are sold in over the counter pills and powders and are sometimes used as ingredients in food products, may be harmful when extracted, but beneficial when a component of the whole food.

The United States is one of the world's top soybean producers, in select years producing as much as 50% of the global soybean crop. This means that soy, like corn, is readily available and relatively inexpensive in the U.S. Therefore, it is widely utilized in various forms throughout the processed food industry. In fact, it is believed that over half of all processed foods in the United States contain soy in some form or another. On food labels it may appear as soy flour, soy lecithin, soy protein isolate, hydrolyzed soy protein, protein concentrate, plant sterols, textured vegetable protein (TVP), soybean oil, or simply vegetable oil. With stats like these, it is easy to see how soy may be "overdone" in the United States.

Nonetheless, the research supports soy in moderation as a healthy addition to most diets, and some go so far as to add it to the list of highly respected "superfoods." Some soy suggestions that may be useful for non-dairy consumers are:

~ Focus on whole soy-based foods (tofu, edamame, soy nuts, etc.) and fermented soy products (miso, tempeh, tamari, etc.).
~ Consume soymilk and soy desserts in moderation; incorporating a good selection of nut and grain based milk alternatives.
~ Limit your consumption of processed foods, and cut out any made with hydrogenated oils or unrecognizable ingredients.
~ Make olive, peanut, grapeseed, and safflower your oils of choice in cooking and baking.
~ Keep your diet well diversified. 'Too much of a good thing" applies to just about any type of food, no matter how healthy it may be. Though your doctor may advise 5 to 10 servings of fruits and vegetables per day, it

would sound ridiculous and unwise if he or she simply recommended 5 to 10 servings of oranges per day. Soybeans qualify as a single food that can be an excellent contributor to a healthy diet, but need not overwhelm it.

~ Eat soy foods as a part of a balanced meal or snack, rather than on their own, when possible. The benefits with most foods are best recognized when consumed in combination with a wide variety of nutrients, vitamins, and minerals.

~ If you like soymilk, consider making your own from dried soybeans (p98). This will ensure a good quality product, without the additives or isolates that may be found in some commercial brands. For homemade soymilk, I do recommend purchasing a soymilk maker, as it will greatly simplify the process and quickly earn its keep. You can inexpensively purchase dried soybeans in bulk, producing quarts of homemade soymilk for pennies.

~ Select organic products and/or those made with non-GMO soybeans whenever possible. Most soybeans grown in the United States are genetically modified. Genetically modified foods are still relatively new, so little is known on their safety. Organic soybeans should be non-GMO, and have been grown without the use of toxic pesticides or chemicals.

Additional Considerations:

For some individuals soy can pose additional health problems that may supersede the soy debate. If you are living with one of the following conditions, consumption of soy products may be ill-advised:

Hypothyroidism - Evidence shows that excess consumption of the isoflavones found in soy may disrupt thyroid function, in those individuals who already have a thyroid disorder, or who consume insufficient levels of iodine (not a typical deficiency in westernized countries). Unfortunately, the research is still vague, and a definition for "excess" has not been given. Those who live with hypothyroidism may wish to limit soy consumption, and should regularly have their thyroid levels checked.

Food Allergies - Soy is noted as one of the top eight allergens in the United States. Though not as common of an allergen as cow milk, many people have found that they are in fact sensitive to soy protein. The only widely accepted treatment for any food allergy at this time is elimination from the diet. However, studies show that most individuals who are allergic to soy protein may be able to safely consume soybean oil (not cold pressed, expeller pressed, or extruded oil) and soy lecithin, as these products rarely contain soy protein. If you suspect a soy allergy, consult a physician.

When Gaining Weight is a Good Thing

The topic of weight loss dominates our society, but for millions of people, weight gain is a more pressing issue. When it comes to growing toddlers in need of nutrition, athletes, and anyone who can't spare to shed another pound, too little fat and protein can be a concern with dairy-free diets. Especially since western societies do tend to use consumption of cow milk products as a "shortcut" to weight gain. Intended for rapid growth of calves, the milk from dairy cows is rich with fat, protein, and hormones that can easily pack the pounds on our significantly smaller species. In fact, most people do not realize that cow milk contains three times the protein of human breast milk.

Of course, eggs, fish, and meat can easily fill the fat and protein void, but there are many other options for those who forsake these animal products, whether for religious, social, health, or taste preferences.

"Healthy" Sources of Dietary Fat

Many argue that the fatty acids from plant sources (such as the monounsaturated fat in olive oil and the Omega-3's in nuts) are not only less harmful to our bodies than the saturated fat from animal sources, but that they could actually be a healthy addition to most diets.

<u>Coconut "Meat," Milk, and Oil</u>
18g of fat per ounce of dried coconut / 25g of fat per 1/2 cup regular coconut milk / 14g of fat per tablespoon of coconut oil
Here we have another controversial item, but really, what food isn't? Coconut is quite high in saturated fat, however, some experts purport that the saturated fat in plants (most foods have some amount of saturated fat, no matter how little) is quite different from the saturated fat found in meat and dairy products. In fact, some even tout the fatty acids in coconut oil for antiviral, antibacterial and antifungal health benefits. At the time of writing, the jury was still out on this topic, but I do believe that enjoying some coconut products in moderation can be worthwhile.

Let the truth be told that I am on the pro-coconut side, but partially because I love the stuff. Coconut milk is a fantastic natural stand-in for cream; shredded coconut offers that tropical flare to smoothies and baked goods; and coconut oil provides a rich, almost buttery flavor. For those who have an aversion to coconut, do not immediately shy away from the milk and oil. When used in recipes, the coconut flavor tends to vanish with great frequency.

<u>The Oil Spectrum</u>
14g of fat per tablespoon of oil
Before cooking entered my personal repertoire (beyond the reheat and serve method that is), I thought oil was oil. I grew up with that big jug of multi-purpose vegetable oil, always ready to report for duty. Of course, using any oil will help to ensure adequate fat in the diet, but there really are so many flavorful oils to choose from. A few that I always keep on hand are grapeseed oil (for baking, cooking, and general purpose), coconut oil (for spreads and specialty recipes), extra virgin olive oil (for dressings and drizzling), peanut oil (for stir-fries and Asian dishes), and sesame oil (for drizzling on Asian dishes). See the chapter on butter alternatives (p109) for more information on the various types of oil available, and how to use them.

<u>Avocados</u>
30g of fat in 1 medium avocado
It's a vegetable; no it's a fruit ... who cares? Avocados are nutritious and delicious, and that is really all that matters to me. They are loaded with monounsaturated fat (the kind that shot olive oil to world class health fame), and very versatile. Chop up the flesh and enjoy it on salads and in sandwiches, or blend it up to create a creamy base for dips. Avocados can even be snuck into recipes as a thick cream or binder.

<u>Tree Nuts and Peanuts</u>
Nuts range from 13g of fat per ounce (cashews) to 21g of fat per ounce (macadamia nuts)
For those who don't have a peanut or tree nut allergy, nuts are excellent options for supplying "healthy" fats. Plus, the selection goes far beyond peanuts; enjoy walnuts, almonds, Brazil nuts, hazelnuts, pecans, pistachios, and pine nuts as a general snack on their own or tossed into a homemade trail mix blend. In recipes, add some chopped nuts to baked goods; stir them into rice or other grain dishes; grind them to use as coatings for meat, fish, or vegetables; use them for structure and flavor in veggie burgers; or simply sprinkle them atop a salad. You can also find most nuts in nut butter form, but if not, you can make your own by grinding the nuts in a food processor until a paste forms, adding oil to thin if needed. Yes, it is that easy.

<u>Seeds</u>
Seeds range from 9g of fat per ounce (chia seeds) to just over 13g of fat per ounce (sunflower seeds)
This often-overlooked food category can jump right into any nut's role, and raw versions (not roasted) may be safe for some nut allergies (always check with our physician before trialing seeds on someone with a nut allergy). You can choose from sunflower seeds, pumpkin seeds, hemp seeds, chia seeds, flax seeds, and sesame seeds. Sunflower and pumpkin seeds are sizable enough for snacking, but the other varieties are best used in recipes, either ground or whole. Both chia seeds and flax seeds actually make great egg replacers in baked goods when ground and combined with water (p137). Though a bit harder to find than nut butters, seed butters are gaining in popularity. You can often find pumpkin seed butter and hemp seed butter in natural food stores. Sesame seed butter, otherwise known as Tahini, is much easier to find, due to its important role in hummus.

<u>Olives</u>
4.5g of fat in 4 kalamata olives
Just like its oil, this finger food packs in a good dose of those "healthy" fats. Olives are a fun food for kids too. To this day my grandfather comments every time I see him about how I used to head straight to the olive appetizer each time we visited, popping an olive on each finger, and enjoying them one by one when I was very little. Beyond straight snacking, olives add wonderful flavor to savory recipes. In place of Parmesan, I typically dice olives (green, black, or Kalamata) and use them as a flavorful topping on pasta dishes.

<u>Chocolate</u>
Chocolate ranges from 9g of fat per ounce (semi-sweet) to 15g of fat per ounce (unsweetened)
Last time I checked, chocolate ranked as a health food. Well, that's my story and I'm sticking to it anyway. Rich with cocoa butter, good quality chocolate is an excellent source of fat and indulgence in my personal opinion. Use caution, as many brands of chocolate are made on shared equipment with milk chocolate. For most dairy-free dieters, trace quantities off milk will not be a problem (most (but not all) companies do a thorough cleaning of equipment between milk and non-milk chocolate batches), but for some who are highly sensitive or allergic, even the minute amount of "parts per million" could spell disaster.

Alternate Sources of Protein
Let's start with a little background on protein, shall we? Technically, humans have a biological requirement for amino acids, the "building blocks" of protein, rather than protein itself. We are unable to internally produce certain amino acids, so we must obtain them from the consumption of food. These are referred to as essential amino acids.

<u>Complete Proteins</u>
Meat, fish, eggs, and milk are often referred to as "complete proteins" because they contain all 8 to 10 essential amino acids (two are essential only in certain cases) in sufficient quantities. Luckily, there are also a few good plant sources of complete proteins. Plant foods that are frequently labeled as complete proteins include spirulina, quinoa, soy (soymilk, tofu, tempeh, etc.), buckwheat, hempseed, and amaranth.

<u>Incomplete High Quality Proteins</u>
Several plant-based foods are labeled "incomplete proteins" simply because they are low in one or more of the essential amino acids. Yet, as one might expect, the incomplete protein sources do add up. A varied diet will allow certain foods to fill in with an essential amino acid that another food may be lacking. Contrary to prior beliefs, these complimentary foods need not be eaten together either. The various essential amino acids will jump into their role whether or not their companions have yet to arrive. Thus, a food can be a good source or protein even if it is not "complete."

Various grains, legumes, nuts, and several vegetables can provide our bodies with a good dose of incomplete proteins and assist in meeting those essential amino acid requirements. Most notably, spinach, broccoli, peas, lentils, and beans are relatively high in protein. One cup of cooked spinach actually provides 13g of protein. Most other nuts (almonds, walnuts, cashews), seeds (sesame, sunflower), and grains (brown rice, bulgur, wheat bread) follow closely behind with at least 2-4g of incomplete protein per reasonable serving size.

Protein Powders
The protein powder world tends to be dominated by dairy in forms such as whey, but as the demand rises, new types of dairy-free protein powders are gradually emerging. Soy protein powder is a long-time contender that is readily available, but one need not feel limited to the bean alone. In recent years, several brands of rice protein powder have emerged, so much so that little packets can often be found near the checkout stands in health and natural food stores. Some other little-known vegan, gluten-free, and food allergy friendly options include hemp protein powder from companies such as Manitoba Harvest (www.manitobaharvest.com) and pea protein powder from Kirkman® (www.kirkmanlabs.com). See the product lists available via www.godairyfree.org for a current list of dairy-free protein powders, shakes, and related food products.

As a side note, AHD International (www.ahdintl.com) patented a cranberry protein powder. It is not available for consumers to purchase directly, but it is being sold to food manufactures as a food allergy-friendly, protein boosting ingredient. I imagine we will see more of this product in dairy-free, soy-free meal replacement beverages, energy bars, and other protein-rich foods to come.

Along this line, protein powders are frequently purchased by food manufacturers to be used as ingredients in their products. Due to an increasing demand for "functional foods," you may find energy bars, cereals, beverages, or other convenience-based products that are fortified with one of the above mentioned protein powders or concentrates. However, be vigilant when considering packaged foods that boast a good dose of protein. Though non-dairy sources are growing in popularity, most of these products will still use milk in some form as the primary protein source.

Skincare, Supplements, and Medication

Lotions, sunscreen, soaps, make-up and other skincare items frequently contain food-based ingredients, including milk in various forms. Since topical applications of food allergens are of less concern than their ingestion, labeling isn't quite as stringent. Yet, some people do have reactions to these products when applied, and others prefer not to support the dairy industry for environmental or social reasons. In the U.S., the FDA does require cosmetic manufacturers to list the ingredients on the product label, but trade secrets (including certain fragrances) do not have to be specifically listed.

Since it is odd to see skincare products that are labeled as dairy-free I look for those that are touted as vegan. Not only are vegan products made without milk, but they also tend to contain "natural" ingredients that are easier to decode. Otherwise, be prepared to translate the chemically worded ingredient labels into plain English, and contact the manufacturer to verify ingredients and processes. A customer service phone number should typically be listed on each package. Even if you feel "safe" with the product, do a mini patch test on your elbow, and wait 24 hours to see if a reaction occurs before liberally applying it.

Supplements and medications are an even trickier minefield since they are in fact ingested; yet still relatively unregulated in terms of food allergen labeling. Lactose and various other milk-based ingredients are often added to those little pills as fillers without warning. In fact, lactose is used as the base for more than 20 percent of prescription drugs and about 6 percent of over-the-counter medicines and vitamins. For most people, the small amount of lactose in these pills may not be a problem, but it is good to use caution, since it can be for some. If you have a milk allergy, consult your physician to discuss if a lactose-containing medication may be safe for you since your nemesis is milk protein rather than lactose, and such a small amount might not pose a risk. If you have severe lactose intolerance and the small amount of lactose in a particular medication causes discomfort, seek another brand, or if this isn't possible, ask your physician if it would be safe to take a lactase enzyme with the medication. Keep in mind that while lactose is the most commonly used milk ingredient in medications, some medications may contain milk protein or other milk-based ingredients.

When ordering a prescription, be sure to ask your pharmacist if the medication is milk-free before they fill it. They should have a list of ingredients for each medication on hand. With over-the-counter medications, all non-active ingredients should be listed on the packaging to alert you to any dairy-containing filler. Allergy sufferers may have a particularly hard time locating dairy-free antihistamines, as many of the brands and generics do harbor lactose. While ingredients in medications can change at any time, at the time of writing, I found lactose-free options with Allegra® (fexofenadine) and several antihistamines in liquid form.

Like food and cosmetics, the ingredients in supplements should be listed on the label, but may change without warning. Once again, seeking out vegan brands of supplements is a good first step. Yet, whenever there is a concern, scour the label and contact the manufacturer. I would like to briefly address two of the most common supplements taken by dairy-free consumers, calcium and probiotics.

Calcium itself, whether in the form of carbonate, citrate, phosphate, etc., is not a dairy product. While calcium is found in milk, calcium pills should not be derived from milk, as that would be a rather laborious and unnecessary process. However, like other supplements, it is possible to find brands with milk ingredients used as fillers, so double check the ingredient statements.

As for probiotics, I have spoken with the customer service lines of many manufacturers, and unfortunately, the staff members are frequently under-informed on the source of their company's probiotics. In their purest form, probiotics are simply bacteria, but many are cultured or "produced" on dairy. The result is a product that may contain trace amounts of casein, whey, or other milk allergy aggravators. This may not be a problem for those with less severe allergies or lactose intolerance, but you might not choose to take this risk. I seek out probiotics specifically touted as dairy-free and/or vegan. When a severe milk allergy is of concern, I would take it a step further and contact the manufacturer, to verify their dairy-free claim if possible.

You will see several types of probiotics that begin with the term Lactobacillus. They are named as such for their ability to convert lactose and other sugars to lactic acid, not because they are derived from dairy. This does not give the green light to all bacteria in the Lactobacillus group, as some may be cultured on dairy, but it also means that you may find this type of bacteria in a "safe" probiotic.

For both skincare and supplements, I have included some of my favorite brands below, as well as recommendations from the helpful people at Vegan Essentials (www.veganessentials.com), Cosmo's Vegan Shoppe (www.cosmosveganshoppe.com), and Ethical Planet (www.ethicalplanet.com). These three online shops (each with a retail location) offer hard to find vegan / dairy-free grocery items, supplements, and skin care products, and are consequently very familiar with the various product lines. Keep in mind, these suggestions are not all-inclusive. Odds are you can find at least a few dairy-free products among most skin care, cosmetic, and supplement lines, but I wanted to offer some recommendations to get you started. Most of the products listed below are available in both the U.S. and Canada, and some are sold internationally.

Skin Care & Color Cosmetics
For those with multiple food allergies, keep in mind that many dairy-free and vegan skin care products may use other "natural" allergens, such as nuts, coconut, soy, gluten, or citrus, so proceed with caution. Vegan products should be free from milk and egg-based ingredients, but always check with the manufacturer first, as ingredients and processes can change, and as mentioned, those labels can be tricky to read.

Alba Botanica™ (www.albabotanica.com, (888) 659-7730) – This is a 100% vegetarian company that offers a broad (easy to find) product line of skin, hair, lip, and sun care products. They do have a few non-vegan products (lanolin or beeswax), but at last check all of their products were dairy-free. I frequently purchase their sunscreens, face products, and lip tints.

Avalon Organics® (www.avalonorganics.com, (888) 659-7730) – This 100% vegan / dairy-free company offers a long-standing line of skin and hair care products, along with a full line of baby and sensitive (fragrance-free) skin care products.

Bare Escentuals (www.bareescentuals.com, (888) 795-4747) – Their bareMinerals® line, like most mineral make-up, is an excellent natural option for sensitive skin that is made without top food allergens, including dairy.

Beauty Without Cruelty (www.beautywithoutcruelty.com, (888) 674-2344) – This 100% vegan company offers a full line of skin, sun, and hair care, plus a full line of color cosmetics.

Blue Lizard® (www.crownlaboratories.com, 423.926.4413) – This "Australian sunscreen" is actually made in Tennessee. The Chemical-Free version has been recommended to me as good for sensitive skin and also multiple food allergies, since it is made without the coconut oil, almond oil, or shea butter that some may react to.

California Baby® (www.californiababy.com) - This line of infant hair, skin, and sun care products is free from gluten and most common allergens, including milk, eggs, peanuts, tree nuts, soy, wheat, and (as I would hope for anything I was slathering on a child's body) fish. Just a couple of their products contain non-vegan ingredients.

Cetaphil® (www.cetaphil.com, (817) 961-5000) - Though this one doesn't qualify as a "natural" brand, in my (extremely sensitive skin) experience, this is the brand most recommended by dermatologists and allergists for those who have sensitive skin. They primarily offer lotions and cleansers.

Desert Essence® (www.desertessence.com) - Their organics line of skin and hair care includes products that are 100% vegan / dairy-free and gluten-free.

Dr. Bronner (www.drbronner.com, (760) 743-2211) – It is hard to match the simplicity of this 60+ year old company. Over the years they have added skin, hair, and lip care products, along with a complete line of sensitive skin / baby products. Nonetheless, the Magic Pure Castile Soaps are still their claim to fame. These mild, oil-based soaps are organic, fair trade, environmental, economical, and can be used for everything from general skin care to house cleaning.

Earthscience® (www.earthessentials.com, (805) 684-4525) - This line of skin and hair care is mostly vegan (a few products do contain beeswax, lanolin, or silk proteins), and it appears to be free from milk ingredients.

Ecco Bella (www.eccobella.com, (877) 696-2220) – This line of cosmetics, and skin and hair care is made without any dairy ingredients, and is mostly vegan with the exception of some of their cosmetics. Their cosmetic line is gluten-free / casein-free (GFCF).

JASON® (www.jason-natural.com, (877) 527-6601) - This is not an exclusively vegan company, but they do sell many vegan / dairy-free products. Plus, in addition to their skin, hair, lip, oral, and sun care products, they have an Earth's Best® 70% Organic Baby Care product line that is touted as hypo-allergenic, and appears to be completely vegan and dairy-free.

Kiss My Face® (www.kissmyface.com, (800) 262-KISS) – Most of their products are vegan; at the time of writing, just a handful contained beeswax or honey, and one contained Lactic Acid (Peaches & Creme 8% AHA), which I presumed was derived from dairy, based upon their site. Kiss My Face® offers skin, hair, lip, oral, and sun care products plus a kid's line.

Nature's Gate (www.natures-gate.com, (818) 882-2951) – This is a 100% vegan / dairy-free producer of skin, hair, oral, and sun care.

Origins (www.origins.com, (800) ORIGINS) - A few products in the Origins line contain beeswax or honey, but the rest are vegan, and all appeared to be dairy-free, at least at the time of writing. They offer a wide range cosmetics, skin and hair care, typically sold in department stores.

Pangea Organics (www.pangeaorganics.com, (303) 413-8493) – I had the opportunity to trial run some of the uber-environmental and socially aware products from this skin and lip care producer, and I was impressed. To the best of my knowledge this is a vegan / dairy-free manufacturer.

Supplements & Probiotics
Vegan products should be free from milk and egg-based ingredients, but always check with the manufacturer first, as ingredients and processes can change, and as mentioned, those labels can be tricky to read.

Amazing Grass® (www.amazinggrass.com, (415) 441-3326) – Their Superfood line is a drink mix that is packed full of vitamins, minerals, pre- and probiotics, and digestive enzymes, and the chocolate version is pretty tasty, I might add. They also offer a Kidz Superfood product. All of their products are vegan, dairy-free, and gluten-free.

DEVA™ Nutrition (www.devanutrition.com, (508) 519-9199) - This is a 100% vegan / dairy-free company offering vitamins, minerals, herbs, and some additional select supplements.

Freeda® Vitamins (www.freedavitamins.com, (718) 433-4337) - This is a very allergy-friendly vitamin, mineral, and probiotic company, offering a wide range that includes children's and prenatal supplements. All of their products are dairy-free and free from most foods of concern (gluten, eggs, yeast, etc.). Most of their product line is vegan, though a few items have a shellac glaze on them.

HealthForce Nutritionals (www.healthforce.com, (760) 747-8822) – This is another 100% vegan manufacturer of vitamins, minerals, herbs, and supplements. Though they do not seem to offer probiotics specifically, they do have probiotic blends within some of their formulas.

Udo's Choice (www.florahealth.com, (800) 446-2110 (U.S.), (888) 436-6697 (Canada & Beyond)) – This is the brand of probiotics that I regularly purchase. Their product line is touted as dairy-free, and to date, I have not had any problems with them. Their core company, Flora Health, offers a good range of vitamins and supplements, many of which are labeled as vegan and dairy-free.

Veglife® (www.affordablesolaray.com, (732) 477-3088) - This is a completely vegan /dairy-free brand of vitamins, supplements, and probiotics from the supplements giant Nutraceutical Corp. You can find many other dairy-free options scattered among their other brands, but the VegLife line makes it easy. The VegLife line also includes a line of vegan shakes / powders sold under the label Peaceful Planet™.

Sequel Naturals (www.sequelnaturals.com, (604) 945-3133) - Their Vega line comes in powder form, and is promoted as a meal replacer. It is vegan, dairy-free, and gluten-free, and it contains a good dose of protein, along with vitamins, minerals, digestive enzymes, and probiotics.

Section 2

Eating Away From Home

CHAPTER 6:
RESTAURANT DINING

Though home-cooked meals are making a big comeback, who doesn't crave a night out? Visiting a restaurant can be a fun social outing, offer a much needed break from the kitchen, and provide sustenance when traveling or in a rush. With some helpful tips and an open mind, you can easily indulge in a night (or two) on the town, without sacrificing your health or non-dairy lifestyle.

Before moving on, I must include an upfront disclaimer. A good portion of this chapter is geared toward those who need not fear potential cross-contamination. Restaurant kitchens are notorious for shared knives and equipment that are not always properly cleaned. For example, while your meal may be made without milk, it may have come in contact at some point in the process with your friend's lasagna. If you are dealing with a severe food allergy then you must exercise extreme diligence when dining in restaurants. You can never be too careful.

When it comes to coping with severe food allergies away from home, my idol is Sloane Miller, aka "Allergic Girl." Sloane has life-threatening food allergies (EpiPen® and all), but she refuses to let them get in her way of living. In fact, she eats out in New York most days of the week. Sloane shares food allergy advice and restaurant stories on her blog (allergicgirl.blogspot.com), and she was kind enough to offer a checklist of "to do's" for managing severe food allergies in restaurants:

~   Bring your medications.
~   Bring allergy cards.
~   Make sure someone at the table knows you have allergies and how to help you in case of an emergency.
~   Call ahead and speak with the manager, always.
~   When ordering talk slowly, calmly, and clearly.
~   Make eye contact.
~   Relax.
~   Be assertive and clear not aggressive and scary.
~   Talk with the highest-level person you can, such as the manager and/or chef.
~   Ask the kitchen's comfort level with your allergies; if they hesitate go elsewhere.
~   Repeat your needs after every course.
~   Thank your server.
~   Tip well.
~   Thank the manager.
~   Go back; re-patronize a restaurant that is able to deal with your needs.

If you are dealing with a child with severe food allergies, I also recommend picking up a copy of *How to Manage Your Child's Life Threatening Food Allergies* by Linda Coss. She touches on many different challenges to be faced in the "real world."

Ordering Off the Menu

When jotting down tips for choosing potential dairy-free menu items, I stumbled across a strange coincidence. The advice for dining dairy-free looked remarkably similar to healthy eating words of wisdom. What fantastic news! Diners who choose dairy-free options will also open themselves up to healthier restaurant habits ... perhaps freeing themselves (at least a bit) from that post-meal sluggishness and belly bulge.

Remember, these suggestions will be most applicable to those who can tangle with a stray cheese shred or two without a trip to the ER, but should offer some general guidance to anyone seeking dairy-free menu items. As always, use your best judgment, and take all necessary precautions.

~ *Ask Questions* - This is by far the most important tip. Don't be afraid to inquire on the ingredients of a dish, or to ask for any changes to a menu item. Any good server will be able to help, or will not hesitate to go ask the chef. Food allergies are growing at a rapid pace, low carb dieters are demanding bun-less burgers, and weight loss fanatics are requesting smaller portions. The hospitality industry recognizes the need to respect those with special diets as a key to success. In fact, research shows that an increasing number of restaurants are providing flexibility in food preparation methods, varied portion sizes, and expanded menu offerings.

~ *Avoid Fried Foods* – If general health isn't reason enough for you to stay away from the deep fryer, then keep in mind that milk (and egg) products may linger within coatings and deep fryers are often a major source of food allergen cross-contamination.

~ *Choose Heart Healthy Oils* - The menu will usually specify if a dish is cooked in oil or butter, but if in doubt, just ask. Most kitchens will have vegetable and olive oils on hand. Also, when ordering meat, fish, pasta, or vegetables, request that butter is not added. Some chefs add a pat to grilled or steamed foods for flavor.

~ *Go Mediterranean* - When ordering pasta dishes, look for tomato and olive oil based sauces rather than cream sauces. You will save yourself loads of saturated fat, and the tomato sauce can even be counted as a serving of vegetables.

~ *Dress Lightly* - Oil & vinegar, honey mustard, French, and vinaigrettes are often suitable dairy-free salad toppers. Avoid the heavy ranch and blue cheese choices. Mustard, ketchup, BBQ sauce, and mayonnaise (contains eggs) are usually dairy-less, but use a light hand to limit your sugar and fat load.

~ *Everything On the Side* - Ask that your condiments and salad dressings come on the side. This is a very common request that most women have made more than a few times. Benefits include portion control and the ability to give the condiment a once over before it comes in contact with your entire meal.

~ *Soup or Salad* - Salads are an excellent way to get your greens. Mind the salad dressing tips above, order it without cheese and you will usually be good to go. Although several appear obvious (chicken noodle, vegetable, chili, split pea), your best option is to ask what dairy-free soups are available. Many restaurants even serve up vegan "cream" soups.

~ *Take a Meat Break* - Most restaurants have added a vegan option or two to their menus over the past few years. Although the entrées may be noted as "vegetarian" (meatless), the growing trend in cutting out all animal products has turned many vegetarian dishes into vegan ones (meat, egg, and dairy-free).

~ *Unload That Potato* - Skip the sour cream, butter, and cheese customarily found on a "loaded" baked potato or blended into your typical mashed potatoes. Salsa, non-dairy salad dressings, or a touch of salt and pepper can add ample flavor to a baked potato. Better yet, choose roasted, steamed, or boiled potatoes.

~ *Get Out of the Butter Rut* - Many restaurants offer fantastic dips and spreads for your bread, appetizers, and meal. Experiment with flavored oils, sweet and savory salsas, tapenades, fresh guacamole (checking to make sure that sour cream has not been added), or hummus.

~ *Cook It Right* - Selecting menu items that are baked, grilled, dry-sautéed, broiled, poached, or steamed will yield the healthiest food as well as better odds at a dairy-free plate.

~ *Keep Recipes in Mind* - However your mother or grandmother used to make it is probably how they are making it in the restaurant kitchen. Pancakes, waffles, scrambled eggs, mashed potatoes, and other traditional fare are typically made with a good helping of milk.

- ~ *Watch for Diet Fads* - Many of the new diet and health options listed on menus are cream-, butter-, and cheese-less.
- ~ *Take It Black* - Have your coffee and tea sans milk and cream. Ask if they have soymilk, you will be surprised how many places do. If you are concerned, bring along your own packet of soy or rice based creamer.
- ~ *Save Dessert for Later* - Still craving dessert? Head home for one of your own dazzling recipes or store-bought treats. Restaurant desserts are typically quite heavy (translation, full of cream and butter). If you must, fruit and sorbet options are usually safe.
- ~ *Read the Menu* - No, I mean, really read the menu. Most restaurants will provide a slightly detailed description of the entrées. This will allow you to narrow down your options, and ask specific questions on the remaining choices.
- ~ *Inspect the Dish Upon Arrival* – Okay, this doesn't have much to do with the actual ordering process, but make sure that the meal arrives as you order it. I have ordered many entrées without cheese, only to find a slice or two lurking within by mistake.

And my absolute FAVORITE tip...drum roll please....

- ~ *Go Ethnic* - That's right, we dairy-free consumers eat like well traveled food connoisseurs, even if we have never left the continent. The following pages include some general guidelines for international cuisine ...

Around the World in 80 Restaurants (Give or Take)

Expand your menu of options with tastes from around the world ... but remember no restaurant follows exactly the same recipe. In fact, many "Americanize" their recipes to make them inexpensive to prepare and more appealing to less worldly taste buds. There are no guarantees of authenticity; you must always ask the chef! For example, while a traditional Thai curry would be made with coconut milk, some restaurateurs might use cow milk (yuck!)

With that said, the following are merely suggestions, a baseline of ideas to get you started if you will. Use your own due diligence and perhaps some of these ideas will materialize into deliciously "safe" restaurants that you can enjoy frequenting.

Green Light Cuisine - Many Dairy-Free Options
Most Asian restaurants will provide an abundance of dairy-free menu items ... but, once again, always double check with each restaurant and exercise precaution whenever there is cause for concern.

Chinese
Chinese menus can be expansive, and the majority of items listed qualify as dairy-free. Indulge in egg rolls, hot and sour soup, chicken in black bean sauce, moo shu pork, fried rice, beef and broccoli, mixed seafood, or Buddha's (vegetarian) feast. Don't forget about dim sum either. This appetizer sized assortment of dumplings, rice rolls, and steamed buns makes for a fun and delicious meal.

Warnings:
- ~ Crab Rangoon is made with cream cheese.
- ~ Aside from fresh fruit, the dessert menu generally contains dairy-rich items.
- ~ The batter used to deep-fry certain dishes (such as sweet and sour chicken) should be free of milk ingredients, but use caution. Vegans and those with multiple food allergies should take note that the batter is usually made with eggs. If in doubt, take the healthy route and avoid the deep-fried entrées.
- ~ I have spotted a few store-bought Chinese sauces that contain a very small amount of dairy. If concerned, ask to verify the ingredients with the chef.

Japanese

Thank goodness for sushi! Okay, not everyone is a sushi fan, but there is much more to Japanese cuisine than raw fish and seaweed wrappers. Virtually the entire menu, including teriyaki and noodle dishes, is abundant with dairy-free options.

Warnings:
~ Vegans and those with egg allergies should be aware that the batter used in tempura is usually made with eggs, though rarely with milk. Also, egg-based mayonnaise is often used in the spicy sauce or to add richness to some of the vegetarian sushi.
~ Aside from fresh fruit, the dessert menu generally contains dairy-rich items.
~ Some "American Style" sushi rolls may contain cream cheese (i.e. Philly or Boston rolls).
~ Some brands of imitation crab (frequently used in California and other "American-style" sushi rolls) do contain a dairy ingredient or two.

Thai

Thai food is an excellent indulgence. The generous use of coconut milk creates many rich and creamy, yet dairy-free meals. You can enjoy curry, basil, and ginger flavored dishes, and as an added bonus there may be a few items on the dessert menu, such as sticky coconut rice, that get the go ahead.

Warnings:
~ As noted, there are no coconut milk guarantees. Verify that the chef is not using milk or other dairy-based products.
~ As a warning to vegans and the egg allergic, fish sauce is a very common ingredient in Thai cuisine, as are eggs, but many Thai restaurants offer several vegetarian options.

Vietnamese

Aside from the desserts, it would be difficult to find any dairy containing items on a Vietnamese menu. The cuisine includes various noodle and broth dishes, as well as uniquely seasoned meats and vegetables served atop rice. The appetizers can also make a filling meal; sample the various spring rolls, summer rolls, and skewers.

Warnings:
~ Vegans take note, though vegetarian items are readily available, fish sauce is frequently used. Request seasonings utilizing soy sauce, lemon grass, and lime.

Yellow Light Cuisine – Proceed with Caution

Since dairy products are quite prevalent in these establishments, there is a higher probability of cross-contamination.

Mexican

Okay, they do love cheese and sour cream, but the "finer" and more authentic Mexican establishments are generous with meat, fish, and vegetables and lighter on the grease. Also, I like to think of Mexican food as assembled rather than prepared. Sour cream and cheese are often added as condiments, but rarely make up the base of the meal.

Suggestions:
~ Choose the green and red sauces, and ask to make sure they are not prepared with cream or butter. These are usually tomato and pepper blends that are free of milk ingredients.
~ Try fajitas, burritos, tamales, wraps, or tacos, but "hold the cheese and sour cream, please." Any Mexican restaurant should easily be able to accommodate this, and almost all of the dishes can hold

their own without the added fat. If you are craving some richness, ask to substitute avocado slices or non-dairy guacamole.

~ Ask for "Mexican guacamole." It is almost always dairy-free. However "American guacamole," which is often served at Mexican establishments along with or in place of the authentic variety, may be blended with sour cream.

~ Tortilla soup is delicious and may be dairy-free. Ask if it is made without cream, and request chopped avocado instead of the usual cheese topping.

~ Enjoy some seafood Vera Cruz. This delightful fish preparation is loaded with tomatoes, olives, and capers. Try other grilled seafood and meat entrées (such as carne asada), and request that they are cooked in oil rather than butter.

~ Enjoy the Spanish influenced entrées such as paella. Spanish cuisine has a strong Jewish (kosher) influence so many of the cheese-less Spanish tapas are prepared without any milk ingredients.

~ Skip the horchata. Though it is traditionally a rice milk drink, horchata is often made with cow milk.

~ House made chips and salsa typically get the go ahead.

~ Skip the custard and cream based desserts.

Greek

Greece is at the heart of the Mediterranean diet, which means olive oil is used abundantly. Yet, yogurt, feta cheese, and Béchamel (white sauce) are major dairy culprits at Greek restaurants.

Suggestions:

~ Hold the tzatziki. This yogurt and cucumber-based sauce is a common topping for gyros and a dip for other traditional dishes. Ask if they have a dairy-free tahini sauce or hummus instead.

~ Though it is possible, the flatbreads used in Greek cuisine are often quite simple, and should not contain dairy derivatives. This means gyros, sans feta and tzatziki, may serve as delicious and hearty alternatives to the "wrap."

~ Trial an authentic Greek salad; they are typically made with a blend of oils, vinegar, lemon juice, and fresh herbs. The eggplant (aubergine) salads and the beet or beetroot salads are two great selections. Some salads may contain fresh mozzarella or feta, so be sure to ask.

~ Chickpea, lentil, bean, and vegetable soups are very popular at Greek restaurants. Most are prepared with olive oil and vegetables as the base. Just a few may utilize butter or cheese, though cream is rarely used. Inquire at the restaurant; they will likely have a few dairy-free options.

~ Ask about the fillo-wrapped items. Though many may be stuffed with only spinach, chicken, or ground meat, feta could lurk within.

~ Enjoy some traditional dishes, including hummus, souvlaki (meat or fish grilled on a skewer, hold the sauce), dolmades (stuffed grapevine leaves), and falafels (deep-fried croquettes of ground chickpeas or fava beans). Moussaka (eggplant casserole) may be dairy-free, but it may be made with a cream sauce and topped with cheese; always check on this one.

~ In traditional Greek cuisine, the meat sauce is tomato based, and the garlic sauce is rich in olive oil. Check with your server, but these should be free of milk ingredients, and good alternatives to Béchamel.

~ Olive oil is used with great abundance in good Greek cuisine. This means the meat dishes and even some of the casseroles are free of milk ingredients. Since the recipes for most Greek dishes are simple in terms of ingredients, the restaurant should be well aware of which entrées contain butter or cheese.

~ The desserts (butter cookies, cakes, baklava, and custards) are typically off limits, as they are usually rich in butter. Halva is one option that should be dairy-free. Also, if they have loukoumades (Greek style donuts) ask if they are made with butter or oil; you may just get lucky on this one.

African

Africa is an enormous continent, and the cuisine can vary widely by region. While traditional African food tends to be rich in milk, curd, and whey, dishes that reign from the more tropical regions are often dairy-free. These non-dairy options are typically abundant in grains, vegetables, and flavor. Don't hesitate to call around and ask about the cuisine; you may find a unique new restaurant to frequent.

Caribbean

Because many small islands have limited access to dairy products, their cuisines have adapted to the use of local spices, herbs, oils, and flavors. This is also region dependent, but worth calling around. One of my favorite restaurants in San Francisco was French Caribbean; the entire menu was fragrant, delicious, and completely open to my special diet.

Red Light Cuisine – Be on High Alert

Though possible, extra diligence may be required to unearth non-dairy dishes in the following types of restaurants.

"American"

Butter, cream, and cheese are practically staples in American-style restaurants, from greasy spoons to upscale "continental" cuisine. Mashed potatoes are whipped with butter and milk, sauces are indulged with cream, pastas are coated in cheese, eggs are scrambled with milk, and even the basic steak may be grilled with butter.

Suggestions:
~ Order salads, hold the cheese, and get the dressing on the side. Ask the server if there are any non-dairy dressing options.
~ If you can, avoid breakfasts out. Most omelets, scrambled eggs, French toast, and pancakes are made with milk. If you must, ask for your eggs poached, hard-boiled, or soft-boiled, or see it they can scramble them without milk. Though not particularly healthy, the meats are most often non-dairy, including breakfast sausage and bacon. Dry toast or bagels (you can top it with jam or honey) may be another option if you are not highly sensitive to potential dough conditioners in bread. Of course, the fresh fruit is always a good selection.
~ Order steamed vegetables, herbed potatoes, or a dry baked potato. Request salsa, salt and pepper, or oil and vinegar for added flavor.
~ Stick to grilled meats and fish. Request that they are prepared with oil rather than butter.
~ If you are not super-sensitive to milk, hamburgers, chicken burgers, and other sandwiches, hold the cheese, may be good options. Assuming the burgers and chicken are not cooked in butter, only the bun/bread should have a small risk of containing whey or other milk-based ingredients. Just make sure to request a dry bun, as most restaurants give it a quick toasting with butter for added flavor. Another option is to skip the bun altogether and order a low carb burger salad.
~ Look for a good international option. Many fast-casual bar and grills have a good selection of not so traditional entrées. On most, I can find Italian pasta dressed with tomato sauce or olive oil and/or a Chinese style stir fry.
~ Skip dessert. Unless you spot sorbet or fresh fruit, American style restaurants tend to hide milk ingredients in what would appear to be dairy-free desserts. The cobblers and crumbles most certainly harbor loads of butter. The cakes and pies are typically made with cream and milk. Plus, a homemade brownie may be made with oil, but in the restaurant world, it likely has some creamy ingredients to up the indulgence factor.

Irish / English Pubs

In general, the above suggestions for "American" cuisine carry over quite well to Irish and English pubs. Cream, butter, and cheese are mainstays on their menus, so care needs to be taken when ordering, and substitutions or changes to the entrée may need to be requested. However, Irish pubs typically offer a few hearty stews, such as the traditional Corned Beef and Cabbage, which are typically dairy-free, though obviously not vegetarian.

Indian
If you are craving a curry, then Thai food is certainly a better option. Nonetheless, there are a few potential selections from the Indian menu, particularly if you are willing to ask questions or if butter, ghee, or yogurt is well tolerated.

Suggestions:
~ Many Northern Indian curries are made with cream. However, a few may be made without dairy, or potentially just with some ghee (clarified butter). These include Channa Masala (chickpeas in a tomato curry); Gosht Vindaloo (spicy lamb curry), and Jhinga Masala (shrimp in coconut curry). Some people believe that ghee is completely safe for both the milk allergic and the lactose intolerant, as it is in essence, purely butter fat. However, many argue that it still contains trace amounts of lactose and casein, and that it is still in fact a dairy product. If this is not a concern for you, then the above listed curries may be a good choice.
~ Skip the tandoor and kabob entrées. Though they may look completely dairy-free, these specialties are typically marinated in yogurt.
~ Try some Southern Indian cuisine. Dosas are vegetable filled crepes that are frequently free of milk ingredients, and may also be gluten-free (always check). They may be prepared using ghee or oil, so be sure to ask if you have a preference.
~ Steer clear of any entrée with the word "paneer". Paneer is an Indian cheese that is the highlight of many well-known dishes.
~ Inquire on samosas. They are deep fried little triangles with a stuffing of meat, potatoes, or other vegetables. A small amount of ghee may be used, and the occasional variety stuffed with cheese is always a possibility.
~ Sorry, the desserts are definitely off limits. Somehow I think cheese balls in sweet cream may be dairy-loaded.

Italian
When I think of the Italian food of days gone past, it brings to mind rich lasagna and manicotti stuffed and topped with mounds of cheese. Sad, but true, these dishes will be a no go, unless you find one specifically labeled "vegan." Cream, vodka, and pesto sauces are also best to avoid. Though some pesto sauces may be free of milk ingredients, most include Parmesan, and may also be thickened with cream.

Suggestions:
~ So many pizzas are becoming elaborate creations. Pepperoni is out; Thai peanut chicken and sun-dried tomato with basil are in! If the pizza toppings sound bold enough to stand on their own, order it without cheese. Just ensure that the sauce they are using is not a cream sauce and that the crust does not harbor milk or cheese.
~ Most plain pasta varieties are safe, though raviolis are more often than not stuffed with cheese. Check on the gnocchi, some may be made with Parmesan, though the plain varieties are often dairy-free.
~ Peruse the menu for fresh tomato sauces, arrabiata (a spicy tomato sauce), or pasta dressed simply with olive oil.
~ Try an upscale Italian restaurant; many will use flavorful vegetables and grains in place of the cheese, for a more "impressive" creation. After all, anyone can throw cheese on a dish to make it taste good.
~ Order a chicken, steak, or fish entrée, and request that it is cooked in olive oil, not butter. This should be an easy request, as any good Italian restaurant should have an abundance of olive oil on hand.
~ Try one of the many green salads, and request a dairy-free dressing on the side.

French

When I think of French restaurants, I envision stylishly thin brunettes nibbling on billowing salads at an outdoor café. In reality, French cuisine can be very heavy, after all, the French love cheese...and cream, and butter, and... well you get the point.

Suggestions:
~ Ask about the regional influence. While cuisine from the northwest of France uses a lot of butter and cream, in the southeast they favor olive oil and fresh herbs and vegetables. Most other regions rely more heavily on animal fat for cooking and flavoring.
~ Order the "whole food" items, such as herbed potatoes rather than mashed, steamed vegetables rather than purees, and fresh fish. Request that the items are cooked in oil or other non-dairy fat if you prefer.
~ Enjoy the French salads. Salade niçoise, mixed greens, and the various vinegar based vegetable salads are lighter and often dairy-free.
~ Avoid the soups, as they are primarily cream based.
~ On the dessert menu, it is best to stick to the sorbet. Though the mousses, custards, tiramisu, and fruits a la crème may be tempting, they are most certainly dairy-rich.
~ On the appetizer menu, forgo the escargot, but enjoy the salmon or beef "tartare" if not following a vegan diet.
~ For a touch of indulgence, enjoy the aioli, it is in essence a flavored mayonnaise, and thus typically dairy-free, but not egg-free or vegan.

German / Swiss

Cream, butter, and cheese, oh my! My last dining experience at a German restaurant left me with one item on the menu to order. It was delicious, but limiting nonetheless.

Suggestions:
~ Though the schnitzels may be dairy-free, they are often cooked in butter. Inquire on the ingredients and request that your entrée is cooked in oil.
~ Fondue is the most popular way to enjoy Swiss food in the U.S. The cheese fondues are always off limits, for obvious reasons. However, the meat and vegetable fondues are typically cooked in a mixture of broth and oil. Also, ask if the chocolate fondue is milk-based. The finer restaurants often prepare a rich dark chocolate version.

Use Caution - Remember, the above tips are general guidelines, but there are no dairy-free guarantees when dining out. Ask questions, survey your meal, and when in doubt, move on.

Fast Food

We all have those moments when sustenance is essential, but we find ourselves trapped in an airport food court, in a late night conundrum looking for food, or simply "allergic" to the kitchen. When easy and inexpensive is the only way to go, utilize these tips to navigate the fast food maze:

~ *Go Green* - Opt for the salads, sans cheese, and reach for the vinaigrette, honey mustard, and French dressings. With fast food, dressing almost always comes on the side. Ask what your options are, check the ingredients where readily available, or go without!
~ *Eat Real Food* - Choose the most "whole" looking options. If it is fried, and thus unrecognizable, it is probably in a coating with numerous unknown ingredients.
~ *Head East* - Asian fast food eateries, as well as Asian menu options, are everywhere. Avoid the fried dishes if you can, this should still leave you with a myriad of choices.

~ *Think South of the Border* - The "Fresh Mex" trend grew rapidly in the '90's and may still benefit you today. Enjoy homemade salsas and tortillas stuffed with a mix of creations; hold the cheese, sour cream, and special sauce, please. Ask about the guacamole, it may in fact be free of dairy ingredients.

~ *Pick the Best* - Sandwich shops and delis vary in quality, but a good sandwich needs no cheese. Though you may want them to use a light hand, mayonnaise is almost always dairy-free (but not egg-free or vegan). Avoid the croissants; there is enough butter in these to make anyone's stomach churn.

~ *Keep Kosher* – Jewish dietary rules forbid mixing milk and meat, making kosher delis an excellent lunchtime resource for dairy-free dieters. Plus, the staff should be fairly knowledgeable on non-dairy offerings.

~ *Check the Soup Board* - Most fast food places have daily soups, but you may have to look around to spot them. Bean, tomato, vegetable, Mexican tortilla, split pea and the ever so popular chili are often excellent options.

~ *Splurge on a Slight Upgrade* - Thank goodness for the growing trend of "fast-casual" chains. They work to offer the quality foods of nicer sit-down restaurants in a fast food atmosphere.

~ *Always Ask* - Never hesitate to ask at the smaller or fast-casual chains if a particular menu item contains dairy. If you inquire at the golden arches, you are likely to get a blank stare, but many emerging fast food eateries are targeted more specifically at the health conscious consumer and the special dieter. If they don't know, most fast food eateries (including the golden arches) have a handy book or poster of ingredients.

~ *Educate Yourself in Advance* – Many fast food eateries now post their ingredients and allergen charts online, so that you can have a little advanced notice on your best menu options.

~ *Take a Look* - Never assume there are no dairy-free options. Even my local smoothie shop offers soymilk upon request or pure fruit smoothies.

~ *Use Good Judgment* - For the majority, a dairy-free lifestyle is very straightforward. Scan the menu for your best, and most enticing, options. It is likely that you will quickly learn to pick the winners.

Use Caution - If you are severely allergic or intolerant, very few fast food joints will be accommodating. Though many may have non-dairy dishes, they are typically prepared in the same kitchen, using the same equipment as dairy-based products. Restaurants that receive "pre-prepared" and packaged foods run a slightly lower risk of cross-contamination. Nonetheless, more vigilant measures must be taken for severe food allergies. Plus, ingredients and processes change very often at fast food eateries. A "safe" item last month may contain milk this month. When in doubt, move on.

CHAPTER 7:
SOCIAL EVENTS & TRAVEL

Dining with Friends and Family

Whether you are invited to a fancy dinner party, a holiday get together, or a potluck, it is never out of line to alert the host of any special diet needs you may have. Here are a few simple suggestions for making the event more enjoyable:

~ *Take All Necessary Precautions.* If lactose intolerance is your nemesis, be sure to have some lactase enzymes stashed in your purse or pocket. If milk allergies are a concern, double check that your medicine is in tow. Just because it may be a casual event doesn't mean that the usual precautions should not be taken.

~ *Schedule Your Personal Menus.* If you are able to follow a rotation style diet, where a little dairy is okay, be sure to plan your "on" day for the day of the get together. This will offer you more flexibility.

~ *Bring an Entrée and Preferably a Dessert to Share with Everyone.* Even if it isn't a potluck, ask your host if you may bring something that accommodates your needs and may be enjoyed by others. This could actually take some burden off of the host. Also, if the guests are eating some of the same foods as you, then you won't feel as out of place.

~ *Load Up on the Non-Dairy Offerings.* Most good dinners or potlucks will have some salads, vegetables, or breads that are likely dairy-free. Ask the person who made the dish to double check on the ingredients. If you can't eat it, they will be less offended knowing that you weren't simply snubbing their dish, and they may be more inclined to accommodate your needs at a future event.

~ *Give the Host Some Advance Notice if Your Diet Needs are Special.* They may easily be able to put cheese or salad dressings on the side for guests to add on their own. This way additional menu items may not need to be prepared. Also, by giving them as much notice as possible, it may help them to make that final decision between lasagna and chicken cacciatore.

~ *Ensure Ample Serving Utensils.* I can't count the number of times that I have spotted the serving spoon for something like lasagna double-dipped into a nice bowl of dairy-free pasta salad. Help the host by putting a proper serving utensil in each dish to help prevent cross-contamination.

~ *Bring Some Back-Up Food.* It is possible that not a single item will be dairy-free at the party. Bring a back-up meal or package of snacks, just in case.

On the Road

Whether you are running errands around town, or heading out on a cross-country road trip, keeping adequate supplies of snacks on hand can be a life saver. At home or when fixated in a particular destination, taking your time to select meal options can be quite feasible. But when traveling from here to there, good options may not appear when hunger strikes. The following foods are some of my personal non-dairy suggestions for quick, safe and easy foods to pack along. After all, you don't need to leave your healthful eating plan in the driveway when you hit the highways ...

- ~ Single-serving boxes or homemade baggies of dairy-free cereal, trail mix, energy bars, granola bars, cereal bars, dried fruit, mixed nuts and seeds, cookies, or crackers.
- ~ Bagels, muffins, or other baked goods (preferably homemade, otherwise, check the label to ensure dairy-free).
- ~ Raw fruit and vegetables including carrot and celery sticks, grapes, apples, peaches or bananas.
- ~ Single-serve applesauce
- ~ Peanut butter or other nut butter (for sandwiches or with celery and apples).
- ~ Jerky, regular or vegan.
- ~ Bottled water and juice boxes.

"Safe" Travel

If dairy-free, vegan, or even GFCF living is your concern, then investigate the dining options at your destination(s) before you head out. Many cities, particularly large ones, will have restaurants that cater to a variety of special diets. A quick search online may reveal some delicious raw eateries (typically dairy-free, vegan, and gluten-free), vegan restaurants, or simply dining spots that go to extra lengths to accommodate special diets.

However, if you are dealing with severe and/or multiple food allergies and intolerances, or you simply can't find good restaurant options at your destination, then dining out on the road can feel like more stress than it is worth. For suggestions on traveling with dietary restrictions I went straight to the expert, Loretta Jay, the President of Parasol (www.parasolservices.com), a consulting organization that specializes in the management of food allergies and celiac disease. In her family of four, three live with celiac disease and both kids have extensive food allergies. Yet even with the challenge of multiple food allergies and gluten-free living, they travel and experience the culture of wherever they visit, thanks to some special planning by Loretta. In the May 2008 issue of *Foods Matter* magazine, Loretta offered the following tips:

Hotel - For weekend trips, ensure that at least a microwave and a mini-fridge are in your room. For longer trips, book a room with a kitchen or kitchenette.

Packing - Consider shipping a box of food ahead to your hotel for emergencies, rather than risking your food in the maze of lost luggage. The box should include a 2-3 day supply of non-perishable "must-haves" that may be difficult to find at your destination. If perishable items are needed, pack these last, in an insulated bag, which you then pack in a hard-sided suitcase for your checked baggage. The bag should also include a signed letter from your physician explaining any allergies, just in case the contents of the bag come under question. If traveling abroad, don't forget to check on international customs regulations, as certain types of foods may not be permitted to cross borders.

Air Travel - Since quick 5 hour flights can easily turn into 2 day adventures with delays, cancelations, and rerouting of flights, carrying on an ample supply of snacks to cover a full day of meals can be worth its weight. Be sure to check the current airline restrictions for carry-on baggage, though. You may be limited on the types of foods you can pack, or a note from a physician may be needed. Food allergies are considered a hidden disability, so accommodations can often be made with some pre-planning. Also, [this is my own tip] call ahead to the airline, as they might be able to accommodate you with a special meal, should they serve food. Many airlines offer vegetarian, kosher (often dairy-free), and other special meals for dietary restrictions.

Shopping - Most regions of the world provide basic foods such as potatoes, rice, onions, legumes, salt, and olive oil. Plus, roadside vendors and local markets can be great places to learn more about the culture while stocking up on local whole foods. While shopping, don't be afraid to strike up a conversation and ask about favorite recipes. You may discover some popular local fare that you can easily prepare and customize to your diet.

Cooking - Loretta's family doesn't eat in restaurants when traveling, but she still wants her family to experience the culture of the land they are visiting, including the food. Before leaving home she does some pre-travel homework (online or at the local library) to learn the types of food and mode of cooking indigenous to the region they will be visiting. For example, in the Caribbean she might add a tropical twist to plain old pancakes by preparing them with coconut milk and serving with plantains; and in Spain some homemade tapas are perfect for a take along lunch while a Spanish tortilla can serve as a native dinner. To avoid getting too overwhelmed with cooking, Loretta also suggests creating simple side dishes (rice, local vegetables, etc.) and going with basic desserts, like some chocolate brought from home, melted, and served with some native fruit for dipping.

Kids: Back to School & Celebrations

Caring for your own special diet needs is one thing, but having to watch out for what a child eats (when you may not be there to help them!) brings a whole new level of challenges. Play dates, birthday parties, and school all present opportunities to breach your child's dietary requirements. Here are a few tips and considerations for navigating the food aspect of these situations:

School Lunch
Lunch programs are often government subsidized and odd as it may sound, this could mean your child is *forced* to take milk if they participate in the program. They can of course discard the milk, but they may not be given another beverage option. Some schools may not be as strict as others, but if your child's is, you have two additional options. One is to pack their lunch, and avoid the school program altogether. The other is to obtain a note from a physician to "excuse" your child from drinking or taking milk.

Luckily, it appears the options for dairy-free children in school lunch programs might be expanding. At the time of writing, The United States Department of Agriculture (USDA) was kicking around the idea of offering soymilk as an alternative to cow milk (with a note from a parent or guardian) for children receiving National School Lunch Program meals. If such a policy takes hold, then it could be a step in the right direction, but still a problem for those children with soy intolerances, or who would simply prefer juice. Parents and guardians interested in finding out if soymilk or other beverage options are available to their child, should contact the food service program at their school.

No matter what option you choose, alert your child's teacher of their needs to help prevent food mishaps. Also, if your child is participating in their school's lunch program, make sure you have a way to confirm the ingredients used. With the increase in food allergies, many schools now have this information readily available.

Birthday Parties
Sarah Hatfield (nowheymama.blogspot.com) has learned many tricks for navigating special events with her milk-allergic daughter. Rather than allowing her to feel left out, she is always armed with cookies, cupcakes, and "ice cream" sandwiches in the freezer. The cookies are usually unfrosted sugar cookies and chocolate chip. As for the cupcakes, after baking and allowing them to cool, she peels back one side of the cupcake wrapper and slices the cupcake almost in half horizontally (as you would a hamburger bun). She then spreads frosting in the middle of the cupcake, so that it is technically frosted, yet easy to freeze and ready for the road. To store, she rewraps the cupcake and places it in a freezer bag with several others. When her daughter attends a birthday party, Sarah sends her off with one ice cream sandwich and one cupcake, so that she can join in the festivities.

Since school birthdays and celebrations can come up without warning, Sarah suggests asking your child's school if you can store "safe" treats with them. Her daughter's school permits them to keep cookies and cupcakes in a freezer in the nurse's office for class parties.

Field Trips, Daycare, and Play Dates

It is important to be prepared for unexpected outings or prolonged daycare and play dates. Beyond any allergy "safety" equipment you may need (such as an EpiPen®), always keep a stash of snacks on hand. See the "On the Road" suggestions on p73 for some ideas. Sarah once again has a nice tip for food and snack storage when away from home, "'Unappealing' adjectives like 'dairy-free' and 'wheat-free' plastered all over the storage containers seem to keep food thieves away." For dairy-free adults, this advice should carry over well in the workplace too!

Also, don't forget about inedible or project-related sources of dairy in a child's environment. The following are a few items that you might find in a preschool, daycare, or early school environment that may contain milk: M&M's® or similar foods that may be used for counting and learning activities, pudding finger paint, shaving cream used for projects, general hygiene products for "clean up time" (soaps, lotions, etc.), and empty milk cartons for projects.

Since your child may feel shy about their diet, make sure to tell any adults who will be at a particular event about their needs.

Dealing with children and anaphylaxis is not my area of specialty, but I know many moms who are real life experts in this field. For more information on keeping a food allergic child "safe," see the Online Resources for Multiple Food Allergies on p258, and consider looking into the book, *How to Manage Your Child's Life Threatening Food Allergies*, by Linda Coss.

Section 3

Grocery Shopping & Preparing Your Kitchen

CHAPTER 8:
DECODING FOOD LABELS

I used to spend so much time worrying about fat and calories that I would completely bypass the ingredient statements ... you know, what is actually in the food. After scanning thousands (no exaggeration) of food labels I was amazed to uncover the countless products that utilize dairy in one (unnatural) form or another. Though deciphering the "secret code" used on ingredient statements was a mind-boggling experience, it allowed me to collect some excellent information to help simplify the process for others.

Dairy-Free vs. Non-Dairy

As you will note throughout this guide, I use the terms non-dairy and dairy-free interchangeably. According to my definition, both equate to 'made without dairy ingredients,' including lactose, casein, whey, and any of their constituents. However, in the food labeling business, they can take on very different meanings.

Non-Dairy – The FDA has created a regulatory definition for the term non-dairy, but amazingly, it does not equate to milk-free. A product labeled as non-dairy can contain 0.5% or less milk by weight, in the form of casein / caseinates (milk protein). This is why you may spot non-dairy creamers, non-dairy whipped toppings, and other non-dairy products that note milk on the ingredient statement. This does not mean that all products labeled as non-dairy contain milk, but it is a word of warning to always read the ingredient statement.

Dairy-Free – On the contrary, there is no regulatory definition for dairy-free, yet I find it to be a much more accurate indicator of milk-free products. Even though the FDA has not established regulations for this term, they do have a blanket policy that forbids the use of false and misleading terminology in general on food labels. This seems to be enough of a fear tactic, as I have yet to stumble across a food item that is promoted as dairy-free, but contains milk ingredients. However, the misleading use of the term dairy-free could easily exist, so always read the label, and contact the manufacturer when cross-contamination may also be a concern. Even if a product is free from milk ingredients, it could contain trace amounts of milk from the manufacturing processes.

The Food Allergen Labeling and Consumer Protection Act (FALCPA)

Otherwise known as the "plain language" labeling law, the FALCPA went into effect for all foods manufactured on or after January 1, 2006, which are intended for sale within the United States. The FALCPA requires that the top 8 allergens (including milk) be declared on food labels using easily recognizable names. There must also be a disclaimer below the ingredient list that states which, if any, of these top allergens are contained in the product. The government has made it clear that even a 7 year old should be able to read and understand the new food labels. However, I recommend that these labels be used only as a first line of defense. Companies are not exempt from error, and I fear that this regulation may sometimes offer a false sense of security. Even though the law has been in effect for some time now, I still occasionally come across food labels that make no specific mention of milk, when I can clearly see some form of milk in the ingredient statement, most often plain old butter.

It is also important to mention that companies are not required to site if their products may contain traces of an allergen due to cross-contamination in manufacturing. While many manufacturers do choose to include "may contain ..." or "processed in a facility with ..." type notes, it is still voluntary, unregulated, and can actually cause more consumer confusion. Since the wording is not standardized (over 30 different ways of saying "may contain" have been noted on various ingredient statements) or quantified, consumers are left wondering how great the risk of cross-contamination for each product really is. If you have a severe food allergy or intolerance, it is essential to check directly with the manufacturer prior to consumption of any processed food.

At the time of writing, Canada was in the midst of adopting a similar food allergy labeling policy, and both the U.S. and Canada were working together toward a long term goal of clearing up the "may contain" confusion with some policies for standardization.

The European Community has adopted similar regulations on the disclosure of top food allergens for pre-packed foods. On their food labels, ingredients derived from milk must be adequately identified (along with 13 other top food allergy and sensitivity offenders) in all cases, with the following exceptions: whey used for making distillates or ethyl alcohol of agricultural origin for spirit drinks and other alcoholic beverages and lactitol. These ingredients are believed to be so far removed from milk that they are not at risk for eliciting a reaction. The EC is struggling with the same "may contain" difficulties as North America.

Utilizing Kosher Certification

Kosher certification is a system of labeling that was originally created for spiritual purposes. However, over the years many individuals have also found it to be a handy way of identifying foods for special diets.

First, I believe it is important to address an ongoing debate regarding the safety of Kosher "Pareve" products for those with milk allergies. Based on policies of the Orthodox Union, the world's super power of kosher certification, those individuals with a severe milk allergy should not rely completely on kosher certification when selecting foods:

> "The trace nuts and dairy disclaimer that is now printed on many products is there to warn consumers that although there are no nuts or dairy in the ingredients of the product itself, there is a possibility of parts per millions floating in the air and 'contaminating' the product.
>
> The 'contamination' would only affect consumers with extremely severe allergies who can detect even the most trace amounts of the substance that they are reacting to. A product that is labeled OU (and thereby certified kosher parve) is halachically (by Jewish Law) parve. The parts per million does not affect the status of a product, because parts per million are negligible and have no halachic significance.
>
> As an example, a factory might produce dairy and parve products on two separate production lines. Nonetheless, air-born particles of milk or whey powder might float onto the parve production line. Though a person might suffer an allergic reaction, the product is still halachically parve."

Fortunately, for most individuals who choose to cut dairy from their diet for religious, personal, social, or medical reasons, kosher labeling can be a very useful tool.

If a product is kosher certified, then a kosher symbol will typically be found near the product name. That symbol may stand alone, or it may state "pareve," "parev," or "parve." In any of these cases, it indicates that the product was made without dairy ingredients. In most (but not all) circumstances, this would also indicate that separate production lines or thorough cleaning processes have been utilized to minimize cross-contamination.

If the kosher symbol contains or is accompanied by a "D," "DE," or the word "Dairy" then the product either contains dairy within its ingredients, or it is simply manufactured on equipment that is shared with dairy containing products and not thoroughly cleaned to pareve standards in between production runs. If your concerns do not lie with cross-contamination, then check the ingredients. It may still be a suitable product for you. There are other notations such as "M" and "Glatt" which note a kosher product that contains meat, or "F" which indicates a kosher product that contains fish. These do not necessarily indicate the presence of dairy.

Kosher certification is issued by a number of different organizations throughout the world. For this reason, various organization-specific symbols are utilized to identify kosher products. Also, each kosher certifying organization may have varying standards. This is another reason why kosher labeling is not highly recommended for strict diets. Nonetheless, it can be a quick and handy tool for a non-dairy or vegan lifestyle.

Dairy Ingredient Lists

When all else fails, consult the following lists to verify if the product you are considering is free of dairy ingredients. If any of the ingredients from the Red Alert List are within the product, then it likely contains dairy in some form.

Definitely Dairy Ingredients

~ Acidophilus Milk
~ Ammonium Caseinate
~ Butter
~ Butter Fat
~ Butter Oil
~ Butter Solids
~ Buttermilk
~ Buttermilk Powder
~ Calcium Caseinate
~ Casein
~ Caseinate (in general)
~ Cheese (All)
~ Condensed Milk
~ Cottage Cheese
~ Cream
~ Curds
~ Custard
~ Delactosed Whey
~ Demineralized Whey
~ Dry Milk Powder
~ Dry Milk Solids
~ Evaporated Milk
~ Ghee (see p109)
~ Goat Milk
~ Half & Half
~ Hydrolyzed Casein
~ Hydrolyzed Milk Protein
~ Iron Caseinate
~ Lactalbumin
~ Lactoferrin
~ Lactoglobulin
~ Lactose
~ Lactulose
~ Low-Fat Milk
~ Magnesium Caseinate
~ Malted Milk
~ Milk
~ Milk Derivative
~ Milk Fat
~ Milk Powder
~ Milk Protein
~ Milk Solids
~ Natural Butter Flavor
~ Nonfat Milk
~ Nougat
~ Paneer
~ Potassium Caseinate
~ Pudding
~ Recaldent
~ Rennet Casein
~ Skim Milk
~ Sodium Caseinate
~ Sour Cream
~ Sour Milk Solids
~ Sweetened Condensed Milk
~ Sweet Whey
~ Whey
~ Whey Powder
~ Whey Protein Concentrate
~ Whey Protein Hydrolysate
~ Whipped Cream
~ Whipped Topping
~ Whole Milk
~ Yogurt
~ Zinc Caseinate

Potentially Dairy Ingredients

~ *Artificial or Natural Flavors/Flavoring* – These are vague ingredients, which may be derived from a dairy source. A few of particular concern are butter, coconut cream, and egg flavors.

~ *Fat Replacers* - Brands such as Dairy-Lo® and Simplesse® are made with milk protein.

~ *Galactose* – This is often a lactose byproduct, but it can also be derived from sugar beets and other gums.

~ *High Protein or Protein* – Ingredients noted with no further details may be derived from milk proteins (casein or whey). This is particularly true in "High Energy" foods.

~ *Hydrolyzed Vegetable Protein* - The processing phase may use casein, but only trace amounts would likely remain.

~ *Lactic Acid Starter Culture* - These cultures may be prepared by using milk as an initial growth medium.

~ *Lactobacillus* – This term is noted often as a probiotic. It is in fact bacteria, not a food byproduct, and is named as such for its ability to convert lactose and other simple sugars to lactic acid. Though often utilized in milk products to create lactic acid, on its own, this ingredient is not always a concern. However, in some cases it may have been cultured or produced on dairy, and thus have the potential to contain trace amounts.

~ *Margarine* - Milk proteins are in most brands, though not all.

~ *Prebiotics* – A newcomer on the digestive health scene, these are indigestible carbohydrates. They are quite different from probiotics, which are living microorganisms. Prebiotics, such as galacto-oligosaccharides, lactosucrose, lactulose and lactitol may be derived from milk-based foods.

Rarely Dairy Ingredients

~ *Calcium or Sodium Stearoyl Lactylate* – Stearoyl lactylates are derived from the combination of lactic acid and stearic acid. They are generally considered non-dairy and safe for the lactose intolerant and milk allergic. However, the stearic acid may be animal derived, which could be a concern for vegans.

~ *Calcium, Sodium, or Potassium Lactate* - Lactates are salts derived from the neutralization of lactic acid, and are rarely a dairy concern. For example, it was noted that the lactate found in one brand of orange juice was made from sugar cane.

~ *Caramel Color* – Anything with caramel in its title may sound like a dairy red flag, but caramel color is typically derived from corn syrup and occasionally from potatoes, wheat, or other carbohydrate sources. While lactose is a permitted carbohydrate in the production of caramel color, it is rarely if ever used.

~ *Lactic Acid* – Lactic acid is created via the fermentation of sugars, and can be found in many dairy-free and/or vegan foods. Most commercially used lactic acid is fermented from carbohydrates, such as cornstarch, potatoes or molasses, and thus dairy-free. Though lactic acid can be fermented from lactose, its use is generally (I said generally) restricted to dairy products, such as ice cream and cream cheese.

Surprisingly Dairy-Free Ingredients / Foods

~ Calcium Propionate
~ Calcium Carbonate
~ Calcium Citrate
~ Calcium Phosphate
~ Cocoa Butter
~ Cocoa Powder
~ Coconut Butter
~ Coconut Cream
~ Cream of Coconut
~ Cream of Tartar

~ Creamed Honey
~ Fruit Butter (Apple, Pumpkin, etc)
~ Glucono Delta-Lactone
~ Lecithin Oleoresin
~ Malted Barley or other Grain-Based Malts
~ Malt Liquor
~ Malt Vinegar
~ Milk Thistle
~ Nut Butters (Peanut, Almond, etc.)
~ Shea Butter

Where the Dairy Hides

So, where might one find dairy ingredients? There are the obvious foods such as cow milk (chocolate, whole, skim, malted, evaporated, etc.), buttermilk, half and half, cream, butter, cheese, ice cream, milk shakes, milk chocolate, and yogurt. However, did you know that the majority of processed foods also contain dairy? Some are fairly easy to spot, such as macaroni and cheese or creamy ranch salad dressing. While others, may be more elusive. Below is a partial list of manufactured foods and non-food items where dairy ingredients may be hiding. A few just might surprise you…

~ *Baby Formula and Baby Food*– If you are seeking a non-dairy baby formula due to milk allergies, check with a physician. Babies can have much more serious reactions to allergies and sensitivities than adults.

~ *Bakery Goods* – It can be difficult to verify the ingredients of freshly baked goods. In general, muffins and quick breads frequently contain milk or buttermilk; scones are almost always rich with cream, buttermilk, or butter; and cookies typically contain butter and may contain milk chocolate. Though yeast breads appear safe, one of the most common dough conditioners utilized in bread is whey, a milk protein. As well, some loaves and rolls may contain milk, dry milk powder, cheese, or buttermilk.

~ *Baking Mixes* (pancakes, cakes, biscuits, etc.) – Dry milk powder, buttermilk powder, and other milk solids are common in these products.

~ *Bath Products* – Though your cleansers, hair products, and lotions are not food products, those who tend to have skin reactions to milk products (i.e. eczema) may want to avoid topical application (see p59).

~ *Beer* – 'Milk' beer has been around for some time, and may linger in breweries under the code name of Sweet Stout. Quite often it makes itself known with a more obvious title, such as Milk Stout or Cream Stout. These beers contain lactose, which adds sweetness, body, and calories to the finished beer.

~ *Breathe Mints* – Not all, but a few do contain casein related ingredients.

~ *Candy* – Much of the candy world (of the non-chocolate variety) is free game from a dairy-free point of view, but a surprise milk ingredient does pop up on occasion.

~ *Canned Tuna Fish* – A few contain hydrolyzed caseinate.

~ *Caramel* – This is a suspicious food and ingredient. It may be made from sugar and water or milk.

~ *Cereal* - Dry and instant cereals vary significantly in ingredients. One type may contain milk ingredients in the brand name, but not in the generic.

~ *Cheese Alternatives* – Some brands of cheese alternatives (whether soy, rice, or almond based) are lactose-free, but still contain milk protein (casein) to create a more cheese-like consistency and texture.

~ *Chewing Gum* – Some brands do contain milk proteins.

~ *Chicken Broth* – Several brands use milk proteins or solids.

~ *Chocolate* – Milk chocolate is a given, but some semi-sweet and dark chocolate brands also contain milk ingredients … even though they really shouldn't in my opinion.

~ *Chocolate Drinks* – Even the non-milk varieties may contain a bit of dairy to make them more substantial.

~ *Clothing* – It is not yet in the mainstream, but a few textile producers have come out with eco-fabrics that use milk fiber. Some clothing manufacturers are in the "testing" phases with the products.

~ *Coffee Whiteners / Creamers* – Milk is certainly white and creamy, and it has many uses in these foods.

~ *Cookies and Crackers* – It's common to find milk ingredients or byproducts in processed foods such as these.

~ *Cream Liqueurs* – These may possess solid milk ingredients or caseinates.

~ *Custard / Pudding* – Most of the prepared puddings, and a few of the dry mixes, contain milk ingredients.

~ *Drugs / Medications* - Lactose is sometimes used as a filler/base for prescription drugs and OTC medications (including antihistamines). Be sure to ask the pharmacist to review the ingredients of any prescription medications you will be taking before they fill it.

~ *Egg Substitute* - Some brands of egg substitute contain or are made from whey.

~ *Eggnog* – This is typically richer in milk and cream than eggs. Try some "soy nog" or Coco-Nog (p165).

~ *Fondue* - Doesn't this mean cheese in Swiss?

~ *Fried Foods* – The breading on fried foods may contain cheese or any number of mysterious substances.

~ *Granola & Nutrition Bars* - Just like cookies, various milk additives may be utilized.
~ *Gravies* - Some contain, milk, milk powder, or milk solids for flavor and texture.
~ *Hot Cocoa Mix* - The best varieties are pure cocoa and sugar, but some may contain milk ingredients for a creamier drink.
~ *Hot Dogs* - What isn't in hot dogs?
~ *Imitation Crab Meat* – I admit it, my family loved [past tense] homemade California rolls, but we banished them after discovering that most brands contain a milk ingredient or two.
~ *Imitation Maple and Other Syrups* – Pure maple syrup is typically a safer selection.
~ *Instant Potatoes* – Many varieties contain milk products, most notably the Au Gratin or Sour Cream.
~ *Kosher Parve Desserts* - Most parve foods are okay, but it is said that those with highly sensitive milk allergies may have a problem with the desserts in particular.
~ *Latex Gloves* – Some disposable latex gloves have milk protein (casein) in them. Interestingly enough, the use of such gloves has been found in skin prick testing, potentially causing false-positive reactions and hives for those who are allergic.
~ *Lactose-Free Milk* – Lactose-free does not mean dairy-free, these will still be loaded with milk proteins.
~ *Processed Meats & Sausages* - Some "meat allergies" are actually dairy allergies in disguise. Lactose and milk protein (caseinates) are fairly common in processed meats, and milk powder is sometimes used as filler. Lest you think I am only speaking of the shaped and formed meats, a colleague alerted me to the various dairy ingredients she discovered in whole turkeys sold for the holidays. Since kosher dietary laws do not permit milk and meat in the same meal, seeking out kosher meats may be a good option. They should be stamped with a kosher symbol, but they will not be labeled as parve, since parve foods cannot contain meat.
~ *Margarine* – A few contain dairy derivatives, and most are rich in hydrogenated oils (trans fats).
~ *Meal Replacement/Protein Powders & Beverages* – Whey and dried milk powder are the two most common dairy ingredients in these drinks.
~ *Potato Chips* – Be extra cautious with flavored varieties, which may harbor buttermilk, whey, or cheese.
~ *Salad Dressings* – Milk components or cheese may be added for flavor or thickening power to any dressing or vinaigrette.
~ *Sherbet* – This is different from sorbet, which is typically dairy-free. Sherbet almost always contains some amount of milk and/or cream.
~ *Soup* - Obviously the creamy varieties are of concern, but even some of the tomato and chicken based soups are not dairy-free.
~ *Soy "Meat" Products* – Veggie hot dogs, sausages, and patties may harbor milk proteins, lactose, or even cheese for flavor and texture.
~ *Spice Mixes* – Some contain whey powder.
~ *Sugar Substitutes* – Some sweeteners, such as tagatose are derived from dairy foods (lactose in this case). Also, certain forms of some sugar substitutes, such as Splenda®. Minis and certain brands of Stevia, contain lactose (in very small quantities) as a filler ingredient.
~ *Toothpaste* – Recaldent is a casein-containing ingredient that is sometimes added for cavity prevention.
~ *Wax Coating on Fruits & Vegetables* – Small amounts of soy or milk protein (casein) are often added to the wax in the production process. The FDA classifies the final fruits/vegetables as "safe," and they are still considered kosher parve by most, if not all, certifiers.
~ *Whipped Topping* –Within FDA regulations, the term "non-dairy" may be utilized on some foods, such as whipped toppings and creamers, which do in fact contain casein.
~ *Wine* – Yes, I'm sorry, but milk protein is sometimes used in the fining process of wine, which could trigger an allergic response. I have been told that vegan and kosher wines are a good place to start when seeking milk-free wines. Kosher certification looks at the process in addition to the ingredients, so kosher certified wines are typically produced without milk, but they may contain eggs. For a good directory of vegan wine and other alcoholic beverages, visit Barnivore, an online vegan drink directory (www.barnivore.com), or Vegans are from Mars (www.vegans.frommars.org) to view their vegan wine guide.

CHAPTER 9:
SHOPPING LIST INSPIRATIONS

It never hurts to have a few ideas in your head before embarking on a supermarket trip; particularly when you have a special diet to consider. The following is a general list of suggestions to "inspire" your quest for dairy-less meals. Products do vary significantly by manufacturer, so always read the label on packaged foods to ensure that the ingredients are in fact dairy-free, and contact the manufacturer whenever necessary to verify manufacturing processes.

Departments with Unlimited Potential

Produce
Go crazy in the produce department! I couldn't even begin to create a list for this category. Fresh fruits and vegetables should always be dairy-free (well, almost always, read about waxed fruit and vegetables on p83), and the choices are endless. As a dairy-free consumer, I am a big fan of the avocado for luxurious dips, the potato for creamy soups, and apples for a classic homemade crisp. Berries, salad greens, kiwis, squash, eggplant, peppers, whatever your fancy…try a new fruit or vegetable each week.

Meat
If you do not follow a vegan diet, this department also has a great deal to offer, but go for the real stuff: unadulterated chicken, beef, turkey, pork, buffalo, etc. Try to limit purchases of hot dogs, deli meats, and other processed options, as many brands contain dairy and/or nitrites. Pork and chicken are free of hormones by law (though they may have been treated with antibiotics). However, beef may have been treated with hormones and/or antibiotics. Whenever your budget permits, opt for organic selections. Always check the ingredients if you are considering a marinated cut.

Seafood
Wild salmon, halibut, tuna, crab, prawns, oysters … in fact, the whole seafood case is open for dairy-free business. As with meats, read the label carefully when looking for marinated seafood or processed selections, such as imitation crab meat.

Cook's Corner

Bottled Sauces
~   *American Tradition* – Mustard, mayo, relish, and ketchup are almost always dairy-free, although egg-free consumers may want to seek out vegan mayonnaise. I highly recommend some of the natural mayonnaises, organic ketchups, and whole grain mustards. The quality can take your burger, or veggie burger, to the next level.
~   *Asian* – Most Chinese, Japanese, Vietnamese, and Thai sauces will be dairy-free. Teriyaki, black bean, hoisin, soy, fish, chili garlic, sweet chili, sweet & sour, and oyster sauces can be found easily in most major grocers, and are all great for stir-fries. Thai curries, satays, and peanut sauces are other tasty considerations.

~ *Mexican* – Hot sauce! Need I say more? Okay, I will anyway … I also like the wide variety of milk-free enchilada sauces and salsas of the green and red variety.
~ *Italian* – Most unadulterated tomato sauces will be free of milk ingredients, unless cheese is in their descriptive title. However, there are a few that hide some cheese or cream, so do read the ingredients.
~ *Salad Dressings* – Highly processed anything is likely to contain milk ingredients, but if you choose from the better quality options, you will likely find many variations of vinaigrette, French, thousand island, and honey mustard salad dressings that are a go.
~ *Chutneys* – Mango is the most popular, but there are various other chunky flavors on the shelves.
~ *Brand Specific* – There are many brand name condiments, from pesto to BBQ sauce to creamy dressings, which are free of milk ingredients. Read the ingredient statement to unearth your own healthy finds.

General Cooking
~ *Vinegar* – Red wine, white wine, rice wine, white, apple cider, balsamic, raspberry, malt, rice (red, brown, white, seasoned), did I get most of them?
~ *Oil* – All plant-based oils, including grapeseed, coconut, olive, avocado, peanut, flax, you name it, are dairy-free. Plus, they are ideal for cooking and baking.
~ *Herbs & Spices* – Experiment with plain herbs and spices; the flavors can offer restaurant quality meals. Season with cinnamon, oregano, basil, rosemary, thyme, coriander, fennel … I could go on all day, but I think you get the picture.
~ *"Pastes"* – Miso, curry, tamarind, and wasabi are very popular flavors throughout Asia. These selections are sometimes found in the refrigerated section and other times in the shelf-stable aisles.
~ *Brand Specific* – Seasoning packets and spice mixes are frequently dairy-free, but some may contain milk ingredients. Check the labels.

Basic Pantry Stocking
~ *Beans (dried or canned)* - All varieties of beans (pinto, garbanzo, butter, black, etc.) are dairy-free and many are a good source of calcium and protein.
~ *Olives* – Sample the many varieties, which are perfect for adding bold flavor to cheese-free meals.
~ *Coconut Milk* – The versatility of coconut milk extends far beyond curries (although I have nothing against curries). I have seen a couple of powdered coconut milks that do contain casein, so watch those labels.
~ *Lentils* – These are easily found in the bulk department, or bagged with the grains. Go with the plain brown, quick cooking red, or French green lentils for a cheap, tasty, healthy, and very filling meal.
~ *Chili* – Most (but not all) hearty canned chilies are dairy-free and will soothe any savage beast.
~ *Canned Vegetables and Fruit* – These are good in a pinch, and most kids (and husbands) enjoy canned fruit cocktails. Personally, I would be lost without some canned pumpkin and crushed pineapple on hand.
~ *Brand Specific* – Soups come in so many varieties from so many manufacturers. Assess them individually.

Baker's Delight

Baking at Home
~ *Flours* – White is out (but still dairy-free); wheat, brown rice, oat, amaranth, quinoa, and garbanzo flours are in. These nutrient dense flours will also add unique flavors to your sauces, coatings, and baked goods.
~ *Sweeteners* – Natural sweeteners, such as honey (not for strict vegans), molasses, agave nectar, and pure maple syrup can be excellent options. However, most sweeteners including granulated sugar, brown sugar, dark brown sugar, evaporated cane juice, and corn syrup are free of milk ingredients. Be wary of sugar substitutes, these may be dairy-derived or could contain milk as a filler ingredient.
~ *Coconut* – Both the sweetened and unsweetened varieties
~ *Chocolate* – Cocoa powder as well as semi-sweet, dark, baking, and bittersweet chocolate (chips, chunks, etc.) should in theory be dairy-free. However, a few manufacturers may slip milk products in, usually in the

form of milk solids or butterfat. Also, most chocolates are at high risk for containing trace amounts of dairy as they share equipment with milk chocolate production. There are a few excellent "safe" brands though.

~ *Baking Agents* – Thickeners, starches, yeast, baking soda, and baking powder should rarely cause a problem.
~ *Pure Flavor* – Real vanilla, almond, anise, cinnamon, rum, and other natural extracts are dairy-free.
~ *Marshmallows* – Not quite nutritious, but these fluffy white sugar pillows (vegan or regular) are handy for kids or holiday baking.
~ *Brand Specific* – Baking mixes, pancake/waffle mixes, and breadcrumbs are great for quick meals and treats, though many do contain dry milk ingredients.

Bakery Fresh
There is an abundance of dairy-free baked goods on the market, but no single category stands out as mostly dairy-free. Breads (sandwich, bagels, English muffins, pita bread, etc.), tortillas, cookies, cakes, pastries and other sweets should always be checked for milk ingredients. Don't hesitate to read the labels on freshly prepared foods or ask the baker.

Snack Time!

Fresh Dips
~ *Guacamole* – Thick, creamy, indulgent, and yes, it is almost always dairy-free. Beware of a few brands that may mix in sour cream.
~ *Hummus* – This spread made the garbanzo bean famous! Other bean dips are sometimes dairy-free, but check the ingredients to be sure.
~ *Salsa* – Okay, this one is a given, but it is still great stuff.
~ *Brand Specific* – Ingredients in dips vary widely, but you may discover some pâtés or spreads that are free from dairy ingredients.

Spreads
~ *Nut Butters* – From natural peanut to almond, cashew, and sesame seed (tahini), nut and seed butters are all the rage. Many are now spiked with honey, fruit, and savory flavors. I have even spotted a few chocolate blended nut butters that would be approved as non-dairy. Use them for their oil and flavor in baking; prepare dips, marinades, and sauces; or spread them on your favorite bread, rice cakes, or English muffins.
~ *Other "Butters"* – Pumpkin butter is my favorite, but there are many varieties, such as apple, fig and cherry.
~ *Jams & Jellies* – It may be out there, but I have yet to find a jam or jelly which isn't dairy-free. Go traditional with strawberry, or jazz things up with some cloudberry preserves.
~ *Honey* – Most grocers now carry a variety of honeys; eucalyptus and blackberry are two intriguing ones. Honey may not be suitable for strict vegans.

Handy Snacks
~ *Dried Fruit* – Dried apples, cranberries, mango, cantaloupe, and even kiwis have been spotted in the bulk food section and snack aisles (for a "convenience price"). Almost any fruit can be dehydrated, and manufacturers have certainly been putting this to the test.
~ *Nuts* – All nuts are dairy-free by nature, including almonds, walnuts, cashews, pecans, and macadamias. Choose raw, roasted, salted, or unsalted, and always check flavored varieties for added ingredients.
~ *Seeds* – Flax, pumpkin, sesame, sunflower, etc.; follow the nut guidelines above for seeds.
~ *Gelatin* – Jell-O® gelatin is in fact dairy-free, but not suitable for vegans.
~ *Applesauce* – Try the regular snack packs for kids, or pick a flavored variety.
~ *Fruit Bars and Leathers* – These aren't just for kids, they are a good way to address adult-sized sugar cravings too.

~ *Popcorn* – Very few microwave brands are dairy-free. Try purchasing the far more economical bag of popcorn kernels and pop it up the old-fashioned way, in a pan with a touch of oil and salt. You can also buy special microwave bags to pop those regular popcorn kernels in a jiffy.
~ *Rice Cakes* – The plain varieties are always dairy-free, but only some of the flavored ones are.
~ *Pickled Vegetables* – From old-fashioned dill pickles to spicy cocktail vegetables, these can make a nice snack or party addition.
~ *Brand Specific* - Granola bars, snack bars, cereal bars, and energy bars abound on store shelves. Though many contain dairy, a good selection do not. In addition, several brands of trail mix, crackers, pudding mixes, and unflavored chips (baked or fried) are also suitable for a non-dairy diet.

Great Grains

For Sides and Meals
From bulk foods to the ethnic centers, all grains (without seasoning, stuffing, or sauce) are dairy-free.
~ *Gluten-Free* – Reach for quinoa, amaranth, buckwheat, millet, teff, brown rice, white rice, or wild rice.
~ *Gluten-Containing* – Wheat, oats, barley, couscous, rye, kamut, triticale, spelt, etc. Though some gluten-free consumers may be tolerant of oats.
~ *Pastas* – Choose from the traditional dried semolina pasta shapes, or mix things up with one of the new blends, such as rice, spelt, wheat, or kamut noodles.
~ *Polenta* – Seek out the "chubs" of premade polenta that look like they should be refrigerated, but are in fact shelf-stable. These are usually dairy-free and packaged conveniently for "slice and heat" preparation.
~ *Brand Specific* – Pre-seasoned, ready-to-cook pasta and rice dishes are a nice shortcut. Also, the potato-pasta hybrids known as gnocchi are delicious, and sometimes free of milk and cheese ingredients.

Cereal Aisle
~ *Hot Cereals* – Those big tubs of oats are healthy and a very cheap breakfast option. The unflavored Cream of … (wheat, rice, you fill in the blank) hot cereals are also good choices. When you start looking at pre-flavored varieties, check the ingredients.
~ *Brand Specific* – Cold cereal options are numerous, however, the ingredients do vary widely by brand.

Keep It Cool

Dairy Case
~ *Eggs* – Although they are located in the "dairy case," eggs come from chickens, and are not related to milk.
~ *Milk Alternatives* –Soy and rice milks have been spotted in quart-sized containers in the refrigerated section.
~ *Dairy Alternatives* – Soy yogurts, dairy-free shortenings, cheese-less cheeses (watch for casein), butter lookalikes, and truly non-dairy creamers are popping up right next to their dairy counterparts.

Vegan Options
~ *Tofu* – Soft, firm, extra-firm, silken, pre-baked, lightly fried, dessert style … there are so many choices and an abundance of ways to use them in cooking, smoothies, and baking.
~ *Brand Specific* – There are many "Meatless-Meats" on the market, but several do contain casein, lactose, or straight up cheese. Look for those options specifically labeled as "vegan."

Fresh Pastas
~ *Asian Style* – Won ton and gyoza wrappers, rice paper, and spring roll pastry are becoming more readily available. Some do contain eggs, but if you search around a few vegan options will likely appear.

~ *"Un-Stuffed"* – Fresh linguini or angel hair is always a deserved treat, but these do typically contain eggs.
~ *Brand Specific* – Though many are cheese stuffed, dairy-free raviolis and perogies can be found.

The Deep Freeze
~ *Soy, Coconut, & Rice "Ice Creams" and Novelties* – Unlike soy cheeses, all of the soy-, rice-, and coconut-based frozen desserts I have found to date are made without milk.
~ *100% Juice Bars & Sorbets* – These fruit based desserts are naturally dairy-free and oh-so refreshing.
~ *Frozen Fruit* – A fantastic option for homemade smoothies, baking, or a cool snack.
~ *Frozen Vegetables* – What a great invention, nicely chopped up vegetables ready for cooking with or without defrost. Be aware, there are some "creamed" varieties out there, which most likely contain dairy.
~ *Asian Meals* – Check the labels, but thus far all of the frozen wontons, gyozas, and egg rolls (except for the Mexican flavored ones) that I have spotted in the freezer section without sauce, have been non-dairy. For a healthy twist, try steaming the gyozas and dumplings, boiling the wontons in soup, or baking the egg rolls with a dusting of heart healthy oil.
~ *Brand Specific* – If you are a convenience lover, then you are still in luck. Numerous non-dairy frozen entrées are available these days. Yes, there are even dairy-free pizzas.

Thirst Quenchers

~ *Juice* – Juice is quick, hydrating, and often nutritious, especially the 100% pure and fresh squeezed varieties. Plus, the selection is multiplying… orange, pomegranate, pineapple, blueberry, carrot, cherry, etc.
~ *Bottled Water* – Just a reminder in case your tap water is undesirable.
~ *Milk Alternatives* – Packaged in aseptic containers, these soy, almond, rice, nut, and grain milks are shelf stable, and typically have expiration dates for a year out. Load up on your preferred varieties when on sale.
~ *Tea* – Some favorites are green, white, chamomile, and jasmine, but any variety will do.
~ *Coffee* – Another naturally dairy-free beverage.
~ *Brand Specific* – When you are short on time, and need a little extra energy, there are some meal replacement beverages, energy drinks, and smoothies that are free of milk products.

Prepared Foods

Unless you have very sensitive food allergies, you need not write off the convenience deli. Look around; most grocers will list the ingredients on the packaging or on a label near the foods. Seek out a natural food grocer that specializes in various diet requirements. Those with severe food allergies should note that deli departments are at high risk for cross-contamination due to the use of shared equipment (i.e. that multi-purpose cheese/meat/vegetable slicer).

Remember, simple and legible ingredient statements equate to *real food*. For some brand-specific, dairy-free (made without dairy ingredients) foods suggestions, see my personal recommendations throughout the Recipe Section of this guide (beginning on p139). For more grocery shopping help, product lists are available via www.godairyfree.org. They include everything from cheese alternatives to soups and breakfast cereals.

CHAPTER 10:
ALISA'S RANDOM GROCERY TIPS

Let's cut to the chase: I am frugal. I make it a point to buy the best quality possible, but I loathe paying too much for anything. Therefore, my collection of tips focuses on money saving ideas and maximizing quality for a pocketbook-friendly yet delicious, dairy-free transition ...

Don't Forget the Basics – My first instinct when I began to cook dairy-free was to find recipes created specifically for "free-from" diets. These are helpful, but I completely overlooked the simple dishes that I loved as a kid, and which are traditionally, without substitutions, dairy-free. Meals such as Spanish rice, spaghetti, and chili are now weekly staples in our home, and each dish is so versatile that I can literally add whatever we have in the pantry.

Don't Think About What it Is; Think About What it Could Be – Dairy-free experimentation helped me to unlock the potential of the produce department. When I see a good deal on cauliflower, I don't think about how my husband loathes this cruciferous vegetable. Instead, I imagine how much he will love the creamy soup I will make with it as the base (recipes on p183 and p187). Likewise, an abundance of in-season (and consequently cheap) zucchini prompts several loaves of his favorite zucchini bread (p150).

Venture the International Markets – Coconut milk and rice noodles run over $1 and $2 respectively at my local grocery stores. Yet, a quick trip the Asian market almost always yields these ingredients for half or less than half of these prices. Likewise, tortillas at the neighborhood Mexican market and tahini from my local Middle Eastern food dealer seem to be more authentic in taste and more affordable. Plus, most countries tend to rely less on dairy products than Western nations, resulting in specialty markets filled with interesting dairy-free options.

Reach for Bold Accent Flavors – Cooking without the fatty flavors of cream, cheese, and butter means that I must compensate in other areas to keep the meals interesting ... hmm, flavor perhaps? I splurge on spices, sun-dried tomatoes, olives, and Asian pastes and curries. Luckily a little goes a long ways when it comes to these powerful additives; so even though they tend to appear more costly upfront, one jar typically lasts for quite a while.

Keep an Eye on Organic – Yes, I am a penny-pincher, I swear, but I have a few great reasons (beyond the obvious) to consider organic foods. First, they are sometimes cheaper than their conventional counterparts, if not pretty close in price. Since most people habitually purchase organic *or* conventional, it is easy to overlook when the organic versions sink lower in price than the pesticide products, but it actually happens quite a bit in both the produce department and the packaged food aisles. Secondly, many organic packaged foods (but definitely not all) seem to be free of dairy. It is my theory that some organic manufacturers skip milk ingredients whenever possible as the organic versions tend to be very expensive. Be sure to check the label though, as a few extravagant companies will undoubtedly splurge on organic dairy. Finally, "surprise" dairy ingredients are less likely since organic food labels are usually easy to read and tend to contain mostly "whole food" ingredients.

Don't Rely on Mainstream Grocers for Specialty Products – Many of the "big guys" have added beautifully manicured natural food sections, and are consequently charging an arm and a leg for those "upscale" products. In most cases, it is actually cheaper to shop on the manufacturer's website or at a natural food store. However, I always do a quick cruise through those specialty aisles whenever we visit our local mega-grocer. Because their natural food sections are seldom popular, I occasionally strike gold with closeout items. I once scored 3lbs of nutritional yeast (the most enormous bag you have ever seen) for just $2.99 per pound.

Look for the Vegan Label – By definition, the vegan diet is free from all animal products, including dairy in all of its forms. While some products may be at risk for cross-contamination in manufacturing (always check!), the word vegan stamped on a food label gives you a good head start to finding some suitable dairy-free products.

Consider Homemade "Milk" - I hear many complaints about the cost of purchasing milk alternatives, but really, how many dairy consumers can whip up a batch of cow milk at home for mere cents? The oat, almond, and cashew milk recipes in this guide are my personal favorites, but rice milk is equally easy and inexpensive.

Buy In-Season – When in-season, produce is typically at its peak of quality and abundance, and harvested relatively nearby, rather than traveling thousands of miles before reaching your plate. Less transportation and greater availability equals a good price. Go with the seasons and your grocery budget will thank you. For those items you must have year round, find a reliable store with fair prices.

Go for Whole Foods - As a general rule of thumb, processed food, unless it is processed junk, will almost always cost more and will not contain the same level of nutrients as fresh, whole foods.

Support Local Farmers – Great prices and fresh food abound at farmer's markets, where you can usually find everything from just-out-of-the-ground vegetables to free range meats and local honey. Also, don't forget to visit local u-pick farms for a fun afternoon activity and bushels of inexpensive fruit.

Rather Than Buying Complete Meals, Buy Meal Helpers - Obviously, making everything from scratch isn't feasible for everyone. I like to buy helpers that make cooking easier, but don't break the budget, rather than buying the complete meal (i.e. frozen dinners). Soups and chili are wonderful for this. Pour them over rice or other grains and include your own add-ins (vegetables, last-night's chicken, etc.) for a quick and nutritious meal.

Get the Most for Your Money - To save money and preserve quality, I never purchase light coconut milk. It often contains additives, and is essentially regular coconut milk thinned with water. When I need 1 cup of a light version, I simply use 1/4 cup of regular coconut milk plus 3/4 cup water. For a slightly richer version, I increase the coconut milk to 1/3 cup and reduce the water to 2/3 cup. In essence, I get 3 to 4 cans of light coconut milk for the price of one. I love a good deal.

Freeze Ingredients, Not Leftovers - Having all necessary components ready to go in the freezer is a recipe for easy meals that are healthier than frozen entrées. Not to mention, you can stock up on frequently used foods when they go on sale. You may choose to purchase the ingredients pre-frozen, or buy fresh and freeze them yourself. Some foods that freeze well include fruit (berries, mango, bananas, peaches, etc.), broccoli, spinach, green beans, corn, peas, ground flaxseed, ground nuts (in flour or "butter" form), wonton or gyoza wrappers, and fillo pastry

Bulk Up - I scoop giant bags of organic rolled oats in the bulk foods section for a fraction of the cost I would pay for non-organic packaged oats. Spices and specialty grains are also excellent foods to purchase in bulk. If you do get hooked on bulk, make sure the bags are labeled to help tell those seeds and grains apart.

Don't Assume That Bulk is Cheapest - Before you go wild filling your pantry with bags of bulk items, check the prices. There are many items, such as quinoa, that I often find for a cheaper price pre-packaged, even in Whole Foods! It is not uncommon for retailers to mark larger packages or bulk foods for a higher per ounce price than smaller packages; deceptive, but true.

Coupons! – Yes they do exist, even for specialty items. While you may occasionally spot soymilk discounts in your local paper, some of the best discounts are offered directly from the manufacturers themselves. I sign up for all of the e-newsletters from my favorite manufacturers, in order to receive coupons and other discount offers.

Chapter 11:
The Well-Equipped Kitchen

Having a good supply of kitchen tools can be quite fun, but personally, I think many of the small appliances out there are simply overkill. Here are my recommendations ...

"Necessities"

These are items that perhaps I could live without, but I really wouldn't want to. Each of these little appliances sees some mileage in my kitchen every week, if not every day, yet they were purchased for less than $30 each.

Blender – This handy gadget is your key to creamy smoothies, shakes, and soups. Honestly, it seems as though my blender gets pulled out for some small task almost daily. That said, in the past few years we have gone through four different blenders, including two higher end models, only to discover that the cheap 10-speed blender works just as well, if not better. It has less "juice" then some of the fancier brands, but because of this, the motor doesn't tend to blow up (like our "high-end" experiences), and it is quieter than most brands. And yes, it really does blend up every last bit of ice. However, I do recommend splurging on the glass jar, as plastic versions tend to crack very easily.

Spice/Coffee Grinder - Since we are a household of two, I find that my spice grinder does just about everything I would need a food processor for, and with insanely quick clean up. Of course, I use it to grind down those cumin seeds, and some may like it for coffee beans (I am a tea girl myself) but it also works in a pinch to grind flax seeds for a nutritious boost to my smoothies and meals, to grind nuts (even into a butter / paste), and to make oat flour in an instant from my supplies of whole oats. Some may dislike doing things in batches, but since I can make 1/3 cup of oat flour in 30 seconds of whirling with a quick "wipe it out with a dry paper towel" clean-up, 1 cup is easily ready with my workspace clean in less than five minutes. Plus, spice grinders can be had for just $10 to $20 at the supermarket. The lower wattage grinders do work well in general, but if you jump up to 150 Watts, you will be rewarded with a better nut butter grinder.

Rice Cooker – In my opinion, the key to living dairy-free is to have some quick and easy meals in your repertoire that contain everyday ingredients. Thanks to the basic 6-cup rice cooker this is completely feasible. It cooks up grains (brown rice, white rice, millet, quinoa, etc, etc, etc) with a quick flip of the switch, and if you get one with a steamer basket, it can cook the rest of your meal simultaneously. I can throw just about any vegetable (including potatoes) in the top basket of my rice cooker, and my meal is ready when I hear the "click." You can even steam fish or chicken along with the vegetables for a quick and healthy dairy-free meal.

 Hand Mixer - Want some nice toned arms? Skip the clunky stand mixer and go for a cheapo hand mixer. Don't think for a minute that these don't pack enough power, mine is actually a little too turbo charged. Just make sure you pick out one that has a good range from low to high in power. I actually mix most things up by hand, but for whipping and creaming, a trusty little mixer is quite useful, and can be taken out and put away with ease.

"Luxuries"

As I write this, I do not own any of the items mentioned below, but I can admit to their usefulness in many kitchens. In fact, I have been keeping an eye out for sales on an immersion blender, and after borrowing my friend's ice cream maker to test some of the recipes in this guide, I am seriously considering investing in a small one myself.

Food Processor - I confess, food processors are quite useful, considering you can do anything from chopping to pureeing with the simple push of a button. Shopping for food processors can be difficult though. Power, reliability, versatility, and ease of cleaning are all important factors to consider; higher end models are often worth the splurge. Be sure to read reviews before investing in a food processor.

Immersion Blender - With the amount of soups I make, I really should invest in one of these. An immersion blender allows you to puree foods right in the pot or bowl. No messy moving to the blender and pureeing in batches.

Soymilk Maker - This is another "life simplifier." It is important to note that it is very difficult to replicate the taste of store-bought soymilk at home. However, soymilk makers can be used to make almost any type of dairy-free milk, including almond, rice, quinoa, and many more.

Yogurt Maker - I have heard from many people that homemade dairy-free yogurt is far better than store-bought, so if you are a true yogi, then this may be a good purchase. You can put together your own yogurt making set-up at home, but yogurt makers are a nice, inexpensive, and clean way to get the job done.

Ice Cream Maker - If you really love ice cream, then do consider purchasing an ice cream maker. These gadgets can allow you to whip up your own dairy-free frozen desserts from coconut milk, nuts, fruit, and other everyday ingredients. While I have had good success in making cool and creamy treats without an ice cream maker, it does take "ice cream" to another level of luxuriousness.

Bread Maker - I know ... this is a trendy item that tends to gather dust on the shelves, but dairy-free living may give you some extra motivation to dust it off. So many retail breads contain dairy that I find it easier (and tastier) to make my own at home. If you are a serious bread connoisseur (or your little ones devour two loaves a week), then this is definitely a nice piece of equipment to have.

Section 4

All You Ever Wanted to Know About Dairy Substitutes

CHAPTER 12:
SO MANY "MILKS," SO LITTLE TIME

Every time someone complains that they (and I quote) "could NEVER go without milk" simply because they just don't like soymilk, I nearly explode with commentary and questions. How many different brands of soymilk have you tried? What about rice, almond, or oat milk, have you tried any of these? For die-hard moo juice fans, I certainly won't promise that there is an identical twin to your old favorite just yet. But, I can almost guarantee that some brand of some milk alternative will suit your palate.

When I dove into the dairy-free diet, my selections were limited. Silk brand soymilk worked for my household just fine, but really, what choice did we have? Now the non-dairy beverage section is brimming with options, and you may be shocked to discover just how unique each brand is. For years I purchased almond milk, and always the same label, but one day I stumbled upon a good sale on a competing brand. I stocked up, assuming that it would pretty well be the same product. While I was still very pleased with it, I was surprised at the variation in ingredients, flavor, and even thickness. The differences may have been subtle in reality, but they were obvious to my taste buds, which were thrilled with the mix-up.

After I finally opened my eyes to the unique qualities of each milk alternative, I began sampling every brand of rice, soy, nut, hemp, potato, and oat "milk" I could find. After years of taste testing, I would like to offer the following observations and words of advice before you head off on your dairy-free shopping spree ...

Milk Alternative Observations

~   *Less Sugar* - My best discovery yet! Although plain and unsweetened varieties of milk alternatives are typically a bit sweeter than cow milk, most are amazingly lower in sugar. Be sure to look at the labels though; I have seen some brands and flavors (especially chocolate) with sugar levels at around 19 grams per serving. For the healthiest options, opt for the "Unsweetened" or "Light" varieties; these typically have only 0 to 4 grams of sugar per 8-ounce serving. Cow milk has a whopping 12 to 16 grams of sugar per serving for your basic regular, low-fat, and skim varieties!

~   *Dairy-Free* - To the best of my knowledge, all of the alternatives I have found to date are made without any milk ingredients (lactose or casein) whatsoever. Some milk alternative brands may be produced on shared equipment with dairy products and thus subject to cross-contamination (though the equipment is typically rigorously cleaned between runs), but a few brands are made on dedicated dairy-free equipment. If cross-contamination is a concern, call the manufacturer before consumption to find out their processes.

~   *Heart-Healthy* - All of the milk alternatives that I have come across to date are plant-based, and thus free from trans fats and cholesterol. With the exception of coconut milk they are also free of saturated fat.

~   *Vitamins and Minerals* - Check the labels; most varieties of soymilk, and many of the rice, oat, hemp, and nut milks are fortified to rival the Vitamin D and calcium available in cow milk. You may also find several brands that are fortified with nutrients such as Vitamin B12, which can be helpful for the vegan diet.

~   *Gluten-Sensitive* - Most non-dairy beverages are gluten-free, but caution is noted with grain milks, such as oat and rice. Just in case, be sure to read the packaging carefully before consuming any milk alternative, and contact the manufacturer when in doubt.

~   *Milk vs. Beverage* – For legal purposes, the makers of almond, oat, and rice "milks" will most often label these products as "non-dairy beverages." Soymilk (all one word) and coconut milk have created their own identities.

~ *Shelf Life* - Always check the expiration date on refrigerated, canned, and aseptic packages ... they do eventually expire, albeit not for quite a long time. Although aseptic packages do not require refrigeration until opened, popping them in the refrigerator a little early does create that nice cool "milk" taste.

~ *Shake it up* – Yes, it is true that ingredients can settle. There is nothing worse than dousing your cereal in almond water, trust me. Give that package a quick shake (use caution as the tops on those aseptic packages often leak when you shake them), pour, and enjoy. This will help to disperse any fortified vitamins and minerals, as well as the creamy texture and flavor.

In addition to a wealth of information on each milk alternative, this chapter includes recipes for making your own "milks" at home. For those who thought the bread maker was the best kitchen invention ever, investing in a soymilk maker may be worthwhile. They can be used to make any of the milks listed in this chapter, and often include a recipe guide.

However, if you do not have a soymilk maker, all is not lost. A blender and a device for straining is all you really need. You can use a fine mesh strainer, a double layer of cheesecloth, a dish/tea towel, or nylons to strain out any stray particles for the smoothest homemade milk alternative.

Also, the recipes in this chapter allow you to flavor the "milks" to taste with your sweetener of choice. This could be agave nectar, maple syrup, evaporated cane juice, or plain white sugar, for example. Should you wish for a sugar-free option, use stevia to taste (beginning with a very small amount) or blend in 2 or more dates (per 4 cups / 1 quart) for natural sweetness.

How to Substitute Milk in Recipes

With the exception of coconut milk, all of the milk alternatives named in this chapter will substitute 1:1 in any recipe that calls for low-fat or nonfat milk (often just listed as "milk" in recipes). For example, if a recipe requires 1 cup of milk, then you can substitute it with 1 cup of plain or unsweetened rice or soymilk.

Substituting milk alternatives in baked goods is fairly seamless; just pretend your aseptic package of non-dairy beverage is cow milk, and you are good to go. This goes for bread, muffins, scones, cakes, and cupcakes. Also, dairy-free milk alternatives can do double duty. If your recipe calls for 1 cup of milk and 1 teaspoon of vanilla, toss them both out and use 1 cup of your favorite vanilla milk alternative instead. In general, flavored milk alternatives such as chocolate and vanilla tend to have more sugar than their plain counterparts (unless specifically noted as unsweetened), and are well-suited to beverages, sweet baked goods, and some desserts.

In cooking you will want to choose your milk alternative carefully, giving consideration to how the fat content and flavor notes may affect your end product. For savory recipes, I always use unsweetened milk alternatives, as even the plain varieties tend to be just a bit too sweet. Also, each type of milk alternative (soy, rice, almond, hemp, cashew, etc.), has its own distinct taste. When experimenting with recipes, you may want to taste the milk alternative both chilled and heated to detect flavor overtones that may affect a particular recipe.

Of course, there is no reason to feel married to milky properties. In baking, feel free to replace the milk with a fruit juice that suits, again, in a 1:1 ratio. Have some fun experimenting with the different flavors that apple, orange, or pineapple juice can impart on your favorite muffin recipe. Keep in mind that you may want to reduce the sugar in your recipe if using fruit juice. For savory dishes, broth offers a wonderful flavor addition, a lighter taste and texture, and it can easily fill the liquid spot that milk leaves behind. In a pinch, when it really doesn't matter, water can replace milk in recipes. This is particularly true in recipes such as yeast breads.

I specified low-fat and nonfat milk above, because if your recipe goes so far as to name whole milk, then you may need a little more fat in the recipe. For whole milk, I have a few suggestions (this again is for 1:1 ratio):

~ If a mild coconut influence will work with the recipe, then try using light coconut milk. It has just a touch more fat than your typical carton of whole milk.
~ Try pureed soft silken tofu. It is just a bit higher in fat than soymilk, and it offers a thicker consistency.
~ Whip up a quick batch of homemade "milk," customized to the consistency you are seeking. For example, some nut milk recipes may call for 4 to 5 cups of water. Simply blend in the lesser amount for a thicker, higher in fat milk alternative.
~ Add a smidgen of oil to the recipe. Just a teaspoon or two whipped into the milk alternative should boost the richness of the dish to the level intended.

Soymilk

Ingredients
Soymilk is made from ground soybeans and filtered water, and it may contain some sweetener, salt, flavors (typically natural), fortification of vitamins and minerals, and/or some additives to improve flavor, texture, or shelf life (such as carrageenan). It is typically fortified to match the calcium levels of milk, but be sure to read the labels, as not all soymilks are created equal. Purists take heart, there are some "unadulterated" brands on the market, which contain only organic soybeans and water, or you can make your own at home.

Allergies, Sensitivities, and Special Diets
Some people do have an allergy or intolerance to soy. If you are one of these people, there is no need to feel trapped by the bean, move onto one of the other varieties of "milk" in this chapter. Soymilk is almost always dairy-free, wheat / gluten-free, nut-free, and vegan. But, as usual, check the ingredients and speak with the manufacturer whenever there is a concern. Also, in the past, a few brands have used Vitamin D3 in fortification, which is not considered vegan.

Taste
In general, soymilk is considered "hearty" among the non-dairy beverages, and is excellent when you are craving something thick and creamy. The plain varieties have a faintly sweet and "beany" flavor that is noticeable by some, but perfectly acceptable to others. Taste and consistency do vary widely among soymilk brands, so take heart if the first one is not to your liking. There is typically a brand and/or flavor out there for even the pickiest "milk" connoisseurs.

Uses
Soymilk can easily be substituted for cow milk in all baking needs, over cereal, for pancakes and waffles, in smoothies, or as a beverage, straight from the glass. Also, in my opinion, the unsweetened varieties work equally well in savory dishes. Even with the invention of so many other options, soymilk is still considered the gold standard of milk substitute versatility. It typically has a slightly higher fat content than the very lean rice milk, for example, allowing it to stand in for milk in more applications. However, soymilk does have a slightly pronounced flavor, so it may not be the top choice for delicate desserts and sauces.

Like cow milk, soymilk has a tendency to curdle when boiled. To avoid curdling, use it in dishes that contain little or no acid, add it at the end of the cooking process, warm-up the soymilk to at least room temperature before pouring it in, and don't let it come to a full boil. Another option is to substitute rice milk (unsweetened for savory applications) for half of the soymilk; this will keep it from curdling as easily, and is a nice blend for cooking.

To Purchase
Soymilk is very easy to track down. It is sold in aseptic packages, refrigerated cartons, and in powdered form. It can be found in most grocery stores in a wide variety of flavors, including plain, light, unsweetened, vanilla, chocolate, fortified, mocha, chai, carob, etc., etc., etc.

If you are new to soymilk, I think the refrigerated Silk® brand (www.silksoymilk.com, (888) 820-9283) is the best option for easing into the flavor. However, there are dozens of brands on the market (including generics), each with their own unique texture and flavor. For example, one colleague recommends the shelf-stable WestSoy® brand of soymilk (www.westsoy.biz, (800) 434-4246) stating that it goes over best with her little food allergic ones, while another prefers the simplicity of EdenSoy® Unsweetened (www.edenfoods.com, (517) 456-7424) for cooking and baking (it contains just organic soybeans and water).

Storage
Soymilk will keep for 7 to 10 days once opened. Packages purchased in the refrigerated section should be refrigerated immediately, while soymilk in aseptic containers is shelf stable, but should be refrigerated upon opening. For optimal taste, go ahead and throw it in your refrigerator a day or so before opening.

My Tips
~ *Choose Organic* - I recommend purchasing only organic soymilk. Soy is a top Genetically Modified product in the U.S., so unless the ingredients specifically state organic or non-GMO, move on. With so many brands to choose from at such a good price, there really is no reason to settle for anything less than the best.
~ *Don't Forget Generics* - Soymilk has become so popular that many stores now carry their own OEM brand. There is no need to feel slighted; these products are likely produced by the big guys, but with the store's generic label slapped on. Just check the ingredients and nutrients to see that it matches up with your expectations, and take home a package for a taste test. If it goes over well, then you may save a bundle by avoiding brand names.
~ *Be Wary of Cross-Contamination* - Rigorous cleaning processes are typically used on products that hold claims of "dairy-free" (but this is not necessarily true for "non-dairy," see p78), which is the case for most brands of soymilk. However, soy is a big industry, and many of the soy products are made by dairy producers or manufactured in dairy facilities. For anyone who may react to the trace amounts of milk from potential cross-contamination in a factory, I advise calling the company to get better acquainted with their processes before considering consumption.

Make Your Own
Unlike most other milk alternatives, soymilk can be a bit of a laborious task to make by hand, and for many people, the taste may never match-up to those palate-friendly, processed varieties found at the grocery store. It's just different. That said, some do love and even prefer the taste of homemade soymilk. For them, I highly recommend a soymilk maker to simplify the process; think of it like a bread maker, but for dairy-free beverage connoisseurs. If you don't yet have a soymilk maker, but would still like to sample some truly homemade soymilk, try the following "authentic" recipe.

Homemade Soy Milk

Yields approximately 16 Cups (1 gallon)

This recipe was shared by Yongkie Hurd, and is originally from China. It requires only a few ingredients and the results are fantastic. You can adjust the sweetness and flavors to your personal taste. As an added bonus, you can view a demo of Yongkie making this soymilk at www.everydaydish.tv.

12 Ounces Dried Organic Soybeans (available in bulk)
14 Cups Water

Pandan Leaf or 1 Teaspoon Almond Extract (optional)
4-1/4 ounces Granulated Sugar (scant 1/2 cup)

In a large bowl, cover the soybeans with a lot of water and soak overnight. The beans will triple in volume. In a blender, combine 1 cup of the soaked soybeans with 3-1/2 cups of water. Blend for two minutes, or until smooth. Repeat the process 3 more times, or until all of the soybeans are blended. If your blender won't hold all 3-1/2 cups of water, then you can do this in 4 batches. Using a double layer of cheesecloth (or a tea towel), strain the blended soybeans into a large pot; make sure to wring all of the liquid from the beans. Repeat until all of the soybean mixture is strained. Skim the foam from the strained soymilk. Strain the soymilk 2 more times to make sure that the liquid is very smooth. Pour the strained soymilk into a large pot.

Add the optional pandan leaf (if using) to the soymilk. Bring the soymilk to a boil over medium heat. Let it simmer for 20 minutes and remove from the heat. Add the sugar, stirring well. Return the pot to the heat, bring to a boil, reduce the heat and simmer for 5 minutes. Remove the pot from the heat. Let the soymilk cool completely. Once the soymilk is cooled, remove the Pandan leaf, if using. If you would like to add some almond extract, this is the time to stir it in. Pour the soymilk into a clean glass pitcher and refrigerate. This soymilk will last refrigerated for up to 1 week.

Cook's note: The soybeans can be de-hulled after soaking, but prior to blending, to reduce the "beany" taste. This involves rubbing off the outer seed coat, and will add a little more time to the process.

Alisa's Note: After preparing the soymilk you will be left with a beany mass that may appear like waste. These leftovers actually have a name, okara, and can be used in recipes as a high-fiber ingredient with a good amount of calcium. A quick online search for "okara recipes," should yield quite a few results.

Almond Milk

Ingredients
Almond milk is made from ground almonds and filtered water, and store-bought brands typically contain one or more of the following: sweetener (several unsweetened varieties are available), salt, starch, natural flavors, fortification of vitamins and minerals, and/or some additives to improve flavor, texture, or shelf life (such as gellan gum or carrageenan).

Allergies, Sensitivities, and Special Diets
Almond milk is always dairy-free, gluten-free, and vegan, to the best of my knowledge. But, as usual, check the ingredients and speak with the manufacturer whenever there is a concern. This milk alternative is obviously not a good option for nut allergies; however, it may be acceptable for soy allergies and sensitivities. A few (but not all) varieties/brands of almond milk do use soy lecithin, though many argue that soy lecithin and soy oil are typically well tolerated by the soy sensitive. Those with soy allergies and sensitivities must of course decide what is best for their health and consult a physician on this topic.

Taste
Almond milk can be described as a light non-dairy beverage with a delicate almond flavor.

Uses
The nutty flavor in almond milk is a plus in various desserts. It has become my personal favorite for smoothies and cereal. Since the advent of unsweetened almond milk, I have found more versatility with this milk alternative in savory dishes. However, like rice milk, it does tend to have a more delicate flavor than heartier "milks" such as soy.

To Purchase
Almond milk is readily available in aseptic packages in most major grocery stores and natural food markets. Plain, fortified, unsweetened, vanilla, and chocolate varieties offer some delicious options. Almond milk is a staple in our household, as we both love the flavor, texture, and versatility. I often purchase Almond Breeze® (www.bluediamond.com, (916) 442-0771) due to its great all around taste and good selection of flavors. However, I have also fallen in love with Pacific's Almond Non-Dairy Beverage (www.pacificfoods.com, (503) 692-9666), which is equally delicious but organic and slightly richer in texture.

Storage
Almond milk is typically sold in aseptic packages and thus is quite shelf stable. However, you must refrigerate almond milk upon opening. It will keep for 7 to 10 days once opened.

Make Your Own
Almonds can be a bit pricey, so I prefer to purchase almond milk. However, there are many recipe options for homemade versions. Plus, it is quite easy to make, and the results are free from additives. The following two are relatively quick and simple, though the almonds may need to be prepared in advance:

Basic Almond Milk
Yields approximately 3 to 4 Cups

1 Cup Raw Almonds (blanched if possible)*
3 to 4 Cups Water, Plus Additional for Soaking

1 to 2 Teaspoons Sugar, Agave Nectar, or Honey or 1 to 2 Tablespoons Raisins (optional)

Cover the almonds with water and allow them to soak for at least 6 hours or overnight. Drain the almonds and place them in your blender, along with 1 cup of fresh water. Blend the almonds on high speed for 2 to 3 minutes, or until the mixture is smooth and creamy. Blend in another 2 to 3 cups of water, depending on your desired consistency. Pour the milk through a fine mesh strainer or a double layer of cheesecloth, squeezing to extract as much of the liquid as possible.** If desired, return the milk to your blender and blend in some sweetener to taste. Refrigerate and use within 3 to 4 days.

No Soak Method: If you need some almond milk in a hurry, skip the soaking time, but use boiling water.

Truly raw almonds may not be available, but just make sure they are not roasted, salted or seasoned in any way. Rather than blanching almonds myself, I often cheat by purchasing sliced almonds that are ready to go.
***The remaining almond pulp can be used in other recipes or skin care (i.e. a facial scrub).*

Almond-Seed Milk

Yields approximately 3 to 4 Cups

This recipe was shared by Meghan Telpner (www.meghantelpner.com), a nutritionist and "healthy cookie" out of Toronto, Ontario. She incorporates seeds into the basic almond milk recipe for an added touch of nutrients.

1/2 Cup Raw Almonds (blanched if possible)*
1/4 Cup Raw Sesame Seeds
2 Tablespoons Whole Flax Seeds

3 to 4 Cups Water, Plus Additional for Soaking
1 Teaspoon Vanilla or Almond Extract (optional)
1 to 2 Tablespoons Agave Nectar or Honey (optional)

Cover the nuts and seeds with 2 cups of water, and allow them to soak for 24 hours. Drain the nuts and seeds, and place them in your blender, along with 2 cups of fresh water. Blend the nuts and seeds on high speed for 2 to 3 minutes, or until the mixture is smooth and creamy. Blend in another 1 to 2 cups of water, depending on your desired consistency. Pour the milk through a fine mesh strainer or a double layer of cheesecloth, squeezing to extract as much of the liquid as possible.** If desired, return the milk to your blender and blend in the sweetener and extract. Refrigerate and use within 3 to 4 days.

* Truly raw almonds may not be available, but just make sure they are not roasted, salted or seasoned in any way. Rather than blanching almonds myself, I often cheat by purchasing sliced almonds that are ready to go.
**The remaining almond pulp can be used in other recipes or skin care (i.e. a facial scrub).

Rice Milk

Ingredients

Rice milk is typically made from brown rice, filtered water, and a wee bit of oil. Since rice milk tends to be a little sweet naturally, it is easy to find brands without added sugar. However, like soymilk, I wouldn't be surprised to find a touch of sweetener, salt, natural flavors, fortification of vitamins and minerals, and/or some additives to improve flavor, texture, or shelf life (such as xanthan gum or carrageenan).

Allergies, Sensitivities, and Special Diets

Rice milk is almost always dairy-free, nut-free, soy-free, and vegan. But, as usual, check the ingredients and speak with the manufacturer whenever there is a concern. Most brands of rice milk are gluten-free, but if it is not specifically noted on the packaging, give the manufacturer a quick call. It is possible that the brown rice syrup used to sweeten some brands has been converted with barley rather than a gluten-free natural enzyme.

Taste

Some say rice milk has that "true milk flavor." It is one of the lightest, sweetest, and most refreshing dairy substitutes.

Uses

With its natural sweetness, rice milk is perfect in desserts and baked goods. When unsweetened, its delicate texture also works well in curries and lighter cream soups and sauces. However, the taste is frequently noted as "off" in heavier, savory dishes.

To Purchase

Rice milk can be found on most grocery store shelves in aseptic packages. You may also stumble across refrigerated quarts of rice milk near the soymilk. Thus far, I have seen plain, fortified, low-fat, nonfat, vanilla, chocolate, and carob versions of rice milk, as well as some "fancier" flavors, such as chocolate chai.

My husband likes plain rice milk, but we tend to shop based on price since his taste buds aren't sensitive enough to detect a major difference in the various brands. In general, this means we usually purchase generic, but on occasion we will pick up one of the more popular brands, such as Rice Dream® (www.tastethedream.com, (800) 434-4246) or Pacific Foods (www.pacificfoods.com, (503) 692-9666).

Storage
Rice milk will keep for 7 to 10 days once opened. Packages purchased in the refrigerated section should be refrigerated immediately, while rice milk in aseptic containers is quite shelf stable, but should be refrigerated upon opening. For that immediate cool and refreshing taste, go ahead and throw those aseptic packages in your refrigerator a day or so before opening.

Make Your Own
Rice milk is cheap, quick to make, and offers the ability to experiment with flavors quite easily. Before you move onto the recipes, here are a few tips:

~ You can make rice milk from many varieties of long and short grain rice, including brown, white, wild, and sweet, as well as combinations such as brown-wild, or sweet brown.
~ Rice milk can be a bit bland, which works well for savory soups and sauces, but I would recommend a bit of vanilla and sweetener if you are using it atop cereal or in desserts.
~ When preparing "cooked" rice milk, use fresh rice that is still hot and hot water for superior results.
~ For smoother milk, re-cook the rice with part of the water until it's very soft. This is an excellent solution for re-using cold or day-old rice.
~ Feel free to flavor or add nutrients to your rice milk prior to blending. Some suggestions include a bit of salt, sweetener (agave nectar, honey, evaporated cane juice, and maple syrup are options with nutrients), chocolate / cocoa powder, cinnamon, almond extract, flax or sesame seeds, and powdered calcium.
~ For a nut-rice milk, substitute almonds or other nuts for up to half of the rice. See the cashew-rice milk option that follows as an example.

Cooked Rice Milk
Yields approximately 4 Cups (1 quart)
This is your basic no-frills rice milk … simple, easy, inexpensive, and reliable. Rice milk made from cooked rice can taste a bit starchy, so I prefer to make the Rice-Cashew Milk option in this recipe for optimal flavor and texture.

1 Cup Hot Brown or White Rice	1 Teaspoon Vanilla Extract (optional)
4 Cups Hot Water	Pinch Salt (optional)
1 Tablespoon Sweetener of Choice (optional)	

Place the rice and hot water in your blender, and puree for 3 to 4 minutes or until smooth.* Let it cool for a few minutes, then pour the milk through a fine mesh strainer or a double layer of cheesecloth, squeezing to extract as much of the liquid as possible. If desired, return the milk to your blender and blend in some sweetener, vanilla, and/or salt to taste. Refrigerate and use within 2 to 3 days.

Rice-Cashew Milk Option: Follow the recipe above, but reduce the amount of rice used to 2/3 cup, and add in 1/3 cup of cashews prior to blending. If you have a spice grinder or food processor, I recommend processing the cashews into a powder or paste prior to blending for a smoother milk alternative.

* Be sure to secure the blender lid when you first turn it on, as you may have an initial kick-back from the hot rice and liquid. If needed, puree in batches.

"Raw" Rice Milk
Yields approximately 3 to 4 Cups
Though not as quick, soaking the rice rather than cooking it can yield rice milk that is closer in taste and consistency to commercial varieties.

1 Cup Uncooked, Short Grain White or Brown Rice
3 to 4 Cups Water, Divided
1 Tablespoon Sweetener of Choice (optional)

1 Teaspoon Vanilla Extract (optional)
Pinch Salt (optional)

Place the rice and 1 cup of water in your blender, and blend for just a minute. Add 2 cups of water, and allow the rice to soak for at least 4 hours or overnight. After soaking, blend the mixture on high for 1 to 2 minutes. For a thinner consistency, blend in up to 1 cup of additional water. Pour the milk through a fine mesh strainer or a double layer of cheesecloth, squeezing to extract as much of the liquid as possible. If desired, return the milk to your blender and blend in some sweetener, vanilla, and/or salt to taste. Refrigerate and use within 2 to 3 days.

Oat Milk

Ingredients
Oat milk is made from oat groats (the hulled grain broken into fragments), water, and a touch of sea salt. You may also find oat bran, sweetener, natural flavors, fortification of vitamins and minerals, and/or some additives to improve flavor, texture, or shelf life (such as gellan gum or carrageenan).

Allergies, Sensitivities, and Special Diets
Oat milk is always dairy-free, nut-free, soy-free, and vegan, to the best of my knowledge. But, as usual, check the ingredients and speak with the manufacturer whenever there is a concern. Gluten-free consumers may opt to purchase certified gluten-free oats and make their own "milk" at home, but I would not recommend store-bought versions for the gluten sensitive or intolerant. I would also be cautious with wheat allergies, as cross contamination is fairly common with oats.

Taste
Unadulterated oat milk is smooth in texture and has a very mild flavor that is lightly sweet. It substitutes very well for low-fat milk since it tends to be a bit hearty.

Uses
Oat milk arrived on the scene with instant praise for its versatility. It has been successfully trialed as a substitute for cow milk in both sweet and savory dishes. In addition to drinking it straight from a glass, oat milk is recommended for your morning cereal, smoothies, baked goods, curries, cream soups and sauces, mashed potatoes, and ...well, you give it a try and see what you think.

To Purchase
Oat milk is currently sold in aseptic packages in the natural foods section of some grocery stores. It has been spotted in plain, vanilla, and fortified varieties. As I write, oat milk is thriving in Europe, with brands such as Oatly (www.oatly.com, Sweden - 46 (0)418 47 55 00) dominating the scene. Yet, the selections have been very limited in North America.

Storage Tips

Oat milk is typically sold in aseptic packages and thus is quite shelf stable. However, you must refrigerate oat milk upon opening. It will keep for 7 to 10 days once opened.

Make Your Own

Luckily, oat milk is very, very easy and inexpensive to whip up at home:

Effortless Overnight Oat Milk

Yields approximately 2 Cups

I have to admit, I was impressed with the results of this simple recipe. The resultant milk is smooth, clean, and tastes like oatmeal in pure liquid form. It can be used in savory recipes, or sweetened for drinking or dessert applications.

1 Cup Rolled Oats

2 Cups Water

1 to 2 Teaspoons Sweetener of Choice (optional)

1/2 Teaspoon Vanilla Extract (optional)

Pinch Salt (optional)

Place the oats and water in a container with a tight fitting lid. Give it a quick shake, and store in the refrigerator overnight. In the morning, shake the container for a good minute (no need to blend), then strain the "milk" through a fine mesh strainer, pressing to extract as much of the milk as possible. If desired, stir or blend in some sweetener, vanilla, and/or salt to taste. Enjoy the leftover oats for breakfast, in recipes, in a smoothie, or for use in homemade bath products (such as a scrub). Refrigerate and use within 2 to 3 days.

"Authentic" Oat Milk

Yields approximately 3 to 4 Cups

Many would argue that to make "proper" oat milk you should use oat groats. These unprocessed grains are exceptionally nutritious, and the end product is tasty, so I see no reason to argue. Look for oat groats at natural food stores, in bulk food departments, or online.

3/4 Cup Raw Oat Groats

3 to 4 Cups Water, Plus Additional for Soaking

1 Tablespoon Sweetener of Choice (optional)

1 Teaspoon Vanilla Extract (optional)

Pinch Salt (optional)

Cover the oat groats with water, and allow them to soak overnight. Drain the oats, and place them in your blender along with 2 cups of fresh water. Blend them on high speed for 2 to 3 minutes, or until the mixture is smooth and creamy. Blend in another 1 to 2 cups of water, depending on your desired consistency. Pour the milk through a fine mesh strainer or a double layer of cheesecloth, squeezing to extract as much of the liquid as possible. If desired, return the milk to your blender and blend in some sweetener, vanilla, and/or salt to taste. Refrigerate and use within 2 to 3 days.

Almond-Oat Milk Option: Follow the directions above, but reduce the oat groats to 1/4 cup, and use 1/2 cup blanched almonds. Soak the almonds overnight, along with the oats.

Coconut Milk

Ingredients
To make coconut milk, finely grated coconut meat is steeped in hot water until it is cool enough to handle. It is then squeezed until dry; the white fluid is strained to remove all of the pulp. Canned coconut milk, as we find it in stores, usually has a stabilizer added, such as guar gum. Some brands may have other additives, but in my opinion this negatively affects the quality.

Allergies, Sensitivities, and Special Diets
For many, coconut milk is a very "safe" food. It is dairy-free, gluten-free, soy-free, and vegan. However, in October 2006, the FDA decided to classify coconut as a tree nut, for the purpose of food allergen labeling. In the past, coconut was rarely restricted for those who had a tree nut allergy, but some doctors may now recommend it. If you are dealing with a tree nut allergy, consult a physician before giving coconut the go ahead, just in case. Keep in mind that coconut allergies do exist, even in some who may have no other known allergens.

Taste
Coconut milk has a strong flavor all its own that is lightly sweet. It is typically a standout in whatever it is added to, from beverages to desserts to the main course.

Uses
Unlike the other milk alternatives listed in this chapter, coconut milk is considered a bit too heavy for sipping on its own. However, the richness of coconut milk makes it a natural born star in Thai and Caribbean cooking. In addition to savory foods, when used in place of cow milk, coconut milk gives a luxurious tropical flavor to desserts, quick bread, and mixed drinks.

To Purchase
Canned coconut milk is readily available in the Asian food section of most grocery stores. It can be found in both light and regular versions. Regular coconut milk is more comparable to a medium-heavy cream in texture, while light coconut milk is closer whole milk or half & half in consistency.

Coconut milk varies from brand to brand in quality and flavor, so be sure to try a few in order to pinpoint your favorite. Good brands of coconut milk will have thick cream floating on top of the can while the milk on the bottom will be much more watery. Brands with milk that appears homogenized tend to have an artificial taste due to excess processing or additives. Whenever possible, I purchase organic coconut milk, as it does seem to be a superior product.

Storage Tips
Canned coconut milk is very shelf stable, but it should be refrigerated once opened. It will keep for up to one week in the refrigerator.

Make Your Own
Since coconut milk is so inexpensive and easy to find, homemade may not be necessary. However, if you would like to give it a whirl, try one of the following ideas:

~ Combine equal parts boiling water and chopped coconut, and allow it to sit for one hour. Strain the coconut water through a double layer of cheesecloth or a tea towel. Squeeze the coconut pulp in the cheesecloth to extract as much of the "juice" as possible. Discard the coconut pulp or use it for another food or skincare application.

~ Bring 1 cup of dried coconut (unsweetened) and 1 cup water to a boil. Remove it from the heat and allow it to cool for few minutes. Mix the coconut water in a blender at high speed, and then strain it through cheesecloth as directed above.
~ Combine 1 cup of coconut milk powder with 1/2 cup of hot water for a shortcut to light coconut milk. Use caution when purchasing coconut milk powder. Several brands will use milk-based ingredients (such as sodium caseinate) to "improve" the product.
~ For "raw" coconut milk, blend 1 cup of raw coconut meat/flesh with 3 cups of coconut water (from the inside of the coconut) in a blender or food processor until smooth. Thin with additional water as needed. Young Thai coconuts work particularly well for this, but feel free to experiment with your favorite variety.

Hemp Milk

Ingredients
Hemp Milk is made from shelled hemp seeds (otherwise known as hemp nuts) and filtered water. While it can now be found unsweetened, most packaged varieties contain some sweetener (such as evaporated cane juice), and they may contain a stabilizer (such as xanthan gum), salt, fortification of vitamins and minerals, and/or natural flavors. Have no fear; while hemp seeds do come from a similar variety of plant, they are not marijuana. Drink and enjoy without fear of breaking the law!

Allergies, Sensitivities, and Special Diets
Hemp milk emerged as a new "savior" for food allergies. Vegan and free from wheat/gluten, dairy, soy, tree nuts, and peanuts, hemp milk offers a second option to those who have felt limited to rice milk. Of course, you should always check with the manufacturer prior to consumption, whenever food allergies are a concern.

Taste
Though there were only two brands of hemp milk on the market at the time of writing, the difference in taste between the two was amazing. Overall, hemp milk has a taste all its own that I can only think to describe as "seedy." While it could be likened to nut milk, without added sugar hemp milk doesn't have that light, naturally sweet taste that you would find in almond or cashew milk. Hemp milk possesses a slightly stronger scent and more of a savory flare. For these reasons, most varieties are sweetened at least a bit to offer more versatility.

Uses
As mentioned, some varieties of hemp milk have a rather strong flavor, so they may tend to overpower more delicate foods and desserts. However, cereal, smoothies, cappuccinos, and heartier applications are quite suitable. Unsweetened hemp milk may find good use in rich savory dishes, particularly since it contains a higher level of "healthy" fats than your average milk alternative. Just be sure not to heat the milk above 350ºF (175ºC), lest some of the Omega-3 benefits be lost.

To Purchase
Hemp milk is quickly making its way onto grocery shelves throughout the U.S. and Canada, where it can be found in aseptic packages. At last check, plain, chocolate, vanilla, and unsweetened flavors were available.

In North America, there are two main brands of hemp milk, both produced in Canada due to the prohibition of growing hemp in the U.S. Living Harvest Hempmilk (www.livingharvest.com, (866) 972-6879) is a milder, fortified brand that is well accepted by sensitive taste buds. Hemp Bliss (www.manitobaharvest.com, (800) 665-4367) contains very few ingredients and is as organic and natural as store-bought hempmilk gets. It has a more pronounced flavor, but I enjoy it in smoothies and recipes. I have written a comparison review of the two brands on www.godairyfree.org, which goes into much more detail that you may find useful.

Storage Tips

Since it is typically sold in aseptic packages, hemp milk is quite shelf stable. However, you must refrigerate hemp milk upon opening. It will keep for 7 to 10 days once opened.

Make Your Own

Shelled (hulled) hemp seed is somewhat soft, so it blends up into a creamy non-dairy "milk" faster and easier than most other seeds and nuts. However, the price of hemp seeds may be a deterrent from homemade; those little nuts can be very expensive! Nonetheless, if you can get your hands on a good amount of those little bits of gold (available at most natural food stores), then don't hesitate to trial the simple recipe below:

Instant Hemp Milk

Yields approximately 4 to 6 Cups

Like most seeds, hemp can have a bitter taste, so I recommend using at least a touch of sweetener for optimal flavor.

1 Cup Shelled Hemp Seeds
4 to 6 Cups Water
1 to 2 Tablespoons Sweetener of Choice, or to Taste

1 Teaspoon Vanilla Extract (optional)
Pinch Salt (optional)

Place the hemp seeds and 2 cups of water in your blender. Blend on high for 2 to 3 minutes, or until smooth. Blend in more water, 1 cup at a time, until it reaches your desired consistency. Pour the milk through a fine mesh strainer or a double layer of cheesecloth, squeezing to extract as much of the liquid as possible. If desired, return the milk to your blender and blend in some sweetener, vanilla, and/or salt to taste. Refrigerate and use within 2 to 3 days.

Many More Milk Alternatives

Aside from the aforementioned, you can make "milk" from spelt, rye, quinoa, flax seeds, hazelnuts, cashews, potatoes, etc. I have even seen a recipe for zucchini milk! Below are a few more milk alternative ideas and recipes, but feel free to experiment once you get comfortable with your favorite flavors.

Whole Grain Milk

This is typically oat milk with other whole grains added for flavor and nutrient value. Store-bought versions are rarely suitable for the gluten-sensitive. However, you can make homemade gluten-free versions using grains such as quinoa and millet. Several homemade recipes will instruct you to cook the grains and then blend. I find that this creates a very thick, gelatinous "milk" that is rather unpleasant, particularly after refrigeration. I prefer to soak and grind the "raw" grains, such as with the oat milk recipes (p103), but you can try cooked or "raw" preparations to see which meets with your taste and texture preferences.

Beyond Almond

Though quite tasty, almonds certainly aren't the end-all-be-all in terms of nut milks. Experiment with different nuts, seeds, and flavors, using the Instant Nut Milk and Seed Milk recipes below.

Potato Milk

A potato-soy hybrid has already hit the refrigerated section in Canada. I trialed the plain version (also available in vanilla and chocolate) and found it to have that same "hearty" flavor as soymilk. In the U.S., there is a popular potato milk powder called DariFree™ (www.vancesfoods.com, (800) 497-4834). As for homemade, potato milk can be a bit starchy, but it is a good option for those with multiple food allergies; you can experiment with the recipe that follows.

Instant Nut Milk

Yields approximately 4 to 5 Cups

I have tested a variety of nuts in this recipe, from cashews to pecans, with surprisingly different results. The three nuts listed below are the ones I recommend for the most reliable and best tasting results. Of the three, cashew "milk" has become my go-to quick recipe for both sweet and savory applications.

1 Cup (5 ounces) Raw Cashews, Hazelnuts, or Brazil
    Nuts
4 to 5 Cups Water

1 Tablespoon Sweetener of Choice (optional)
1 Teaspoon Vanilla Extract (optional)
Pinch Salt (optional)

As an optional first step, blend the nuts in your spice grinder until they pass the powder stage and just begin to clump. Place the nuts and 2 cups of water in your blender, and blend for 2 to 3 minutes or until smooth. Add 2 cups of water, and blend for another minute. If it is too thick for your taste, blend in more water until it reaches your desired consistency. Strain the "milk" through a fine mesh strainer or a double layer of cheesecloth, squeezing to extract as much of the liquid as possible. Return the milk to your blender, and blend in the sweetener, vanilla, and/or salt, if using. Refrigerate and use within 2 to 3 days.

Seed Milk

Yields approximately 3 to 4 Cups

Because seeds can be slightly bitter when compared to nuts, I do not consider the sweetener and vanilla optional in this recipe, but feel free to customize the recipe to your tastes.

3/4 Cup Pumpkin or Sunflower Seeds
3 to 3-1/2 Cups Water, Plus Additional for Soaking
1 to 2 Tablespoons Sweetener of Choice, or to Taste

3/4 Teaspoon Vanilla Extract
Pinch Salt

Cover the seeds in water and allow them to soak overnight. Drain the seeds and add them to your blender, along with 2 cups of fresh water. Blend the seeds for 2 to 3 minutes or until smooth. Add 1 cup of water, and blend for another minute. If it is too thick for your taste, blend in more water until it reaches your desired consistency. Strain the "milk" through a fine mesh strainer or a double layer of cheesecloth, squeezing to extract as much of the liquid as possible.* Return the milk to your blender, and blend in the sweetener, vanilla, and salt. Refrigerate and use within 2 to 3 days.

*On a raw website I discovered an innovative recommendation to save the unsweetened pulp from seed milk and add it to hummus or baba ghanoush (p171).

Potato Milk

Yields approximately 4 to 6 Cups

Potato milk powder yields a more user-friendly consistency, as cooked potatoes tend to be a bit starchy. Nonetheless, this quick and easy milk alternative is quite useful for savory or hearty applications. Alternately, you can sweeten it to taste with your sweetener of choice and add 1 teaspoon of vanilla extract for use in desserts or as a beverage.

4 to 5 Cups Water, Plus Additional for Boiling
1 Large Potato, Peeled and Diced (about 1 cup)
Pinch Salt

1/4 Cup Sliced Almonds (optional, for calcium and flavor)

Place the potato in a medium-sized saucepan, cover with water, and add the salt. Boil for 10 to 15 minutes, or until the potato chunks are quite tender. Drain, and place the potato in your blender, along with 3 cups of fresh water, and the almonds, if using. Blend the potato milk for 3 to 4 minutes, or until it is smooth and creamy. Blend in another 1 to 2 cups of water, depending on your desired consistency. Strain the "milk" through a fine mesh strainer or a double layer of cheesecloth, squeezing to extract as much of the liquid as possible. Refrigerate and use within 2 to 3 days.

Sweet Cantaloupe Milk

Yields 1-1/2 Cups

The idea for this easy milk came from the website www.goneraw.com. I liked the concept of getting some nutrition out of those cantaloupe seeds rather than throwing them away. The taste of this "milk" will vary quite a bit depending on the quality and sweetness of the cantaloupe you use, so do adjust the sweetener to taste. For a quick and light breakfast, I omit the sweetener, and blend in 1 frozen, ripe banana.

1/4 Cup Cantaloupe Seeds (see the instructions)
1 Cup Water
1/2 Cup Chopped Cantaloupe Flesh

1 to 2 Teaspoons Agave Nectar or Honey (optional)
Dash Vanilla Extract (optional)
Generous Pinch Cinnamon (optional)

Scoop out the seeds from a freshly cut cantaloupe, and rinse them off. Add the cantaloupe seeds and water to your blender, and blend on high for 2 to 3 minutes. Strain the liquid through a fine mesh strainer, quickly rinse out your blender to get rid of any remaining seed kernels, and return the liquid to your blender. Add the cantaloupe flesh and the sweetener, vanilla, and cinnamon, if using. Blend for another 1 minute, or until everything is well combined.

CHAPTER 13:
MOVING BEYOND BUTTER

"But you can eat butter, right?" If you haven't heard this question yet, be patient, you will. While it might seem logical to many that butter is in fact a dairy product, to some people it stands alone in its very own food group, far removed from the cow and exalted in purity. Be vigilant when someone tells you that a particular dish doesn't contain dairy. When I inquire further with the more specific question, "Does the entrée contain butter or is butter used in the preparation?" at least 50% of the time, the answer is yes.

Now you may be wondering if butter is really a concern for your particular situation. If you are dairy-free for political, religious, social, or general health reasons then odds are you will avoid all dairy products, including butter. When it comes to milk allergies and lactose intolerance, butter often meets controversy.

Butter is created by churning fresh or fermented cream or milk. It is mostly butterfat (80 to 85%) surrounded by tiny droplets, which consist mostly of water and milk proteins. Yes, butter still contains some of those milk proteins that wreak havoc on the milk allergic. Be warned; as I have actually seen some websites that incorrectly state butter does not contain casein or whey. It is true that butter contains less milk protein than what you will find in milk and cheese, but it is there nonetheless.

If your allergy or intolerance is not hyper-sensitive, then you may be very lucky. Butter is unknowingly slathered on sandwich buns, stirred into fresh pasta, and even used to prepare the grill in many restaurants. The staff may not even realize when they are using butter. If you can tolerate the small amounts of milk protein or lactose that might make their way into your food from these unintentional additions, then your life could be much simpler. However, even these small amounts can elicit reactions in many milk allergic individuals, so use caution. You and your physician must decide what level of dairy, if any, is safe for you or your loved one before risking consumption of any butter.

Contrary to popular belief, butter is not lactose-free, but it is very, very low in lactose. It may contain as low as 0.1% lactose, unless milk solids are added back to the butter, which would pump that level up a bit. Since butter is considered a very low lactose food, it can be consumed by many lactose intolerant individuals without fear of symptoms. Of course, this varies from person to person, and with the severity of the intolerance.

In the milk allergy and lactose intolerant circles we often hear about clarified butter and ghee, so I would like to address these also ...

Clarified butter is produced by melting butter, allowing the milk solids, water, and butterfat to separate by density. The water evaporates, while the whey proteins float on top (and are skimmed off) and the casein proteins sink to the bottom (where they are left behind when the butterfat is poured). In essence, clarified butter is almost pure butterfat. Many cooks like clarified butter because it has a much longer shelf life than butter and it has a higher smoke point for better use in sautéing.

Ghee is basically clarified butter that is brought to higher temperatures. Once the water has evaporated, the milk solids brown, and are then removed, leaving behind the butterfat. This process gives ghee a unique flavor that is popular in the Middle East and South Asia, and produces antioxidants that lengthen its shelf-life to 6 to 8 months.

In theory, clarified butter and ghee should be safe for milk allergies and lactose intolerance. However, those with milk allergies must be warned that these two types of butter may still have a lingering milk protein or two. There is no guarantee that traces of casein or whey won't be left behind, which is why it still makes my dairy ingredient list (p80). While it is possible that trace amounts of lactose may remain, the lactose levels in ghee and clarified butter are typically so extremely low that only in rare instances would it be a problem for lactose intolerant individuals.

When Butter isn't Butter

One of the most common questions I receive is on chocolate, but it isn't what you might be thinking. Milk chocolate or milk added to dark and semi-sweet chocolate is a definite concern, and cross-contamination of milk ingredients in chocolate manufacturing is a big risk, but some dairy-free consumers are unsure if they can even enjoy chocolate at all, regardless of the additional ingredients or manufacturing processes. They fear one of the core ingredients, cocoa butter.

To ease your minds, many foods with the word "butter" in their title are in fact okay for dairy-free consumers, and in pure form, safe for milk allergies and intolerances. When we speak of butter in relation to dairy-free living, we are only speaking of dairy butter, whether it is from a cow, goat, sheep, or other mammal. Luckily, the following buttery foods should be totally vegan, and thus free from milk*:

~   Cocoa Butter (chocolate lovers rejoice!)
~   Coconut Butter
~   Shea Butter
~   Peanut Butter*
~   Tree Nut Butters (almond, cashew, macadamia nut, etc.)*
~   Seed Butters (hemp seed, tahini (sesame seed butter), sunflower seed, pumpkin seed, etc.)*
~   Fruit Butter (pumpkin, apple, pear, etc.)*

* Keep in mind that fancy new versions of foods are everywhere. Always check ingredients on these "butters," as they may have some milk ingredients added for a unique flavor. To date, I have only spotted a couple varieties of peanut or nut butter with milk additions, and have yet to come across fruit butters with dairy added, but it could happen!

Margarine or Vegetable Shortening

Some may abhor the use of margarine, but I can't lie, I really don't have a problem with it ... as long as it is a non-hydrogenated version. I grew up in a household struggling to make ends meet, so we stayed content with the 4 for $1.00 pack of four sticks. Real cream butter wasn't a luxury that my taste buds matured with, so I have never felt slighted by this aspect of the dairy-free diet.

That being disclaimed, I find margarine to be an excellent 1:1 substitute for butter in baking, cooking, or as a versatile spread. Not all brands of margarine are dairy-free, and many do contain trans fats, so choose your margarine wisely. I always keep Earth Balance® Buttery Sticks (www.earthbalancenatural.com, (201) 568-9300) on hand for baking, and when on sale, I pick up a tub of Smart Balance Light (www.smartbalance.com, (201) 568-9300) for general spreading.

Vegetable shortening is best used as a substitute for butter in baking. You may reduce the amount of vegetable shortening to 3/4 to 7/8 cup for every 1 cup of butter that a recipe calls for. This is the standard rule, and seems to work quite well in cakes; however, I have had great success with many recipes when I cut back even a bit more, reducing the fat to just 2/3 cup or even 1/2 cup per 1 cup called for. Like margarine, be careful about the brand you choose. Most (but not all) are made without dairy, but they could be loaded with hydrogenated oils. Be sure to look for one that is labeled as trans fat free, such as Earth Balance® Shortening (contact information above), which is sold in a four pack of sticks in the refrigerated section.

Shortening is also a good option for those who have a soy allergy or intolerance, because there are a few brands that are milk and soy-free. Unfortunately, this is a difficult combo to find in margarine. For a good soy-free, dairy-free, trans fat-free shortening, try Spectrum Shortening (www.spectrumorganics.com, (800) 434-4246). It is sold in tubs and typically placed on the lower shelves in the baking department of natural food grocers.

Cooking (and Baking) Oils

When I discovered the possibilities of oil, I was hooked! Though it might take a bit of experimentation at times, oil can be utilized as an excellent substitute for butter in most applications, even in baking. Obviously oil will work very well as a substitute for butter in sautéing or roasting. However, in baking much less oil is typically required (really, is this a bad thing?), as it will yield a greasy product if you use a 1:1 ratio.

As a fat equivalent, they say that 7/8 cup (3/4 cup + 2 tablespoons) vegetable oil (or other good baking oil) equals 1 cup of butter. I agree that 3/4 to 1 cup of oil substitutes well for butter in recipes such as cake. However, for cookies and bars, I think this is a bit generous. I modified a cookie recipe to use just 1/2 cup of oil in place of the 1 cup of butter called for, and those little chocolate chip morsels are always gobbled up with huge smiles (recipe on p226). Any more oil and the cookies turn out quite greasy. Each recipe varies, but in general, I use 1/2 to 3/4 the amount called for when substituting oil for solid or softened butter in baked goods. As a side note, if a recipe specifically calls for a certain amount of melted butter, then you should be able to replace it with the equivalent amount of oil.

I have included some charts on the following pages that list the smoke points of various oils to help you select the best oil(s) for use in your recipes. The smoke point is the temperature at which cooking oil begins to break down, and literally smokes. When this happens, the oil is essentially burning (not safe!) and losing its nutritional benefits. As you might expect, burnt oil does not leave the best taste on your food either. Keep in mind that this is just a general guide, as smoke points can vary depending upon the refining process and the source of the oil. As you will notice, the more refined the oil, the higher the heat it can take. However, unrefined oils are typically considered much more nutritive.

No Heat Oils
Best for Dressings, Marinades and Dipping

The following oils have a low smoke point and should not be heated. Luckily, these unrefined oils tend to have a nice rich flavor that compliments food nicely when drizzled on as an afterthought.

Type of Oil	Smoke Point °F	Smoke Point °C
Olive Oil, Extra Virgin	200-250°F	93-121°C
Borage Oil, Unrefined	225°F	107°C
Canola Oil, Unrefined	225°F	107°C
Evening Primrose Oil, Unrefined	225°F	107°C
Flaxseed Oil, Unrefined	225°F	107°C
Safflower Oil, Unrefined	225°F	107°C
Sunflower Oil, Unrefined	225°F	107°C

Low Heat Oils
Best for Light Sautéing and Sauces

These oils are suitable for lightly sautéing vegetables, simmering a sauce over low heat, or low heat baking. Of course, they will also suit no heat applications nicely, acting as a base for salad dressings or drizzled atop your meal.

Type of Oil	Smoke Point °F	Smoke Point °C
Corn Oil, Unrefined	320°F	160°C
High-Oleic Sunflower Oil, Unrefined	320°F	160°C
Olive Oil, Unrefined	320°F	160°C
Peanut Oil, Unrefined	320°F	160°C
Safflower Oil, Semi-Refined	320°F	160°C
Soybean Oil, Unrefined	320°F	160°C
Walnut Oil, Unrefined	320°F	160°C
Hemp Seed Oil, Unrefined	330°F	165°C
Canola Oil, Semi-Refined	350°F	177°C
Coconut Oil	350°F	177°C
Sesame Oil, Unrefined	350°F	177°C
Soybean Oil, Semi-Refined	350°F	177°C

Medium Heat Oils
Best For Baking and Sautéing

These oils tend to have a nice neutral or light flavor, making them good all-purpose oils for baking, normal sautéing, or in cold or hot applications acting as the carrier for salad dressings and sauces.

Type of Oil	Smoke Point °F	Smoke Point °C
Macadamia Nut Oil	390°F	199°C
Walnut Oil, Semi-Refined	400°F	204°C
Canola Oil, Refined	400-475°F	204-246°C
Almond Oil, Refined	420°F	216°C
Cottonseed Oil	420°F	216°C
Grapeseed Oil	420°F	216°C
Virgin Olive Oil	420°F	216°C

High Heat Oils
Best for Frying and All-Purpose Cooking
These oils sit at the top of the oil food chain, but as you will notice, most are quite refined. This means that they have undergone a chemical process in most cases to make them more resilient to high temperatures. For this reason, they may not possess the same nutritive properties or full-bodied flavor of lower heat oils. I prefer to use these types of oils sparingly, and only as needed.

Type of Oil	Smoke Point °F	Smoke Point °C
Hazelnut Oil, Refined	430°F	221°C
Sunflower Oil, Refined	440°F	227°C
Corn Oil, Refined	450°F	232°C
High-Oleic Sunflower Oil, Refined	450°F	232°C
Palm Oil, Refined	450°F	232°C
Peanut Oil, Refined	450°F	232°C
Safflower Oil, Refined	450°F	232°C
Sesame Oil, Semi-Refined	450°F	232°C
Soybean Oil, Refined	450°F	232°C
Sunflower Oil, Semi-Refined	450°F	232°C
Olive Oil, Extra Light	468°F	242°C
Tea Seed Oil	485°F	252°C
Rice Bran Oil	490°F	254°C
Apricot Kernel Oil, Refined	495°F	257°C
Avocado Oil, Refined	520°F	271°C

A Few Extra Oil Notes
~   *Canola Oil* - This is also known as rapeseed oil, and is a major crop of Canada. Use caution as canola oil is a common GMO crop; purchase non-GMO or organic canola oil whenever possible.

~   *Coconut Oil* - For those who don't mind the subtle hints of coconut, this oil provides a very rich buttery flavor. It can be rather expensive in stores, but larger quantities purchased online prove to be very cost effective.

~   *Flaxseed Oil* - This is one of the richest forms of Omega 3 fatty acids next to fish, so it can easily double as a delicious supplement for vegetarians or the fish-averse. I like to stir a bit of flaxseed oil into leftover quinoa or rice, along with some cinnamon, a dash of salt, and some fruit when I need a quick, low sugar breakfast that satisfies.

~   *Extra Virgin Olive Oil* - In many foodie circles I have seen extra virgin olive oil recommended for sautéing and stir frying. Some say that the smoke point is actually closer to 375ºF or even as high as 400ºF rather than the 250ºF noted above. This could be true, but the evidence is very controversial. To preserve the most nutritional benefit and flavor, I have chosen to err on the cooler side of the recommendations.

~   *Grapeseed Oil* - I was amazed to discover how inexpensive and multi-purpose grapeseed oil is. It is becoming very easy to find in most stores, and works wonderfully in baked goods (sweet or savory) due to its neutral taste.

~   *Hemp Seed Oil* - Hemp seed oil is gaining in popularity as a health supplement. Though it can tolerate some heat, use it in no heat applications to maximize its benefits.

~   *Sesame Oil* - A little bit of sesame oil goes a long way in adding just the right taste to Asian-inspired meals. Though you can sauté with it, I recommend drizzling sesame oil in near the end of cooking to get the most out of its bold flavor.

~   *Soybean Oil* - Soy oil often hides under the guise of vegetable oil. Like canola, it is a major GMO crop; purchase non-GMO or organic soy and vegetable oil whenever possible.

Fruit Purees

Blend up that apple pulp or a handful of prunes and you have an excellent, healthy butter substitute for baking sweets and quick breads. In fact, pureed bananas, pineapple, and pears also give an excellent "fat" consistency to recipes with an added jolt of health and flavor. Here are a few tips to help maximize your results:

~   Because the fruit will add more sweetness than butter, reduce the sugar in your recipes a touch.
~   Think of the flavor of your recipe to judge which fruit flavor will work best. For example, prune puree blends nicely with chocolate desserts, such as brownies, while pineapple adds a tropical flair to quick breads.
~   Use 1/2 cup of pureed fruit in place of 1cup of butter. You may need to add 1 to 3 tablespoons of vegetable shortening or oil back into the recipe to achieve the best results. Baked goods without any fat tend to be a bit gummy.
~   If you don't have fresh fruit on hand, drained applesauce, strained baby food fruit, or a puree of water with any dried fruit (apples, apricots, peaches, etc.) will work in a pinch. See the Prune Puree recipe below for dried fruit help, or try a mixture of 1/2 cup of applesauce and 1/2 cup of vegetable oil as a replacement for 1 cup of butter in cakes and quick breads.
~   Use a straight blender puree, or get a little fancy with the Apple-Pear Puree recipe below.

Apple-Pear Puree
Use 5 Tablespoons of this substitute plus 2 Tablespoons of oil for every 1/2 Cup of butter in baked goods
The lecithin acts as an emulsifier in this recipe, keeping the ingredients from separating, but you can omit it if it isn't readily available, or if you are following a soy-free diet.

2 Medium Apples, Cored, Peeled, and Cut into Chunks
2 Medium Pears, Cored, Peeled, and Cut into Chunks
2/3 Cup Water

1 Tablespoon Lemon Juice
1 Tablespoon Lecithin (liquid or granules, available in most health food stores) (optional)

Put all ingredients in a saucepan, bring to a simmer, cover, and cook for 40 minutes. Check in on occasion to mash the ingredients as they cook. Press the fruit mixture through a strainer to remove any excess liquid (reserve the liquid to use in other recipes if desired). This recipe will last for several days in the refrigerator, and can be preserved in the freezer for up to 6 months.

Prune (Dried Fruit) Puree
Use 1/4 to 1/3 cup prune puree plus 1 to 2 tablespoons of oil for every 1/2 Cup of butter in baked goods
This substitute will have a strong flavor, and thus is best suited to heavily spiced baked goods (i.e. gingerbread) or chocolate-based desserts. Substitute other dried fruit such as apples, peaches, and apricots for half of the prunes for a flavor and nutrient variation.

1 Cup Pitted Prunes

1/2 Cup Hot Water

Puree the prunes and water in your blender or food processor until smooth.

Coconut Butter & Oil-Based Spreads

The terms coconut butter and coconut oil are often used interchangeably, because coconut oil tends to solidify (much like butter) at room temperature. This unique property and the rich, buttery taste of coconut oil gives me cause to pay a little extra attention to this versatile food away from the general oil guide. The melting point of unrefined coconut oil is 76ºF (24ºC), so it could be a liquid or a solid in your home, depending on your idea of "room temperature." The solid form of coconut oil is very hard, so you may need to melt it before using it in recipes. Also, make sure that the other ingredients you are adding to the recipe are at least at room temperature. A chilly cup of milk alternative will cause little chunks of solid coconut oil to form.

I am usually a purist (read: lazy), so I enjoy a dollop of coconut oil melted into hot rice and sprinkled with some spices ... but ... when I am feeling just a bit more energetic, I like to experiment with buttery spread ideas, including the recipes below. Some incorporate coconut oil, while others can be used with your choice of oil.

Corn Buttery Spread
Yields 3/4 Cup
This buttery blend will be slightly coarse, due to the cornmeal, but it still yields a nice rich flavor.

1/4 Cup Yellow Cornmeal
2 Tablespoons Unsweetened Shredded Coconut
1-1/4 Cup Water
1 Teaspoon Salt, Divided

2 Tablespoons Coconut Oil
1/2 Teaspoon Lemon Juice
1/2 Teaspoon Agave Nectar, Honey, or Granulated
    Sugar, or to Taste

Grind the cornmeal and coconut in your spice grinder until powdered. Add the cornmeal mixture to a small saucepan along with the water and 1/2 teaspoon of the salt. Cook over medium-low heat, stirring often when it begins to absorb the water, until the cornmeal thickens quite a bit. Place the cornmeal mixture into your blender along with the oil, lemon juice, and sweetener. Blend until smooth and creamy. Blend in 1/2 teaspoon of salt, or more to taste.

Carrot Whip
Yields 3/4 Cup
This simple spread comes together quickly, and is pleasant with vegetables or atop toast. It isn't comparable to butter or margarine, but rather is a rich and tasty spread in its own right. I like to use just coconut oil, as it creates a unique "whipped" texture once chilled, however, olive oil can add a nice rich taste that mellows the coconut flavor.

1 Cup Chopped Carrots
1/4 Cup Coconut Oil (or palm oil, p117)
1/2 Teaspoon Salt, or to Taste

2 Tablespoons Extra Virgin Olive Oil or Additional
    Coconut Oil, Plus Additional as Needed
Unsweetened Milk Alternative of Choice (optional)

Boil or steam the carrots until they are very soft, about 20 minutes. Mash the carrots and place them in your blender with the 1/4 cup of coconut oil, salt, and the additional 2 tablespoons of olive or coconut oil. Blend until the mixture is smooth and creamy. Refrigerate the spread for a few hours, and briefly whip it with a fork before using. If it is too thick for your liking, whip in additional oil or unsweetened milk alternative as needed.

Quick Whip Option: Follow the directions for the Creamy Margarine Spread (p116), whipping the carrot spread in an ice bath (after it is pureed) for instant solidification.

Creamy Margarine Spread

Yields approximately 3/4 Cup

Homemade margarine often calls for raw egg yolk as an emulsifier ... I don't know about you, but I always get a bit nervous when working with raw eggs. Luckily, after reading a bit on emulsifiers, I discovered that mustard (including the powder) can also facilitate the merger of oil and water (or in this case, milk alternative). This recipe uses just a touch of mustard powder for binding; it adds a hint of yellow color to the spread, but imparts only a slight influence on the flavor. This spread stays a nice, soft and spreadable consistency when refrigerated.

1/4 Cup Coconut Oil (or palm oil, p117)
1/2 Cup Olive Oil or Extra-Virgin Olive Oil
1-1/2 Tablespoons Unsweetened Milk Alternative of
    Choice

Scant 1/4 Teaspoon Mustard Powder
Salt, to Taste (see instructions)
Optional Add-Ins (p117)

Prepare a large metal bowl of ice water. Add the two oils, milk alternative, and mustard powder to a medium-sized metal mixing bowl (the bowl should be small enough to fit inside the larger bowl with ease, yet large enough to accommodate the beaters of your hand mixer). Place the medium-sized bowl inside the larger bowl of ice water, and begin mixing with your hand mixer on low speed. Within a few short minutes, you should begin to see the spread thicken and whip, right before your eyes. Whip in some salt to taste, beginning with a generous pinch. It is easy to over salt this spread, so proceed cautiously. I usually end up whipping in about 1/8 teaspoon of salt, or perhaps a pinch more. With the bowl still in the ice bath, beat in any "Optional Add-Ins" you would like. For a basic spread, I add a few drops of agave nectar to contrast the slight bitter taste of the mustard powder (up to 1/4 teaspoon), though you can use plain old sugar or omit the sweetener altogether. Store the spread in an airtight container in the refrigerator. This spread may want to melt at warmer room temperatures, so keep it refrigerated between uses.

Whipped Coconut Buttery Spread

Yields approximately 1/2 Cup

Don't let the lengthy instructions below intimidate you; this spread is amazingly fast to prepare ... it takes just five minutes from the measuring cup to perfectly whipped pillows. This spread will solidify just a bit in the refrigerator, so you may want to whip it with a fork before each use.

1/4 Cup Coconut Oil (or palm oil, p117)
1/4 Cup Olive Oil or Extra-Virgin Olive Oil

Salt, to Taste (see instructions)
Optional Add-Ins (p117)

Prepare a large metal bowl of ice water. Add the two oils to a medium-sized metal mixing bowl (the bowl should be small enough to fit inside the larger bowl with ease, yet large enough to accommodate the beaters of your hand mixer). Place the bowl with the oils inside the larger bowl of ice water, and begin mixing with your hand mixer on low speed. Within a few short minutes, you should begin to see the oils thicken and whip, right before your eyes. Whip in some salt to taste, beginning with a generous pinch. It is easy to over salt this spread, so proceed cautiously. I usually end up whipping in a scant 1/8 teaspoon of salt. With the bowl still in the ice bath, beat in any of the "Optional Add-Ins" from below that you would like. Scrape the bowl to ensure that no coconut oil has solidified to the sides and give it one last whip with the beaters. Store the spread in an airtight container in the refrigerator; it should keep for quite a while. Since this spread will tend to melt readily at room temperature, keep it refrigerated between uses.

Optional Add-Ins: For the "Creamy Margarine Spread" and the "Whipped Coconut Buttery Spread" you may choose to whip in one or more of the following to customize the spread to your tastes or your meal …

~ Generous Pinch Turmeric (for color, unnecessary if using palm oil)
~ 1 to 2 Teaspoons Nutritional Yeast Flakes, Ground in Your Spice Grinder
~ 1/4 Teaspoon Agave Nectar, Honey, or Granulated Sugar, or More for a Sweet "Butter"
~ 1/4 Teaspoon Garlic Powder, or to Taste
~ Herbs and/or Spices, to Taste
~ A Few Drops of Lemon Juice

Basic Olive Oil Spread

Pour some olive oil into a small container. Cover, and place it in your freezer for several hours or overnight. After it has solidified, whip it and season it as desired (salt, garlic, herbs, nutritional yeast, or a pinch of turmeric for color). This does melt very quickly at room temperature, so return it promptly to the freezer when not in use.

Homemade Coconut Butter

You can make thick, but spreadable coconut butter by toasting grated coconut and whizzing it in your blender, food processor, or spice grinder.

To toast in the oven, spread the grated coconut out on a cookie sheet, and toast it at 300ºF, until the coconut is light brown in color (but not burnt), and you can smell the sweetish scent. This will take just a few minutes.

To toast in a pan, place the coconut in a dry skillet over low heat, and toast it while shaking (keep those flakes moving) until light brown in color.

Once toasted, puree the coconut in your blender or food processor until it takes on the consistency of a smooth paste. Add a little oil if it appears to need some moisture.

Palm Oil Alternative

If you aren't a fan of coconut oil, or if you are allergic to it, then palm, palm kernel, or red palm oil is a good alternative to coconut oil when making homemade buttery spreads. Palm oil has similar properties to coconut oil, as a semi-solid at room temperature, and it is rich in beta-carotene. Due to this high Vitamin A status, palm oil has a reddish hue that will lend color to your homemade margarines. If desired, use palm oil in place of the coconut oil in the preceding recipes using a 1:1 ratio.

Unfortunately, though palm oil is one of the most commonly used oils in commercial products (next to soybean oil), it isn't very easy to find on store shelves. Look for food grade palm oil online, at Asian markets, or ask for it at your local natural food store.

CHAPTER 14:
CHEESY IDEAS

Store-Bought Dairy-Free "Cheese"

In the past ten years, the world of dairy-free cheese has not only risen, it has flourished. A variety of vegan soy-, rice-, and nut-based "cheeses" are now available both in stores and online. Does this mean that finding the perfect cheese substitute is no longer a problem? Well, no. Unfortunately, mimicking cheese without the use of casein ... the all-powerful, super-binding milk protein ...is a great challenge. Nonetheless, manufacturers are getting closer with every attempt, and most people are able to find a cheese alternative or two that they enjoy.

Lactose intolerant individuals will likely find a few good options in lactose-free cheeses since lactose isn't really required to give cheese its signature texture. If you do come across a "cheese" that slices and melts perfectly atop your pizza, give that ingredient label another once over just to be sure; there is a good chance some casein (milk protein) is hidden within. Yes, cheeses that contain casein and don lactose-free labels sit right alongside dairy-free "cheeses," so read the ingredient statement carefully at all times. A good rule of thumb is to make sure the label specifically says vegan. This is the 'no dairy ingredients added' guarantee. That said, vegan cheese gets better every year, and some of the latest varieties do in fact "melt."

Because I knew you would want a few recommendations, I solicited my dairy-free and vegan comrades for their favorite brands of dairy-free "cheese." The following names seemed to pop up with regularity:

~ *Galaxy Nutritional Foods*® (www.galaxyfoods.com, (407) 855-5500) - Use caution with this brand as they have cheese alternatives that contain dairy (casein) which look very similar to their dairy-free line. This isn't one of the best alternatives on the market, but they have a rice "cheese" line that is soy-free, and a parmesan alternative that is very popular.
~ *Parma!* (www.eatintheraw.com, (541) 665-0348) – This simple Parmesan substitute is a healthy blend of nuts, nutritional yeast, and salt. It comes in an easy-to-sprinkle package.
~ *Sheese*® (www.buteisland.com, UK - 01700 505357) - They offer a variety of hard and spreadable vegan cheese alternatives (even Cheshire), and I must admit, they are pretty tasty.
~ *Teese* (www.teesecheese.com, (630) 629-9667) - This cheese alternative hit the market with rave reviews for its excellent flavor and versatility in cooking and snacking.
~ *Tofutti*® (www.tofutti.com, (908) 272-2400) - Better Than Cream Cheese® from Tofutti is a truly amazing replica. Even if it doesn't manage to pull one over on you when slathered on a bagel, try it in recipes (such as the Mini Icebox "Cheesecake" on p242), it works seamlessly as a substitute for dairy cream cheese. Do look for the Tofutti version which is made without hydrogenated oils.
~ *Vegan Gourmet*® (www.followyourheart.com, (818) 725-2820) - Known for its ability to melt (sometimes), this brand has long been a favorite of many dairy-free foodies. They offer both sliceable and "cream cheese."
~ *VeganRella* - Due to their lack of web presence, I have read few comments on VeganRella, yet I know so many people who purchase this brand.

For a complete list of brands, product lists are available from www.godairyfree.org.

Homemade Dairy-Free "Cheese"

Before we head into the recipes, there are a few special ingredients that you should be familiar with:

Agar

Otherwise known as agar-agar, this is a vegetable gelatin made from algae or seaweed. It comes in powder or flake form, and is useful not only in place of gelatin in vegan recipes, but also in the creation of sliceable dairy-free "cheese." It replaces some of the binding power provided by casein in dairy cheese. Agar is sold in Asian stores and in many natural food stores, but it can also be found online. While the agar powder is the most useful, you can easily grind the flakes in a spice grinder until a powder forms.

Miso

This rich, salty, fermented condiment is very popular in Japanese cooking. It comes in many colors, ranging from creamy white to red and dark brown, and it may be made from soybeans, rice, chickpeas, or barley. Look for tubs of miso in the refrigerated section of Asian markets and natural foods stores. Though perishable, it will keep in the refrigerator for many months.

Nutritional Yeast

I hate the name but love the versatility. Cheesy in taste and loaded with B vitamins, nutritional yeast has become a staple ingredient for non-dairy and vegan recipes. It can be found in flake or powder form in large bulk food departments, natural food bulk food sections, or pre-packaged near the baking supplies in natural food stores. If you can't find it in your area, nutritional yeast is available to purchase via many online retailers. Don't confuse nutritional yeast with brewers or baker's yeasts, which are quite different.

Tahini

Otherwise known as sesame seed paste or butter, tahini typically has a very sharp, bold, and often bitter taste that makes it a poor option for slathering on bread. However, when just a bit is added to recipes, it frequently serves as the special ingredient that makes the flavor pop. Such is the case with hummus, and often with dairy-free cheese. Luckily, a little goes a long ways, so a single jar should last you quite a while. You can find tahini at most grocery stores, in Middle Eastern markets, or online.

Tofu

Tofu is very versatile in dairy-free recipes, and it comes in two primary types, silken and regular (pretty much the tofu that isn't designated as silken). Silken tofu ranges from soft to extra-firm, and will produce the creamiest product when processed. This is great for whipped "creams", "cream" cheeses, and some cheesy sauces. The most popular line of silken tofu is Mori-Nu® brand (www.morinu.com, (310) 787-0200). It is completely shelf-stable (until opened), but due to market perception, stores will often sell it in the refrigerated section. If you do purchase a silken tofu that is packed in water, make sure to drain it well prior to using it in recipes.

Regular tofu (which will be identified simply as "tofu") also ranges from soft to extra-firm, and is best when a chunkier finish is preferred (i.e. feta). For most recipes, you will want to ensure the tofu is well drained and pressed to remove any excess water prior to use. Tofu is a fairly mainstream product, but should you have trouble finding a specific variety, seek out an Asian food market in your area, or peruse online.

Now, onto the ideas and recipes...

Dairy-Free Feta-ish
Yields 1-1/2 Cups
This cheese alternative takes on flavor and sets up a bit as it chills. Use it in place of dairy feta in your favorite recipes.

1 16-Ounce Package Firm Tofu
1/4 Cup Extra-Virgin or Regular Olive Oil
1/4 Cup Water
1/2 Cup Red or White Wine Vinegar
2 Teaspoons Dried Basil

1 Teaspoon Dried Oregano
1/4 Teaspoon Garlic Powder
1/4 to 1/2 Teaspoon Black Pepper
1-1/2 to 2 Teaspoons Salt

Press the tofu to remove any excess water, and crumble it or cut it into 1/2-inch cubes. In a medium-sized bowl, whisk together the oil, water, vinegar, basil, oregano, garlic, pepper, and salt to taste. Add the tofu, and stir to ensure it is well coated. Cover and refrigerate for at least 2 hours, but preferably overnight. Drain any excess liquid prior to use.

Bryanna's Quick Tofu "Feta"
Yields approximately 3 Cups
Recipe adapted from the blog, Notes from the Vegan Feast Kitchen (veganfeastkitchen.blogspot.com), by Bryanna Clark Grogan – *This feta cheese alternative has a clean taste, is very easy to make, and it keeps very well in the refrigerator. According to Bryanna, "It even melts when heated, so you can grill it in grape leaves, or coat it in breadcrumbs and fry it until crispy on the outside and melty in the middle."*

"Cheese:"
12 to 14 Ounces Firm Tofu (not silken), crumbled
2 Teaspoons Agar-Agar Powder or 4 Tablespoons
    Agar-Agar Flakes
1/4 Cup Water

2 Tablespoons Vegetable or Grapeseed Oil
1 Teaspoon Granulated Sugar
1/2 Teaspoon Salt
6 Tablespoon Fresh Lemon Juice

Brine:
2 Cups Water

2 Tablespoons Salt

Blend the tofu, agar, water, oil, sugar, and salt in your blender or food processor until very smooth. Place the mixture in a heavy-bottomed small saucepan and stir over medium heat until it bubbles for a few minutes and thickens. Alternately, place the mixture in a microwave-safe bowl and microwave it on HIGH for 3 minutes. Whisk briefly, and microwave 2 minute more. Whisk the lemon juice into the cooked mixture (this is added last as the juice interferes with the jelling of the agar if cooked with it). Pour it into a flat container, cover, and chill until firm. Cut into squares.

Make a brine by boiling the water and salt together for 5 minutes, cool, and pour the liquid over the chunks of "cheese" in a glass jar or other covered container to cover. The "feta" will keep for several weeks in a covered container in the refrigerator in this brine. The "feta" will get saltier the longer it sits in the brine, so taste it now and then to get it to your liking, then drain it and refrigerate the squares in a jar of neutral-tasting oil (not olive oil, because it thickens during refrigeration). Make sure all of the cheese is covered in oil, to keep the air out, and screw on the lid. The cheese will keep this way for several weeks. If desired, rinse off the oil under warm water before using.

Herbed "Feta" Option:
Once you have transferred the "feta" squares to the jar of, pack it with sprigs of your favorite fresh herbs and a few garlic cloves (whole, peeled). You may also choose to add a few dry bay leaves, dried red chili peppers for color, or some Greek olives. This keeps in the refrigerator for weeks, and the herb flavors penetrate the "feta" as it stands.

Sliceable Swiss-Style Cheese

Yields 1 3-Cup Loaf

Recipe adapted from the website, The Vegan Chef (www.veganchef.com), by Beverly Lynn Bennett - *This hard "cheese" gets its thickening power from the agar flakes, which can be found in natural food stores and Asian markets.*

1-1/2 Cups Water
1/3 Cup Agar-Agar Flakes
1/2 Cup (2.5 ounces) Raw Cashews
1/3 Cup Blanched Almonds
1 Tablespoon Safflower, Sunflower, or Vegetable Oil
1/3 Cup Plain or Unsweetened Milk Alternative of Choice

1/3 Cup Nutritional Yeast Flakes
3 Tablespoons Lemon Juice
1 Tablespoon Light or Mellow Miso
1 Tablespoon Prepared Dijon Mustard
1 Tablespoon Onion Powder
3/4 Teaspoon Garlic Powder
1/4 Teaspoon Salt

Place the water and agar-agar flakes in a small saucepan, and simmer over low heat to thoroughly dissolve the flakes. Meanwhile, place the cashews, almonds, and oil in your food processor, and process for 1 to 2 minutes to form a smooth paste. Scrape down the sides of the food processor. Add the remaining ingredients and process for 1 minute. After the agar-agar mixture has simmered for 5 minutes, add the mixture to the food processor, and process an additional 2 minutes to thoroughly blend the flavors.

Lightly oil a 3-cup mold, plastic container, or small loaf pan. Pour the cheese mixture into the mold, cover, and chill overnight. Unmold the cheese and use it sliced or shredded in place of commercially made cheese in your favorite recipes, or enjoy with crackers, bread, or fruit. It will keep for 7 to 10 days in an airtight container in the refrigerator.

Sunflower Seed "Cheese"

Yields approximately 1 Cup

Recipe adapted from the website, The Healing Feast (www.thehealingfeast.com) by Janet L. Doane - *Seed cheese can be used in place of sour cream, cottage cheese, ricotta, or yogurt in any of your favorite recipes.*

1 Cup Hulled, Raw Sunflower Seeds, Soaked (see directions)
1/2 Cup Water, Plus Additional for Soaking and Blending

Juice of 1 (or 2) Lemons
1 Tablespoon Unpasteurized Apple Cider Vinegar
1 Garlic Clove
1/2 Teaspoon Salt (Celtic, Himalayan, etc.)

Place the dry sunflower seeds in a 1-quart bowl, and cover with about 2 inches of filtered water. Soak for 6 to 8 hours.

Drain the seeds by pouring the water off through a strainer. Re-cover the seeds with several inches of water. Rub the seeds together between the palms of your hands to remove the seed skins (these will float a bit). Pour the water and skins through a strainer, holding back the seeds as best you can. Repeat several times. This will remove most of the skins. Doing this step improves the texture and color of the seed cheese; without taking the skins off, the seed cheese can turn a grayish color. Drain all of the water from the seeds. They are ready to use, or to store, covered, in the refrigerator for later use. They will keep for about 2 days if they are rinsed and drained each day.

Place the seeds in your blender, and just cover with filtered water to about 1/4 inch higher than the seeds. Add the lemon juice, vinegar, garlic, and salt. Begin to blend on low, increasing the speed of your blender as possible. Add water, if necessary, 1 tablespoon at a time. Blend until the mixture is as creamy as possible.

Port Wine Uncheese [Spread]

Yields 1-1/2 Cups

Recipe adapted from *The Ultimate Uncheese Cookbook* by Jo Stepaniak - *This is just one of the many faux cheese-centric recipes Jo shares in her popular dairy-free / vegan cookbook. According to Jo, this spread has rich undertones of cheddar and wine, with a pleasant plum color.*

1 15-Ounce Can Pinto Beans, Drained and Rinsed
1/4 Cup Red Wine

3 Tablespoons Tahini
1 Tablespoon Light or Chickpea Miso

Combine all of the ingredients in a food processor [or blender], and process until very smooth. Chill for several hours before serving to allow the flavors to blend. Stored in a covered container in the refrigerator, Port Wine Uncheese will keep for 5 to 7 days.

Cashew Crème "Cheese"

Yields approximately 8 Ounces or 3/4 Cup

Mimicking cream cheese is no easy task. Just one look at the dozens of "test" jars in my refrigerator is evidence of that. However, I found that I prefer the mild and slightly sweet flavor of this alternative, which isn't spot on for the original, but pretty tasty in its own right. It also works quite well in cream cheesy recipes.

1 Cup (5 ounces) Raw Cashews
2 Tablespoons Lemon Juice
1 Tablespoon Grapeseed or Vegetable Oil

1/4 Teaspoon Salt, or to Taste
2 Tablespoons Water, Plus Additional as Needed*

In 2 to 3 batches, grind the cashews in your spice grinder or food processor until they pass the powder stage and begin to clump a bit. Place the ground cashews, lemon juice, oil, salt, and 2 tablespoons of water in your blender, and puree until very smooth, about 3 to 4 minutes. Place in the refrigerator to chill overnight or optimally for 24 hours. It will thicken quite a bit as it chills, taking on a nice spreadable consistency. If it thickens up too much, mix in more water 1 tablespoon at a time until it reaches your desired consistency.

* If using right away, blend in just 1 tablespoon of water, adding more as needed to reach your desired consistency.

Rich & Nutty Ricotta

Yields approximately 3/4 Cup

This cheese alternative is incredibly luxurious when used in recipes, like the Eggplant Cannelloni (p197).

1/2 Cup Raw Pine Nuts
1/2 Cup (2.5 ounces) Raw Cashews
1 Tablespoon Lemon Juice
2 Teaspoons Nutritional Yeast Flakes

1/4 to 1/2 Teaspoon Salt
1/8 Teaspoon Onion Powder
1-1/2 Teaspoons Olive or Grapeseed Oil
1-1/2 Tablespoons Water (or more if needed)

If using a blender, grind the pine nuts and cashews in your spice grinder (together) until they are well ground and a paste just begins to form, about 1 minute. Place the nuts along with all remaining ingredients in your food processor or blender, and puree until smooth. If the mixture is too thick, blend in more water, 1 teaspoon at a time.

Tofu Ricotta

Yields 22 Ounces or 2-1/2 Cups

This makes a soft ricotta, ideal for lasagna (p201), stuffing shells, and raviolis (p204). I like the texture of silken tofu combined with regular tofu, but you can experiment with whatever type and firmness you have on hand.

1 12.3-Ounce Package Firm Silken Tofu
8 Ounces Firm Tofu
2 Tablespoons Olive or Grapeseed Oil
4 Teaspoons Lemon Juice
1 to 2 Tablespoons Nutritional Yeast Flakes

1-1/2 Teaspoons Salt, or to Taste
1/4 Teaspoon Black Pepper
1 Teaspoon Dried or 1 Tablespoon Fresh Herbs
    (oregano, basil, thyme, parsley, or whichever
    herbs compliment your primary recipe best)

Firmly press the tofu (especially the regular firm variety) to eliminate any excess water. Combine the tofu (both types), oil, lemon juice, 1 tablespoon of the nutritional yeast, salt, and the pepper in a medium bowl. Mash everything together with a fork or potato masher until all ingredients are well incorporated and the mixture takes on a ricotta-like texture, about 3 to 5 minutes. Give it a taste, and mash in more nutritional yeast, if desired. Stir in the herbs.

Tofu Cottage "Cheese"

Yields 2 Cups

Recipe adapted from The Vegetarian Mother's Cookbook *by Cathe Olson - I can always count on Cathe for easy, nutritious recipes. This one offers a good dose of protein and calcium.*

1 lb Firm Tofu, Pressed to Remove Excess Water
1 Tablespoon Olive Oil
4 Tablespoons Fresh Lemon Juice (1 large lemon)

1 Tablespoon Tahini (optional)
1/2 Teaspoon Sea Salt

Divide the tofu in half. Place 1/2 in your blender or food processor with the remaining ingredients, and puree until smooth. Place the other half of the tofu in a medium-sized bowl and mash it with a fork. Pour the blended tofu mixture into the bowl and stir to mix.

Herbed Cottage "Cheese" Option: Stir in 2 tablespoons minced chives, 1 tablespoon minced fresh herbs (dill, tarragon, thyme, parsley, etc.), and add sea salt and black pepper to taste.

Pineapple Cottage "Cheese" Option: Stir in 1/2 cup crushed pineapple.

Easy Parmesan Substitute

Yields 3/4 Cup or 8 to 12 Servings

Since this basic recipe contains just three ingredients, it can easily be adjusted to your personal tastes. Sprinkle it on popcorn, pasta, or wherever your food could use a cheesy burst of flavor.

1/2 Cup Nutritional Yeast Flakes
1/4 to 1/2 Teaspoon Sea Salt

1/2 Cup Raw Walnuts, Almonds, or Sesame Seeds

Place the nutritional yeast, 1/4 teaspoon of salt, and the nuts or seeds in your food processor or spice grinder, and reduce to a fine powder. Blend in additional salt, if desired (1/4 teaspoon of salt often suffices for the nuts, but I use the full 1/2 teaspoon for the seeds). This should keep for a few weeks in a covered container in your refrigerator.

Definitely Not Parmesan

Yields 1/2 Cup

While in no way an imitation, this flavorful mixture offers just the right taste and texture when sprinkled atop pasta, cooked vegetables, and casseroles.

2 Tablespoons Peanut, Sunflower, or other High-Heat Oil (p111)
1/2 Cup Breadcrumbs (regular or gluten-free), Plus Additional as Needed

1 Garlic Clove, Minced
1/8 to 1/4 Teaspoon Salt, or to Taste

Heat the oil in a large skillet over medium-high heat. Add the breadcrumbs, and keep them moving until they appear lightly toasted. Add the minced garlic and salt. If the mixture is too wet, then add more breadcrumbs 1 tablespoon at a time. Continue to cook and stir until the crumbs are nicely toasted.

More Cheesy Ideas

~   Sprinkle nutritional yeast on popcorn or pasta dishes for a quick cheesy pop.
~   Finely dice kalamata or green olives and sprinkle them over your entrée as you would Parmesan. Though distinctively different in taste, they offer just the right amount of bold flavor that can often seem lacking without a sprinkling of cheese. I frequently purchase the ones stuffed with garlic or jalapeno for an even bigger flavor boost.
~   Thinly slice smoked or baked tofu for a mozzarella or provolone-like experience on sandwiches or with crackers.

CHAPTER 15:
EVEN MORE DAIRY ALTERNATIVES

Do you have a few recipes that you or your family just can't live without? Try the substitutes in this chapter for commonly used dairy products to make your old recipes new again.

Milk, Powdered

Powdered milk alternatives are an easy solution for many recipes, though they can be harder to find. Look for them in natural food stores, at Asian markets, or online.

Many bread machine recipes call for dry milk powder in addition to water. If you are unable to find one of the milk powder alternatives below, use a fresh milk alternative (almond, rice, soy, etc.) in place of any water called for in the recipe (if you will be mixing the dough right away) and eliminate the milk powder, or you can simply omit the milk powder. Dry milk powder may add a bit to the taste and texture of the bread, but it is not integral to the bread's success.

~ *Soymilk Powder* – Use equal parts soymilk powder to replace the milk powder in recipes. Better Than Milk® (www.mybrands.com, (973) 338-0300) is the most readily available brand, though you can sometimes find generics in Asian food markets.
~ *Rice Milk Powder* –Use equal parts rice milk powder to replace the milk powder in recipes. Better Than Milk® (see above) is the most readily available brand.
~ *Potato Milk Powder* – Use equal parts potato milk powder to replace the milk powder in recipes. DariFree™ (www.vancesfoods.com, (800) 497-4834) is a well known soy-, gluten-, and rice-free brand.
~ *Coconut Milk Powder* – Use equal parts coconut milk powder for milk powder. Be cautious, a few brands of coconut milk powder do contain dairy milk in some form (such as caseinate) as an additive.

Milk, Evaporated

Mimicking evaporated milk is really quite easy, since it is simply a lower moisture version of milk.

Store-Bought Soy Creamer
Some people swear by store-bought liquid soy creamer as a 1:1 substitute for evaporated milk. You can read more about dairy-free soy creamer on p129.

Coconut Milk
Depending upon the recipe, you may find regular or light coconut milk to be a very suitable substitute. Light coconut milk tends to have the same level of fat as evaporated milk, and it may provide enough thickness for some recipes. However, for rich desserts, try regular coconut milk. You can use it as is, or allow the can to settle for 30 minutes, and skim off some or all of the coconut cream that comes to the surface, reserving it to use in other recipes.

Homemade Evaporated "Milk"

Since soy creamer can be hard to find in some areas, and I rarely have a carton on hand, I usually whip up a homemade alternative using one of the recipes below. Store any leftovers in the refrigerator.

Old Reliable Evaporated Milk Alternative
Yields 1-1/2 Cups

Since milk alternatives are an easy stand-in for dairy milk in nearly every application, it stands to reason that evaporated milk alternative is also an excellent substitute.

3 Cups Plain or Unsweetened Milk Alternative of Choice

Add the milk alternative to a saucepan, and place it over medium-low heat. Cook, stirring frequently, until the volume has reduced in half. Allow the evaporated "milk" to cool to room temperature before using it in recipes.

Evaporated "Milk" from Powder
Yields just over 1 Cup

Preparing a milk alternative from powder, using a higher ratio of the powder to water, is a quick and easy shortcut to the thicker properties of evaporated milk.

6 Tablespoons Soy, Rice, or Potato Milk Powder   1 Cup Boiling Water

In a blender or a bowl (using a wire whisk) combine the two ingredients until the powder has dissolved completely. Allow the evaporated "milk" to cool to room temperature before using it in recipes.

Milk, Sweetened Condensed

Store-Bought Sweetened Condensed Milk Alternative
Though hard to find, there is a brand or two of sweetened condensed "soya" milk circulating in some countries and online. If you can't get your oven mitts on some, take heart, one of the following recipes should work wonderfully in that pumpkin pie.

Cream of Coconut
Canned cream of coconut is typically sold in or near the liquor department of grocery stores. It is the "special" ingredient used to make tropical drinks such as piña coladas. Do not confuse it with coconut cream. Cream of coconut is very sweet and can be substituted for sweetened condensed milk using a 1:1 ratio. Coconut cream on the other hand is simply the cream skimmed off the top of regular coconut milk, and it will not be sweet enough on its own to mimic sweetened condensed milk.

Homemade Sweetened Condensed "Milk"
Each of the following recipes should be cooled before using, and stored in the refrigerator:

Sweetened Condensed Coconut Milk

Yields 14 Ounces (equivalent to 1 can of sweetened condensed milk)
This is my go-to recipe for a beautifully rich, sweetened condensed milk substitute.

2 14-Ounce Cans Regular Coconut Milk (not light)
1/2 Cup Granulated Sugar or Evaporated Cane Juice

1/2 Teaspoon Vanilla Extract
Pinch Salt

Add the coconut milk and sugar to a medium saucepan, and place it over medium heat. Cook while continuously stirring (until it begins to thicken, you can check in to stir every minute or so), until the volume reduces to 14 ounces or 1-3/4 cups (approximately 40 to 50 minutes). Remove from the heat, and fold in the vanilla and salt.

Soy, Rice, or Light Coconut Milk Option: If you would like to use another milk alternative, such as soy or rice, the above recipe will work, but use 3 cups of the milk alternative and reduce it until the yield is about 1 cup of sweetened condensed "milk." It won't be as thick and rich as the coconut milk.

Sweetened Condensed "Milk" from Powder

Yields 14 Ounces (equivalent to 1 can of sweetened condensed milk)
While I prefer the recipe above, this is a good shortcut recipe when you are in a hurry.

1/3 Cup Boiling Water
1 Cup Rice or Soymilk Powder
2/3 Cup Granulated Sugar, Evaporated Cane Juice, or
   Agave Nectar

3 Tablespoons Dairy-Free Margarine or Shortening,
   Melted
1/4 Teaspoon Vanilla Extract (optional)

Pour the boiling water into a blender. Add the remaining ingredients, and blend for 30 seconds, or until smooth. This should keep for about 1 week in the refrigerator.

Cream, Heavy

For years I completely avoided cream sauce recipes, assuming that a dairy-free equivalent would be impossible. After I finally let my guard down, I discovered a whole world of foods that could provide the feeling of comfort I had been missing. No, they aren't identical, but they are rich, creamy, satiating, and according to my palate, delicious.

Store-Bought Dairy-Free "Cream"
Over the years, I have spotted a few brands of vegan "cream" (not creamer), using soy, nuts, or oats as the base. These tend to be most readily available in Europe, but are becoming easier to find in North America thanks to an onslaught of new "free-from" products and the Internet. A few brands that come highly recommended include:

~   *Mimic Crème™* (www.mimiccreme.com, (866) 486-5495) – This is a nut-based "cream" that comes sweetened for "ice cream" making or unsweetened for sauces. It is made without gluten, dairy, and soy.
~   *Soyatoo!®* (www.soyatoo.de, +49 6 593 99 670 – Germany) - Available in Europe and North America, this soy-based cream alternative comes in both sweetened and savory versions (in small aseptic packages) that are "whippable."
~   *Oatly Dairy-Free Alternative to Cream* (www.oatly.com, +46 (0)418 47 55 00 – Sweden) - Available throughout Europe, this popular brand is oat-based (free from soy), and best used in general cooking.

Coconut Cream

Such a versatile food! Allow a can of regular (not light) coconut milk to rest (no shaking) in the refrigerator for 1 hour or longer. The coconut cream will rise to the top and can easily be skimmed off. Each can of coconut milk yields about 1/2 cup of coconut cream. Substitute equal parts coconut cream for the dairy cream in recipes. This works particularly well in sauces for seafood and poultry, and can also be used in place of the cream in desserts.

Coconut cream in its thickest form will whip, but be sure to purchase an organic brand of regular coconut milk or one without additives to ensure the purest separation. Coconut cream can sometimes be found ready to go in cans at the grocery store, but do not mistake it for cream of coconut, which is loaded with sugar and far too sweet to use in place of heavy cream.

Pureed Tofu

Blend firm silken tofu until smooth or blend together one part extra-firm silken tofu with one part unsweetened rice or soymilk. This works as an excellent substitute for milk and cream when a thickener is needed in sauces and soups. Pureed tofu can be substituted for heavy cream using a 1:1 ratio and is a much healthier, lower fat option.

Pureed Vegetables

White vegetables, such as cauliflower and potatoes, can add a healthy dose of creamy texture to your sauces and soups, without the added fat. Simply boil the vegetables in some water (a ratio of 1/2 lb cauliflower florets or chopped potatoes to 1-1/2 to 2 cups of water works nicely). Once tender, puree the vegetables and cooking water together in your blender or food processor until creamy. Add more liquid as needed to reach your desired consistency.

Thickened Soy, Rice, or Oat Milk

Blend 2/3 cup of rice, oat, or soymilk with 1/3 cup melted dairy-free margarine or oil. If needed, add a bit more milk alternative to reach 1 cup. This will be equivalent to the heavy cream often called "light whipping cream." For the heaviest whipping cream, add 1 more tablespoon of oil or dairy-free margarine. Either version can be used in recipes such as sauces, but they will not whip.

Nutty Crème

Pureed nuts offer a wonderful richness that is perfect for mimicking cream. To get the consistency of heavy cream, I use a 1:1 ratio of water to nuts. For roughly 3/4 cup of slightly sweet cream, I blend 1/2 cup of cashews (pre-ground in a spice grinder) or almonds (soaked overnight) with 1/2 cup of water until smooth and creamy, about 3 to 4 minutes. For roughly 3/4 cup of savory cream that is well suited to lasagna and moussaka, I blend 1/2 cup of pine nuts with 1/2 cup of water until smooth and creamy, about 3 to 4 minutes. Filter the crème through a fine mesh strainer or a double layer of cheesecloth for the smoothest consistency.

Cream, Light

Light cream contains a little more than half the fat of heavy cream, and consequently has a much thinner consistency. As you might expect, leaner versions of the cream substitutes above will work quite well in place of light cream.

Coconut Milk

Shake away; there is no need for separation when using coconut milk to substitute for light cream. Regular coconut milk has a fat content similar to light cream, and will substitute in a 1:1 ratio in recipes. It works surprisingly well in lighter white sauces, creamy soups, and desserts. Be careful not to use light coconut milk, it is far too low in fat and would not be a suitable alternative for the richness of light cream.

Pureed Tofu

Blend soft silken tofu until smooth. This works as an excellent substitute for milk and light cream when a thickener is needed in sauces and soups, but it should also work in baking. Pureed tofu can be substituted for light cream using a 1:1 ratio and is a lower fat option.

Thickened Soy, Rice, or Oat Milk

Blend 7/8 cup (3/4 cup + 2 tablespoons) of rice, oat, or soymilk with 3 tablespoons of melted dairy-free margarine or oil. This will equal roughly 1 cup of light cream for your recipes

Nutty Light Crème

Thinning the heavy nut crème just a bit is an easy short cut to a lower fat "cream." Follow the instructions for the Nutty Crème on p128 but thin the crème with 1/4 cup of additional water to obtain approximately 1 cup of light cream alternative.

Half & Half

Moving down the fat scale, we have finally arrived at the lightest of the three creams, half & half. As you might have guessed by now, several of the substitutes mentioned for light and heavy cream will work for half and half when thinned just a bit further for that lighter consistency.

Store-Bought Soy Creamer

There are a few brands of liquid soy-based creamers on the market. These have the consistency of half & half, and work quite well in coffee, baking, "ice cream," and recipes in general. You can find them in the refrigerated section near the other dairy alternatives or dairy-based creamers. Though I am not a coffee drinker, I have used Silk® brand soy creamer (www.silksoymilk.com, (888) 820-9283) in recipes with great success.

Use caution, many brands of creamer claim to be non-dairy, but they may contain up to 0.5% milk ingredients. Look for brands that are liquid and specifically labeled as vegan.

Coconut Milk

Combine 1/2 cup + 1 tablespoon regular coconut milk (shaken) with 7 tablespoons plain or unsweetened milk alternative to get a half & half consistency. To mimic half & half in thickness, do not reach for light coconut milk, as it is still a bit too lean, and closer to whole milk in consistency.

Pureed Tofu

Blend one part soft silken tofu with one part unsweetened or plain soy, rice, or oat milk to obtain a low fat alternative to half & half.

Thickened Soy, Rice, or Oat Milk

Blend 3/4 cup + 2 tablespoons of rice, oat, or soymilk with 2 tablespoons of melted dairy-free margarine or oil. This will equal roughly 1 cup of half & half for use in recipes.

Nutty Half & Half

Increasing the water to nut ratio in the Nutty Crème, results in a quick creamer. In this case, I use a 2:1 or 3:1 ratio of water to nuts. For roughly 1-1/2 cups of slightly sweet creamer that is perfect for coffee and homemade ice cream, I blend 1/2 cup of cashews (pre-ground in a spice grinder) or almonds (soaked overnight) with 1 to 1-1/2 cups of water until smooth and creamy, about 3 to 4 minutes. For roughly 1-1/2 cups of savory creamer, I blend 1/2 cup of pine nuts with 1 to 1-1/2 cups of water until smooth and creamy, about 3 to 4 minutes. Filter the crème through a fine mesh strainer or a double layer of cheesecloth for the smoothest consistency.

Buttermilk

Just as regular cow milk can be soured to create a quick buttermilk stand-in, milk alternatives can easily be "soured" to create faux buttermilk. Use this easy recipe for a seamless substitute ...

"Buttermilk" for Baking
Yields 1 Cup
I use this foolproof substitute recipe more than any other when baking.

1 Tablespoon Lemon Juice, Apple Cider Vinegar, White Vinegar, or Cream of Tartar

Plain or Unsweetened Milk Alternative of Choice

Place the juice, vinegar, or cream of tartar in a glass measuring cup, and add enough of the milk alternative to make one cup. Stir, and let the solution stand for ten minutes before adding it to your recipe.

Sour Cream

Store-Bought Dairy-Free "Sour Cream"
There are a few of brands of sour cream alternative on the market (mostly soy-based), and they really are quite convincing. If you can't find one at your local store or online, try one of the other ideas below.

Dairy-Free Yogurt
Use a plain unflavored dairy-free yogurt as a 1:1 substitute. This works best in dips and salad dressings. From a texture perspective, dairy-free yogurt will also work in place of sour cream in baked goods, but with a slightly different flavor flare. Soy yogurt is quite easy to find, with several brands and even generics available in many stores. Soy-free options such as rice and coconut yogurt are also becoming available.

Mayonnaise
In dips, natural mayo or vegan mayonnaise (trust me, this stuff is awesome!) is a great substitute for sour cream. Yes, though it looks rich, creamy, and dairy-full, mayo is made via an emulsion of oil and eggs, and thus unless it has some strange milk additives, it should not contain milk in any form. As for vegan mayo, we keep Grapeseed Oil Vegenaise® (www.followyourheart.com, (818) 725-2820) on hand for salad dressings and recipes.

Homemade Dairy-Free "Sour Cream"
While not 100% identical, the following recipes definitely give off that sour cream vibe. Plus, a quick whirl in your blender or food processor is all the work required to whip up an entire batch of these faux sour creams. Use a dollop atop your baked potato, chili, soup, or other dish that is clamoring for a cool and creamy garnish. These sour cream substitutes should also be suitable stand-ins for recipes that call for sour cream:

Silken "Sour Cream"

Yields 1-1/3 Cups

This is an excellent make-ahead recipe. Refrigerating for a few hours (or even overnight) before use gives the flavors some time to "marry."

1 12.3-Ounce Package Firm Silken Tofu
1 Tablespoon Grapeseed or Vegetable Oil
2 to 4 Teaspoons Lemon Juice

2 Teaspoons Apple Cider Vinegar
1 Teaspoon Agave Nectar or Sweetener of Choice
1/2 Teaspoon Salt

Place the tofu, oil, 2 teaspoons of the lemon juice, vinegar, sweetener, and salt in your food processor or blender, and process until the mixture is smooth and creamy. Give it a quick taste test and add up to 2 teaspoons more of the lemon juice (I usually add 1 more), as needed. Refrigerate until ready to use.

Sour Cashew Crème

Yields 8 Ounces or 3/4 Cup

This sour "cream" is a bit different from the traditional when tasted straight, but even my husband admitted that the flavor was spot on when used in recipes. I swirled a large dollop of this into the Quick & Creamy Bean Soup (p185) and we both loved it. I use the full 2 teaspoons of vinegar and 3 tablespoons of lemon juice, but you may want to start with a bit less of each, should it prove to be a bit too tangy for your tastes.

1 Cup (5 ounces) Raw Cashews
1/4 Cup Water, Plus More as Needed*
1 Tablespoon Grapeseed or Vegetable Oil

Generous 1/4 Teaspoon Salt, or to Taste
1 to 2 Teaspoon Apple Cider Vinegar
2 to 3 Tablespoons Lemon Juice

In 2 to 3 batches, grind the cashews in your spice grinder until they pass the powder stage and begin to clump a bit. Place the ground cashews, water, oil, salt, vinegar, and lemon juice in your blender, and puree until very smooth, about 3 to 4 minutes. Place the cashew crème in the refrigerator to chill for at least one hour; it will thicken as it chills. If it thickens up a bit too much, add more water 1 tablespoon at a time until it reaches your desired consistency.

* If using right away and you want to skip the refrigeration, reduce the water to 2 tablespoons, adding additional water as needed until it reaches your desired consistency.

Yogurt

Store-Bought Dairy-Free Yogurt

Soy yogurt has hit the mainstream with almost as much fervor as soymilk. Most of the major grocers I have visited carry their own generic soy yogurt, in addition to several brand name versions. Like most foods, soy yogurt differs quite a bit from brand to brand, so don't hesitate to dare another if your first taste test didn't go so well. However, always double check the ingredients and ensure that the cultures used in the soy yogurt are made without dairy. The soy label is no guarantee that the yogurt is dairy-free. The two brands that have met with my approval thus far are Whole Soy & Co.® (www.wholesoyco.com, (415) 434-3020) and So Delicious® (www.turtlemountain.com, (541) 338-9400), but you may find another favorite.

Soy yogurt typically matches up to dairy yogurt in terms of beneficial bacteria and protein, so once you find one that suits your palate, there will be no need to feel like you are missing out on anything but the milk.

Of course, you may be wondering if there are there any dairy-free, soy-free yogurts. Until recently, I couldn't offer such an alternative, but manufacturers have finally begun to recognize the demand, and are responding with other types of yogurt. The first to hit the shelves was a rice-based yogurt. While it still holds good potential, the first version met with mixed reviews. Then a coconut milk-based yogurt, also by So Delicious® (www.turtlemountain.com, (541) 338-9400), arrived on the scene, and I must say, it really is good. As a matter of fact, I like it better than soy yogurt. It is milder and a bit sweeter, with a slight coconut vibe.

Coconut Cream
This seems to be a dairy-free wonder food. Allow a can of regular coconut milk to settle (about 1/2 hour). The coconut cream will rise to the top and can easily be skimmed off. Depending on your needs, coconut cream may be a nice substitute for yogurt in recipes using a 1:1 ratio. Be aware that coconut cream is much higher in fat than yogurt, and won't provide the characteristic tang of yogurt.

Pureed Tofu
Medium firm silken tofu will puree into a nice consistency, and may be substituted for yogurt in recipes using a 1:1 ratio. It does lack the tartness of yogurt, and thus is most suitable for "heartier" dishes. However, you can add just a bit of lemon juice to the tofu for that yogurt-like tang.

Sour Cream Alternative
Try one of the sour cream alternatives (p130) as a straight substitute (1:1 ratio) for yogurt in salad dressings and dips.

Buttermilk Alternative
Buttermilk alternative (p130) works very well for marinating and cooking purposes, and is also recommended when yogurt is called for in baked goods, dressings, and sauces. It can be substituted using a 1:1 ratio.

Homemade Dairy-Free Yogurt
Some people love to make yogurt at home. It can be a very economical and fun project, and some find homemade results to be tastier than store-bought. To simplify the process, I do recommend a yogurt maker. They are surprisingly inexpensive, and should come with some "how-to" recipes. Simply substitute soymilk for the dairy milk, soymilk powder for the milk powder, and store-bought soy yogurt (as a simple starter culture) for the yogurt wherever called for in the recipes, and you have your own homemade soy yogurt.

Before moving onto some yogurt recipes, I just want to briefly mention starter cultures. Most yogurt recipes call for a starter culture to get the friendly bacteria moving. The most widely used starter culture shortcut is store-bought yogurt. You can use soy, rice, or coconut yogurt purchased from your local grocer as your dairy-free starter culture, or you can purchase dairy-free starter cultures (the bacteria alone). One brand of starter culture that touts itself as dairy-free and gluten-free is GI ProStart™ (www.giprohealth.com, (508) 264-1463), but read up on the product before purchasing, as it does have some "dairy exposure." Another brand carrying the "dairy and casein-free" claim is Custom Probiotics Yogurt Starter (www.customprobiotics.com, (818) 248-3529).

Now, on to the recipes ...

Susan's Soy Yogurt

Yields 4 cups (1 quart)

Recipe adapted from the blog, Fat Free Vegan (blog.fatfreevegan.com) by Susan Voisin – *In this recipe, Susan uses a modest amount of agar for thickening. The results are a bit thinner than your typical dairy yogurt, but her family loves it atop cereal, in smoothies, or served plain with fruit. Susan recommends using a packaged soymilk that is not fat-free (contrary to her bog namesake). She uses Soy Dream® (www.tastethedream.com, (800) 434-4246), but feel free to experiment. If you use a homemade or unsweetened soymilk, add 1 tablespoon of sugar, as the yogurt cultures need some sugar to feed upon. Also, don't forget to save 1/2 cup of the finished soy yogurt to use as your next yogurt starter.*

1. Take 1/2 cup of plain soy yogurt out of the refrigerator and allow it to come to room temperature. [You may use 1 packet of starter culture instead; see p132]
2. Put a kettle or pot of water on to boil. While it's heating, gather your materials:

Dinner Plate	1 Measuring Teaspoon
2 Large Spoons	Agar-Agar Powder
1 Whisk or Hand Blender	1 Quart (4 cups) Plain Soymilk
Large (non-plastic) Microwaveable Bowl	Yogurt Maker (1 quart capacity)
Food Thermometer	

3. When the water boils, scald the dinner plate first, making sure that the whole surface comes into contact with the water. Then scald the other utensils, including the thermometer, and place them on the plate. Be sure you also scald the hand blender or whisk, the bowl, and the yogurt maker's container and anything else that might come into contact with the yogurt. You don't want any stray bacteria growing in your yogurt!
4. Put 2 cups of the soymilk into the bowl and sprinkle it with 1 teaspoon of the agar powder. Allow it to soften for a few minutes. Then place the bowl in the microwave and set it on high power for about 4 minutes. Stir every minute until it reaches a boil.
5. When the soymilk reaches a boil, remove it from the microwave and add the remaining 2 cups of soymilk. Stir well. Put the food thermometer into the milk and wait until the temperature drops to about 115ºF (45ºC). While you are waiting, stir the soymilk every once in a while to keep the agar from gelling.
6. Plug in your yogurt maker to begin warming it.
7. When the temperature of the soymilk drops to 115ºF (45ºC), add the 1/2 cup yogurt [or starter culture]. Blend it in very well using either a whisk or hand blender. Pour it into your yogurt maker's container and place inside the yogurt maker.
8. Check the yogurt after 5 or 6 hours. If it's as tart as you'd like, you may stop then, but normally it will take about 8 hours to reach the right tartness (when I use store-bought yogurt as a starter, it takes much longer, often 12 hours, to be ready). Do not worry if it has separated. When it seems tangy enough, remove it from the incubator and whisk or blend it well with the hand blender. Put it into the refrigerator and chill for several hours. Your yogurt will now be ready to use.

Homemade Coconut Yogurt

Yields 4 cups (1 quart)

Thanks to the advent of coconut yogurt, a soy-free version of Susan's homemade yogurt can easily be had. Follow the directions above for her Homemade Soy Yogurt, but substitute 2 14-ounce cans of light or regular coconut milk plus 1/2 cup of water and 1 tablespoon of sweetener for the soymilk. Also, you can use either store-bought coconut-based yogurt for your starter culture in the first step, or you can use a dairy-free starter culture, as mentioned on p132.

Cathe's Cashew Yogurt
Yields 2 Cups
Recipe adapted from *The Vegetarian Mother's Cookbook* by Cathe Olson - *According to Cathe, "This creamy, non-dairy yogurt just takes a few seconds to mix up. The incubation period is 8 to 24 hours depending on how warm you keep it."*

1 Cup (5 ounces) Raw Cashews   1 Cup Water

Grind the cashews into a coarse powder using your spice grinder or food processor. Place the cashews and water in your blender, and blend until smooth. It should have the consistency of heavy cream. Pour the mixture into a jar and place it in a warm location (70 to 100ºF or 21 to 38ºC). Cover with a light towel or napkin. Start checking the yogurt after 6 hours. First you should notice bubbles forming. When it has formed a thick curd with a layer of liquid (whey) on the bottom, cover and transfer to your refrigerator. Chill for at least 1 hour. When ready to eat, stir the whey and yogurt together. Add a little honey, agave nectar, maple syrup, molasses, fruit, or jam if desired. This yogurt will keep refrigerated for up to a week.

Cook's Note: Choose a place where the temperature will remain constant to incubate your yogurt. I like to fill a small cooler with warm water and place the jar in the water (make sure the water is below the level of the jar). Another good place is on top of the pilot light in a gas stove. As long as the temperature in your house is at least 70ºF, you can place the jar anywhere. Keep in mind, the lower the temperature, the longer the incubation. At 70ºF, it will take about 20 hours.

Chocolate

Traditional milk chocolate is off limits for dairy-free dieters, but there is no need to close the door on chocolate altogether. There are many excellent dark, semi-sweet, and faux milk chocolates that are quite suitable for non-dairy noshing and baking.

For any of the store-bought options mentioned below, always double check the ingredients. Even the darkest of darks may contain milk in the ingredients, particularly if produced by one of the larger manufacturers. Also, always contact the manufacturer prior to consumption whenever you suspect a sensitive or severe milk allergy or intolerance. It is not uncommon to see "may contain traces of milk" on chocolate wrappers, as cross-contamination of milk in chocolate production is very common. Luckily, there are several brands of chips and bittersweet bars that are made on dedicated equipment, and many companies take extra measures in equipment cleaning to make their chocolate as safe as possible for food allergies. Just to clarify, cocoa butter (a key ingredient in many types of chocolate) is a dairy-free ingredient, so enjoy!

Store-Bought "Milk" Chocolate
Oh yes, it is true; a few specialty manufacturers have begun producing chocolate with the luxuriousness of milk chocolate, but using rice milk powder or other milk alternatives to keep them dairy-free. A few brands are readily available online and at select natural food grocers. I did have the opportunity to taste test Terra Nostra's Ricemilk Choco™ Bars (www.terranostrachocolate.com, (604) 267-35050), and they were quite silky and rich. For a food allergy safe brand (made on equipment that is free from dairy, gluten, and nuts), try the Boom Choco Boom™ Rice Milk Bar (www.enjoylifefoods.com, (847) 260-0300), or in the U.K., look up the Dairy-Free line from Plamil® Foods (www.plamilfoods.co.uk, +44 (0) 1303 850588).

Store-Bought White Chocolate
White chocolate does not depend as heavily on dairy ingredients as milk chocolate, so it isn't uncommon to find an obscure generic brand that just happens to be dairy-free. I tend to avoid most brands, as they also contain

hydrogenated oils, but better options are emerging from natural and vegan manufacturers. In the U.K., the Vegan Organica (www.venturefoods.com) line of chocolates boasts a White Bar that is rumored to be quite tasty.

Store-Bought Dark & Semi-Sweet Chocolate
Lets face it, the best quality chocolate is pure, not a mention of milk on the ingredient statement. Unadulterated dark chocolate is real chocolate in my book. For newcomers, I recommend starting with semi-sweet or dark chocolate that contains 50% cocoa or less and working your way up in intensity as your taste buds adapt. Chocolate is much like wine in that respect, begin tasting with the sweetest options, and graduate to bolder flavors with time.

When baking, semi-sweet and bittersweet are typically your best options regardless, as the rich, sweet flavor of milk chocolate can overpower a recipe. For semi-sweet chocolate chips, the brand I purchase most often is generic, but when I need mini-chips, I turn to Enjoy Life® Chocolate Chips (www.enjoylifefoods.com, (847) 260-0300). Not only do they taste excellent, but they are also food allergy-friendly.

As for dark chocolate, I recommend the Scharffen Berger® Home Baking Bars (www.scharffenberger.com, (800) 930-4528) for recipes. There are many brands of dark chocolate I enjoy for snacking, but my husband and I always seem to go back to Endangered Species® dark chocolate line (www.chocolatebar.com, (800) 293-0160). They offer various delicious flavors, but keep in mind that this brand of chocolate (as with most) may contain traces of milk due to the shared equipment used in manufacturing. These are just my personal preferences, but there are dozens of wonderful dark chocolates on the market. You can find many more options from the product lists at www.godairyfree.org.

Homemade Chocolate
No chocolate on hand? Look no further than your basic pantry supplies and the recipes that follow. Unlike other everyday cooking oils, coconut oil solidifies at the low end of room temperature. This makes it an easy stand-in when you need a quick batch of "safe" chocolate chunks. Just be aware that coconut oil melts easily, so these chunks will tend to melt in warm hands or if the temperature in your home is a bit toasty.

White Chocolate
Yields approximately 4 Ounces
Hannah Kaminsky, author of My Sweet Vegan, created this homemade white chocolate recipe, which is remarkably simple. The key is to find food grade cocoa butter. It is sold in some natural food stores, and of course, online. The end result is quite sweet, so Hannah recommends using it in recipes (such as cookies!) rather than for straight snacking.

1/4 Cup Food-Grade Cocoa Butter
1 Teaspoon Vanilla Paste or Extract
1/3 Cup Powdered / Confectioner's Sugar

1/2 Teaspoon Rice or Soymilk Powder
Pinch Salt

Place your cocoa butter in a microwave-safe bowl and microwave it for just a minute or two, so that it liquefies. Be sure to keep an eye on it at all times, as it has a much lower melting point than a bar of finished chocolate. Once completely melted, quickly stir in the remaining ingredients, being thorough so as to break up any clumps of sugar and completely dissolve everything into the molten fat. Tap the molds on the counter lightly so as to remove any air bubbles, and don't even think about touching them again for the next few hours while they set up. I highly recommend parking them in the refrigerator to speed up the process... Just don't forget about them in there!

Quick Chocolate Chunks

Yields approximately 4 Ounces

Coconut oil is much easier to find than food grade cocoa butter, and I find that it works in a pinch for creating easy homemade chocolate. However, coconut oil does have a lower melting point, so it will readily melt at warmer room temperatures and in toasty hands. To keep it nice and solid, store the resultant chocolate in the refrigerator or freezer. If desired, you can substitute food grade cocoa butter for the coconut oil.

1/4 Cup Cocoa Powder

1 to 3 Tablespoons Agave Nectar or Powdered / Confectioner's Sugar (see options below)

1/4 Cup Coconut Oil or Food-Grade Cocoa Butter

1/4 Teaspoon Vanilla Extract (alcohol-free if possible)

Pinch Salt

Lightly grease 6 muffin cups (I use silicone) or some candy/chocolate molds. Sift the cocoa powder and powdered sugar (if using) into a small bowl and set aside. In a small saucepan over low heat, melt the coconut oil with the agave nectar (if using), vanilla, and salt. Remove from the heat and whisk in the cocoa powder and sugar (if using). Pour the chocolate into your prepared molds, and immediately pop in the freezer for 1 hour. If desired, break into chunks for baking or ice cream purposes. Store the chocolate in the refrigerator or freezer; it should keep for a while.

Bittersweet Option: For dark chocolate I use 1 tablespoon of agave nectar. It presents the smoothest texture and seems to work well in small amounts. If you prefer powdered sugar, start with 1-1/2 tablespoons, and adjust to taste.

Semi-Sweet Option: For semi-sweet chunks I usually use 2-1/2 to 3 tablespoons of powdered sugar. It produces a nice firm chocolate. If using agave nectar, use just 2 tablespoons, and be aware that it will be a much softer chocolate.

Sugar-Free Option: Homemade chocolate lends itself well to customization. For a sugar-free chocolate, substitute the sweetener with a very small amount of stevia to taste.

Nutty-Milk Chocolate Option: Melt 2 tablespoons of unsalted creamy cashew or almond butter along with the oil.

Peanut Butter "Chips"

Yields approximately 4 Ounces

These are very sweet, yet quite addictive.

2 Tablespoons Coconut Oil

1/4 Cup Unsalted Creamy Peanut Butter

1/4 Teaspoon Vanilla Extract

Pinch Salt

6 Tablespoons Powdered / Confectioner's Sugar

Lightly grease 6 muffin cups (I use silicone) or some candy/chocolate molds. In a small saucepan over low heat, melt the coconut oil with the peanut butter, vanilla, and salt. Remove from the heat and sift in the powdered sugar. Blend or vigorously whisk until everything is well combined. Pour the mixture into your prepared molds, and immediately freeze for 1 hour, or until solid. If desired, break into chunks for baking or ice cream purposes. Store the peanut butter "chocolate" in the refrigerator or freezer; it should keep for a while.

For serious chocoholics who want to try some "real" chocolate making … from bean to bar … I recommend the website www.chocolatealchemy.com. They cover the entire chocolate making process, host a chocolate forum, sell hard to find ingredients (i.e. food grade cocoa butter), and offer a basic selection of recipes that includes soy "milk" chocolate.

CHAPTER 16:
EGG SUBSTITUTES

Egg substitute ideas are helpful to have on hand when you are dealing with an egg allergy (a common buddy to milk allergies), watching cholesterol and fat intake, following a strict vegetarian or vegan diet, or have simply run out of eggs! Most of the recipes in this guide are made without eggs, but I wanted to offer a quick resource for substituting eggs in baking and cooking to help make the most of your other recipes …

Tofu
Pureed tofu works well as an egg substitute in dense cakes and brownies, and in smooth savory type dishes that call for quite a few eggs, such as quiches and custards. Firm, crumbled tofu (along with some added spices) makes a great substitute for eggs in eggless "egg salads" and breakfast scrambles.
1 egg = 1/4 cup pureed soft or silken (firm) tofu

Applesauce, Mashed Bananas, or Pumpkin Puree
These fruits work well in sweetened baked goods (quick breads, muffins, pancakes, etc.), but make sure you are picking a recipe with compatible flavors. The apple, banana, or pumpkin taste will likely shine through just a bit. For a lighter texture, add an extra 1/2 teaspoon of baking powder to the recipe.
1 egg = 1/4 cup fruit puree

Pureed Prunes
Prunes have a strong flavor, so they are best to use in complimentary, dense desserts, such as brownies and other chocolate rich goodies.
1 egg = 1/4 cup prune puree

Ground Flaxseed
Flaxseed has a wholesome taste that suits heartier baked goods, such as pancakes and bran muffins. It also works quite well as an egg replacer in cookies. Purchase whole flax seeds and grind them fresh in a spice grinder whenever you need an egg or two (1 tablespoon whole flaxseed equals about 2-1/2 tablespoons ground flaxseed). When whisked with hot water, ground flaxseed takes on a gelatinous texture, much like an egg white.
1 egg = 2-1/2 tablespoon ground flaxseed + 3 tablespoons hot water

Chia Seeds
Chia seeds are convenient, because they do not need to be ground, but they are quite a bit pricier than flax seeds. Should you have some handy, they work similarly to ground flaxseed in baked goods.
1 egg = 1 tablespoon chia seeds + 3 tablespoons hot water

Vinegar
As long as the recipe contains another rising agent (such as baking powder), vinegar works well as an egg substitute in general baking.
1 egg = 1 tablespoon white vinegar

Burger Binders

Tomato paste, arrowroot starch, potato starch, cornstarch, flour (whole-wheat, unbleached, oat, or bean), finely crushed breadcrumbs (or cracker meal or matzo meal), quick-cooking oats, cooked oatmeal, mashed potatoes, mashed sweet potatoes, or instant potato flakes can replace the binding action of eggs in recipes such as veggie burgers and meatballs. Start with 2 tablespoons per egg, and work your way up as needed.

1 egg = 2 to 3 tablespoons of a "burger binder" mentioned above

Dairy-Free Yogurt

Soy, coconut, or rice based yogurt is another good substitute for eggs in quick breads and cakes. The plain and unsweetened versions also work well in savory recipes. Yogurt alternatives do impart a slight tang on the finished good that may be overwhelming when used in large quantities. See p131 for more information on dairy-free yogurt options. For a lighter texture, add an extra 1/2 teaspoon of baking powder to the recipe.

1 egg = 3 to 4 tablespoons dairy-free yogurt

Agar Powder

Agar is a vegetable gelatin made from algae or seaweed. It works well in recipes that call for an egg white or two.

1 egg white = 1 tablespoon agar powder dissolved in 1 tablespoon water; whip, chill and whip again

Powdered Egg Replacer

This store-bought product can be a quick and easy shortcut to faux eggs in baking. There are a few brands on the market, but Ener-g (www.ener-g.com, (800) 331-5222) is by far the most popular. It is also a surprisingly good stand-in binder for recipes such as veggie burgers and meatballs.

1 egg = 1-1/2 teaspoons Egg Replacer + 2 tablespoons of water

A few egg alternatives that work similarly to Ener-G include (per egg):
~   1 heaping tablespoon soy flour + 1 tablespoon water
~   2 tablespoons cornstarch + 2 tablespoons water
~   2 teaspoons baking powder + 1 tablespoon oil + 2 tablespoons water

Section 5

Time to Eat!
Recipes & Recommendations

CHAPTER 17:
QUICK RECIPE SECTION INTRO

My Recipe Process

In creating and selecting recipes for this guide I had several goals in mind. Of course, taste was of utmost importance, but there were many other factors to consider:

Recipes for dairy-free cravings - The prior section on dairy substitutes offered many baseline recipes for creating homemade dairy alternatives, but dairy-free goes well beyond straight alternatives. Creamy soups, rich shakes, and flavorful casseroles are all comfort foods that can still be enjoyed without milk products.

Recipes that incorporate "helpful" ingredients - Beyond just giving you substitutes and suggested healthy foods, I wanted to offer some ways that you can enjoy them. You will find several recipes that focus on calcium-rich foods (kale, bok choy, figs, carob, almonds, tofu, etc.), healthy sources of fat and protein (avocados, nuts, coconut, etc.), and that show you how to incorporate some of the dairy alternatives.

Recipes offering a "taste" of other chefs - More than just listing them in the resources section, I have included sample recipes from some of my favorite recipe creators, whether they are cookbook authors or well-respected bloggers. The purpose is to give you some great recipes of course, but also to help you identify blogs and cookbooks that may meet with your own tastes and cooking style. These are all authors from whom I enjoy recipes at home, but they each have their own niche.

> ***Please note:*** *Recipes from other chefs state that they are "adapted." They have been edited as needed to keep the flow of the recipes in order and to keep the ingredient wording consistent throughout this guide, but the recipes themselves (ingredients used, processes, etc.) are true to the creators' originals. Permissions for reprint (in this guide only) have been obtained from the recipe authors.*

Recipes that are friendly to multiple diets - All of the recipes in this guide are dairy-free. However, most are also vegan and egg-free, and many of the recipes are naturally free from various allergens. Plus, whenever applicable, there are tips to make the recipes gluten-free, soy-free, and/or nut-free. Feel free to scan the food allergy index on p277 to quickly identify recipes that can meet with your dietary needs. Keep in mind this is a dairy-free guide. While I point out recipes that *can* be made "free-from" certain allergens, it is up to you to obtain the necessary and proper ingredients to make the dish "safe" for consumption.

Recipes with a budget in mind - For my own family, health, taste, and cost are the three most important factors when it comes to food. Like most, I have my splurges, but for the most part, I use whole foods or minimally processed ingredients to keep both our health and grocery bill in check. I purchase and use dairy substitutes only on occasion, using everyday pantry items whenever possible.

Ingredients Used

Most of the ingredients I use are purchased in the bulk foods department, or are commodity type products that I either purchase generic or feel no particular brand loyalty to. I like to prepare recipes that use as many everyday ingredients as possible. However, there are a few ingredients for which I do purchase specific brands. You may choose to use a similar product or a different brand, but the following are the products/brands I used to create and test the recipes in this guide ...

Almond Milk – Pacific Foods (www.pacificfoods.com, (503) 692-9666)
I switched to Pacific when they came out with an unsweetened, organic line of almond milk that is typically cheaper than non-organic competing brands. This is my go-to milk for smoothies and dessert recipes. For other types of milk alternatives, I typically stick with generics.

Broth – Pacific Foods (www.pacificfoods.com, (503) 692-9666) and Imagine® (www.imaginefoods.com, (800) 434-4246)
 My husband loves soup, so I always keep a good stash of premade broth in the pantry. Some brands surprisingly contain milk, so I stick with the No Chicken (a personal favorite), Chicken, and Vegetable broths from Imagine, and the Mushroom (another favorite), Chicken, and Vegetable broths from Pacific. Both brands are organic, sold in aseptic packages, and seem to go on sale for a decent price with regularity.

Coconut Oil – Nutiva Organic Extra Virgin Coconut Oil (www.nutiva.com, (800) 993-4367)
I am rarely particular about brands when it comes to purchasing oil, but I am addicted to Nutiva's, and purchase it in the bulk sizing online for a fraction of the price of those small jars in stores. This brand does have more prominent coconut undertones than some of the more refined brands.

Dairy-Free "Cream Cheese" – Vegan Gourmet® Cream Cheese Alternative (www.followyourheart.com, (818) 725-2820) and Tofutti Better Than Cream Cheese® Non-Hydrogenated (www.tofutti.com, (908) 272-2400)
Vegan Gourmet boasts all-natural and organic ingredients, while Tofutti is a slightly more "authentic" taste. I use both depending on availability.

Dairy-Free Margarine – Earth Balance® Buttery Sticks (www.earthbalancenatural.com, (201) 568-9300)
There are a few brands of dairy-free margarine on the market, but in the U.S., our selection of non-hydrogenated margarines is slim. Luckily, Earth Balance® saves the day with these non-hydrogenated sticks, which work perfectly in baking applications.

Dairy-Free Yogurt - So Delicious® made with Coconut Milk Yogurt (www.turtlemountain.com, (866) 3TURTLE)
There is no better in my book. Aside from being absolutely delicious, this yogurt works perfectly in recipes and is both dairy-free and soy-free. If you prefer a soy version, there is also a So Delicious line of soy yogurts.

Mayonnaise - Grapeseed Oil Vegenaise® (www.followyourheart.com, (818) 725-2820)
I have nothing against regular (all-natural or organic) mayonnaise, which is almost always dairy-free, but my family actually prefers this egg-free and vegan version.

Shortening – Earth Balance® Natural Shortening (www.earthbalancenatural.com, (201) 568-9300)
Many brands of shortening are hydrogenated, so I prefer to buy this brand, which is non-hydrogenated and comes in easy to measure sticks. For soy-free, I turn to Spectrum® Shortening (www.spectrumorganics.com, 800-434-2406), as it is made with 100% palm oil.

Silken Tofu - Mori-Nu® brand (www.morinu.com, (310) 787-0200)
This shelf-stable tofu exceeds the performance of other silken tofu brands that are refrigerated and packed in water. Since Americans are not used to purchasing tofu off the shelves, many stores will put this brand in the refrigerated section to improve sales, but it doesn't require refrigeration until it is opened, and it will keep for quite a while in your cupboard.

Soy Sauce - San-J Wheat-Free Tamari (www.san-j.com, (804) 226-8333)
We only purchase non-GMO or organic soy products, so I buy this brand, which just happens to be gluten-free.

Vegan "Cheese" – Vegan Gourmet® Cheese Alternative (www.followyourheart.com, (818) 725-2820)
This brand is quite easy to find in my area, and it performs nicely when integrated into recipes.

Product Recommendations

Beyond recipes, I saw this section as a fitting place to share other menu ideas and some of my favorite store-bought products, for when you may not have the time or energy to cook from scratch.

Over the years I have reviewed hundreds upon hundreds of dairy-free products. Among them I have been privileged to taste some truly delicious items, yet I have only found a handful of foods and brands that truly stand out in my mind as superior. Some I now stock regularly and some I purchase for the occasional indulgence. These are included within the appropriate chapters in this section, along with recommendations from some of my fellow Go Dairy Free product reviewers: Barb Nicoletti (food allergy mom), Sarah Hatfield (nowheymama.blogspot.com), Liz Stark (veggiegirlvegan.blogspot.com), Amy (mariposa-whatdoieatnow.blogspot.com), and Hannah Kaminsky (bittersweetblog.wordpress.com).

This is our short list of favorites, but there are hundreds of product reviews on www.godairyfree.org and thousands of great products out there, many of which we have yet to sample.

CHAPTER 18:
BREAKFAST TO BRUNCH

Oatmeal Blender Waffles
Yields 4 to 6 Servings

After sampling the Coconut Waffles Mix from The Vegetarian Express (www.thevegetarianexpress.com, (734) 355-3593), I knew I had to come up with my own version at home. I fell in love with the ease, nutrition, and great taste of these incredibly simplistic waffles. Plus, they freeze quite well for a quick and healthy toaster breakfast any morning.

4 Cups Rolled Oats

3 Cups Water, Plus More as Needed

2 Small, Very Ripe Bananas

2 Tablespoons Grapeseed, Coconut, or Vegetable Oil

2 Teaspoons Vanilla Extract

1/4 to 1/2 Teaspoon Salt

Optional Add-ins (see below)

Place all ingredients in your blender (except the berries "add-in," if using) and blend until relatively smooth. Let the batter sit for 5 to 10 minutes to thicken, while you grease and heat up your waffle iron. When the waffle iron is ready, give the batter another quick pulse. If it becomes too thick to pour at any time, blend in more water, 1 tablespoon at a time, until it is pourable, but still quite thick. Pour the batter onto your waffle iron, and cook according to the waffle iron directions without lifting the lid. Some waffle makers may indicate done when the waffles are still a bit soft. I typically wait for the waffles to stop steaming as a more accurate indicator, but do prepare them as you see fit.

Serve topped with pure maple syrup, fresh fruit and whipped coconut cream (p253), nut butter, jam, or extra bananas, chopped nuts, and maple syrup for a true banana nut bread experience.

Optional Add-Ins:
~   1 to 2 Cups Blueberries, Raspberries, or Other Berries, Fresh or Frozen (stir in after blending)
~   1-1/2 to 2 Teaspoons Ground Cinnamon
~   2 Tablespoons Agave Nectar or Sweetener of Choice (optional)

Coconut Waffle Option: (still my favorite) Substitute 6 tablespoons of unsweetened coconut (shredded or grated) for the banana and add 2 to 3 tablespoons of your favorite sweetener. For an extra dose of coconut, replace the vanilla extract with coconut extract and add 1/4 cup of plain or vanilla coconut-based dairy-free yogurt.

Pumpkin Waffle Option: Use 2/3 cup pureed pumpkin in place of the banana, and add 2 teaspoons pumpkin pie spice (or 1 teaspoon cinnamon, 1/2 teaspoon ginger, 1/4 teaspoon nutmeg, and 1/4 teaspoon allspice) and 1/4 cup of brown sugar or evaporated cane juice.

Home Baked Granola

Yields 7 Cups

Since discovering the ease of homemade granola, I haven't bothered to scour the ingredient label on a single box of premade cereal. My husband loves the fresher taste, and we both love the lower price, especially when I purchase the ingredients in bulk. This is a versatile recipe; customize the flavor with your favorite nuts, dried fruit, and/or spices.

3-1/2 Cups Rolled Oats

1 Cup Sliced, Slivered, or Chopped Almonds

1 Cup (5 ounces) Raw Cashews, Coarsely Chopped

1/3 Cup Light or Dark Brown Sugar, Firmly Packed

1 Teaspoon Ground Cinnamon

1/3 Cup Pure Maple Syrup

1/4 Cup Grapeseed, Extra-Light Olive, or Vegetable Oil

1 Teaspoon Vanilla Extract

1/4 to 1/2 Teaspoon Salt

3/4 to 1 Cup Raisins

Preheat your oven to 250ºF (120ºC). In a large bowl, combine the oats, nuts, brown sugar, and cinnamon. In a separate bowl, whisk together the maple syrup, oil, vanilla, and salt. Stir this wet mixture into the oats and nuts, until everything is well coated. Spread the mixture into two large, ungreased glass baking dishes.* Bake the granola for 1 hour, checking in to give it a stir every 15 minutes. When done, transfer the granola to a large bowl and stir in the raisins. Once cool, store it in an airtight container.

Nut-Free Option: Substitute the almonds and cashews with any combination of additional oats, sunflower seeds, pumpkin seeds, soy nuts, and/or coconut.

If you only have metal pans or cookie sheets, reduce the oven temperature by 25ºF (15ºC) and keep a close eye. Dark metal pans will cause the granola to brown (and consequently burn) very quickly. In a pinch, you can make this entire batch in one 9x13-inch dish; I just find that the granola browns more evenly when two dishes are used.

Cream of Multi-Grain Cereal

Yields 2 Cups or 6 Servings

I love the idea of eating whole grains in the morning, but preparing them can easily take 30 or 40 minutes. This technique allows you to fit in the grains of your choice with just 5 to 10 minutes of cook time. Keep in mind that the grains below are simply a guideline. Feel free to use whatever grains you would like, including quinoa, rye flakes, wheat flakes, barley, buckwheat flakes, buckwheat groats, cornmeal, wheat germ, or wheat bran.

1/2 Cup Brown Rice

1/2 Cup Millet

1/2 Cup Rolled Oats

1/2 Cup Amaranth

Process the grains in your food processor, blender, or spice grinder (in batches), until they reach a medium-coarse consistency (if you prefer a heartier hot cereal) or until powdered (if you prefer a "cream of" type cereal). Store the ground grains in an airtight container in the refrigerator or freezer.

To Prepare 1 Serving: Whisk together 1 cup of cold water, a scant 1/3 cup of the cereal, and a dash of salt in a saucepan. Bring the cereal to a boil, reduce the heat to low, cover and simmer for 10 to 12 minutes (3 to 5 minutes if using powdered grains). Remove from the heat, and season as desired with sweetener, cinnamon, raisins, fresh fruit, margarine, etc.

Toasted Grain Option: You can toast the grains prior to grinding to bring out a bit of their nutty taste. Add the heartier grains (such as the brown rice and barley) to a large dry skillet over medium heat. Toast while continuously stirring for about 5 minutes. Add the remaining grains and toast, while stirring, for another 5 minutes. Proceed with the grinding.

Maple-Pecan French Toast

Yields 1 Serving or 2 Slices

Recipe adapted from Vegan Bites *by Chef Beverly Lynn Bennett - Your basic French toast recipe can be made dairy-free by simply using milk alternative in place of the milk, but why not try a totally different experience rather than settle for a substitution? Beverly's cookbook focuses on easy, small batch recipes for single and two-person households, but you can multiply this recipe by however many mouths you are feeding.*

1/4 Cup Pecans [raw and unsalted]
1/4 Cup Water
3 Tablespoons Pure Maple Syrup
1/2 Teaspoon Vanilla Extract
1/4 Teaspoon Ground Cinnamon

1/8 Teaspoon Ground Ginger
1/8 Teaspoon Salt
2 Slices Whole-Grain Bread of Choice [regular or gluten-free]

Process the pecans in a blender or food processor* for 1 minute, or until they are finely ground. Add the water, maple syrup, vanilla, cinnamon, ginger, and salt and process for 1 minute, or until smooth and creamy. Place the bread slices in a large casserole dish and pour the pecan mixture over them. Flip the bread over to coat the other sides. Allow the slices to soak in the mixture for 1 minute. Lightly oil a large skillet and place it over medium heat. When the skillet is hot, carefully place the soaked bread slices in it and cook them for 1 to 2 minutes or until golden brown on the bottom. Flip the slices over with a metal or heatproof spatula and cook for 1 to 2 minutes or until golden brown on the other side. Serve hot with your desired toppings.

* Alisa's Note: Grinding nuts in a blender can be tricky, and may not always work well with such a small amount. I prefer to grind the nuts in my spice grinder, and then add them to the blender with the other ingredients.

Pillowy Whole-Grain Pancakes

Yields 16 Pancakes

Since so many pancake mixes contain dairy, I turned to whipping them from scratch long ago. Yet, after numerous whole grain flops, I was sure that processed white flour pancakes were the only way to go. But then I came across an inspiring batch of Carob & Date Pancakes from Ricki at Diet, Dessert and Dogs (dietdessertndogs.wordpress.com). With Ricki's version as my guide, I turned out pancakes that were perfectly fluffy and picky husband approved!

1-3/4 Cups Plain Milk Alternative of Choice*
1/4 Cup Grapeseed or Vegetable Oil, Plus Some for
   the Skillet
2 Tablespoons Ground Flaxseed
2 Tablespoons Agave Nectar or Honey
2 Teaspoons Apple Cider Vinegar or Lemon Juice

1 Teaspoon Vanilla Extract
2 Cups Whole-Grain Spelt Flour (may substitute
   whole wheat, white-wheat, or white spelt flour)
1 Tablespoon Baking Powder
1/2 Teaspoon Baking Soda
1/4 Teaspoon Salt

Measure the milk alternative in a glass measuring cup. Stir In the 1/4 cup of oil, flaxseed, agave or honey, vinegar or lemon juice, and vanilla. Set aside for moment. In a large bowl, sift together the flour, baking powder, baking soda, and salt. Add the milk alternative mixture and mix well. Heat a small amount of oil in a large skillet over medium heat. Using roughly 1/4 cup per pancake, pour the batter into the pan. Cook the pancakes until the outside edge begins to look dry, and bubbles break on the surface of the batter, about 3 minutes. Flip and cook the other sides for about 2 to 3 minutes, or until light golden brown. Serve with maple syrup, fresh fruit, or your favorite whipped "cream" topping.

*This makes rather fluffy pancakes. If you like them even cakier, feel free to lower the milk alternative by up to 1/4 cup, or increase it by up to 1/4 cup (2 cups total) for thinner pancakes.

Real Donuts

Yields 12 to 14 Donuts + Donut Holes

Though I know it is probably a blessing in disguise, I become a bit sad whenever I stroll by a donut shop and realize that those soft and squishy indulgences are a thing of the past. Yes, pretty much all of the "Dunkin" varieties are laced with milk, but luckily, for those special occasions, homemade dairy-free donuts are a reality.

1/2 Cup Plain Milk Alternative of Choice	3 Tablespoons Granulated Sugar
1-1/2 Teaspoons White or Apple Cider Vinegar	2-1/2 to 3 Cups All-Purpose (Plain) Flour, Divided
1 Tablespoon Active Dry Yeast	1 Tablespoon Baking Powder
1/2 Cup Warm Water	1 Teaspoon Salt
3 Tablespoons Vegetable Shortening, Melted	3 to 4 Cups Vegetable or other High Heat Oil (p113)

In a small bowl, combine the milk alternative and the vinegar, and set aside for a few minutes. In a large bowl, dissolve the yeast in the warm water and allow it to sit for a few minutes to proof. Once the yeast is a bit bubbly, add the now soured milk alternative, shortening, sugar, 1 cup of the flour, baking powder, and salt, and mix well. Continue mixing in the remaining flour, adding just enough to make a soft ball of dough. Turn the dough out onto a lightly floured surface and knead it several times. Roll the dough out to about 1/2-inch thickness and cut out donut shapes with a 2-1/2-inch donut cutter. If you do not have a donut cutter, use a large biscuit cutter, and if desired, cut donut holes from the center using a smaller round cutter. In a pinch, you can also use the mouth of a drinking glass to cut the donuts out. Place the donuts on a lightly floured surface, cover, and let them rise for about 1 hour or until they double in size.

Add 3 inches of oil to an electric deep fryer or deep stockpot, and heat until the oil reaches 360 to 380ºF (180 to 195ºC). Slowly and carefully place each donut into the hot oil. Cook for about 1 to 2 minutes, or until the donuts take on a light golden color, flip and cook for 1 minute more. Remove the donuts with a slotted spoon and allow them to drain on paper towels. While still warm, dip the donuts in one of the glaze/topping options below, and allow them to cool briefly on a wire rack. For the biggest smiles, serve while still warm.

Optional Glazes / Toppings:
~ Granulated or Powdered Sugar
~ Cinnamon Sugar - Stir together 1/4 cup white granulated sugar and 4 teaspoons ground cinnamon
~ Vanilla Glaze - Whisk together 2-1/2 cups powdered sugar, 1/4 cup plain milk alternative of choice and 1/2 teaspoon vanilla extract. If needed, whisk in more milk alternative 1 teaspoon at a time.
~ Chocolate Glaze - Add about 1/2 cup of semi-sweet chocolate chips (melted) to the vanilla glaze.

Breakfast Parfaits

Yields 1 Serving

Give fast food a run for its money with this allergen-free version of the easy, yet elegant, yogurt parfait. My favorite combination is vanilla (coconut-based) yogurt with blueberries and homemade granola sans raisins.

1 6-Ounce Package Plain or Vanilla Dairy-Free Yogurt	1/2 Cup Fresh Berries (blackberries, blueberries, raspberries, etc.) or Chopped Fruit
1/2 Cup Granola (homemade or store-bought, regular or gluten-free)	

In a glass, layer half of the yogurt, 1/4 cup of the granola, and 1/4 cup of the berries or fruit. Repeat these layers.

Dessert-Worthy Option: Use broken gingersnaps or vanilla wafer cookies in place of the granola.

Mini Crustless Tofu Quiches

Yields 12 Mini-Quiches or 3 Servings

Recipe adapted from the blog, Fat Free Vegan (blog.fatfreevegan.com) by Susan Voisin - Preparing a quiche without milk, cream, and cheese, is no easy task, but Susan is always up to the challenge. These little gems are not only packed with flavor, but they are also quite low in fat, kid-friendly and extremely versatile (packed into lunch boxes or even served for dinner). For parties, prepare the quiches in mini-muffin tins, reducing the baking time accordingly.

Olive Oil Spray
1 Teaspoon Minced Garlic
1/2 Cup Diced Red or Green Bell Peppers
1 Cup Chopped Mushrooms
1 Tablespoon Minced Fresh Chives or 1 Green Onion, Minced
1 Teaspoon Minced Fresh Rosemary or 1/2 Teaspoon Dried, Crushed
Freshly Ground Black Pepper, to Taste

1 12.3-Ounce Package Firm Silken Tofu, Drained
1/4 Cup Plain Soymilk
2 Tablespoons Nutritional Yeast Flakes
1 Tablespoon Cornstarch, Arrowroot Powder, or Potato Starch
1 Teaspoon Tahini (preferred) or Cashew Butter
1/4 Teaspoon Onion Powder
1/4 Teaspoon Turmeric
1/2 to 3/4 Teaspoon Salt

Preheat your oven to 375ºF (190ºC) and grease 12 muffin cups. Lightly spray a non-stick skillet with olive oil and sauté the garlic, bell peppers, and mushrooms over medium heat until the mushrooms just begin to exude their juices. Stir in the chives, rosemary, and freshly ground black pepper, and remove from the heat. Place the remaining ingredients into your food processor or blender, and process until completely smooth. Add the tofu mixture to the vegetables and stir to combine. Divide the mixture between your prepared muffin cups, filling each about halfway. Place the quiches into your oven and immediately reduce the heat to 350ºF (175ºC). Bake for 25 to 35 minutes, or until the tops are golden and a knife inserted into the middle of a quiche comes out clean. Allow them to cool for about 10 minutes.

Cinnamon Roll Biscuits

Yields 15 Small Biscuits

Recipe adapted from What's To Eat? The Milk-Free, Egg-Free, Nut-Free Food Allergy Cookbook by Linda Coss - Linda answered my prayers with "cinnamon rolls" that could be ready in just 30 minutes. She writes, "I remember the first time I tried this recipe. My kids and I sat and ate the entire batch, one biscuit after another ... you can drizzle these with a powdered sugar-and-water glaze after they come out of the oven, but for my taste they're sweet enough as is."

2 Cups All-Purpose (Plain) Flour
2 Tablespoons Granulated Sugar
1 Tablespoon Baking Powder
1/2 Teaspoon Salt
1 Teaspoon Vanilla Extract

1/3 Cup Vegetable or Grapeseed Oil
2/3 Cup Water
1/4 Cup Dairy-Free Margarine, Melted
1/4 Cup Light Brown Sugar, Firmly Packed
1 Teaspoon Ground Cinnamon

Preheat your oven to 450ºF (230ºC). Mix together the flour, sugar, baking powder, and salt. Set aside. In a 1- or 2-cup measuring cup, mix the oil and water together. Add the vanilla and oil-and-water mixture to the dry mixture; mix until blended. Knead the dough 20 to 25 times on a floured board. Roll the dough into a 1/4-inch thick rectangle that is approximately 11x14 inches. In a small bowl, mix the melted margarine with the brown sugar and cinnamon. Spread the brown sugar mixture evenly over the dough rectangle. Roll the dough up jelly-roll fashion, so that you end up with one 14-inch long roll of dough. Pinch the long end of the roll closed so that it doesn't come unrolled. Slice the dough roll into 1-inch wide slices. Place the slices into ungreased muffin cups, 1 slice per hole, so that the spirals show. Bake for 12 to 15 minutes, or until golden brown. Remove to a serving platter; serve warm.

Light Apricot Scones
Yields 8 Scones

This recipe offers a good degree of flexibility. For a heartier scone, substitute whole wheat pastry flour for part or all of the all-purpose flour; for a different flavor, replace the apricots with dried cranberries; or in a pinch, substitute pureed firm silken tofu, dairy-free sour cream, or buttermilk substitute (p130) plus 1/2 teaspoon vanilla extract for the yogurt.

2 Cups All-Purpose (Plain) Flour
1/4 Cup + 2 Teaspoons Granulated Sugar, Divided
2 Teaspoons Baking Powder
1 Teaspoon Baking Soda
1/4 Teaspoon Salt
1/4 Cup Chilled Dairy-Free Margarine or Shortening

1/3 to 1/2 Cup Finely Diced Dried Apricot
1/4 Cup Sliced Almonds (optional)
1-1/2 Teaspoons Almond or Vanilla Extract
1 Cup Vanilla Dairy-Free Yogurt
2 Teaspoons Plain Milk Alternative of Choice

Preheat your oven to 400°F (205ºC). In a large bowl, combine the flour, 1/4 cup of the sugar, baking powder, baking soda and salt. Cut in the margarine or shortening with a pastry blender or fork until the mixture resembles coarse crumbs. Add the apricots and almonds (if using) and mix thoroughly. Stir the extract into the yogurt, and fold the yogurt into the flour just until you can collect the dough. Turn the dough out onto a lightly floured surface, kneading just until it can be shaped, but no more (just a few turns, as over-kneading will make the scones tough). If the dough is too sticky add a little more flour but take care not to add too much as it toughens up the scones. Divide the dough in two, place the dough balls on a baking sheet, and gently press each into a disk that is roughly 1-1/4 inches high. For a light topping, brush 1 teaspoon of milk alternative over each disk, and sprinkle each with 1 teaspoon of sugar. Score the disks into quarters with a long knife by cutting just halfway through the dough. Bake the scones for 20 minutes, or until they are lightly golden. Let the scones cool for 10 minutes before gently breaking them apart.

Cocoa-Nut Scones
Yields 4 Scones

Recipe created by Hannah Kaminsky, author of My Sweet Vegan - Hannah originally created this recipe for her first cookbook, but the chocolaty scones just wouldn't cooperate in front of the camera. Nonetheless, she was determined that this delicious pastry should be in print, and thus offered it for inclusion in this guide.

3/4 Cup All-Purpose (Plain) Flour
1/4 Cup Cocoa Powder
1 Tablespoon Granulated Sugar
1/2 Teaspoon Baking Powder
1/2 Teaspoon Baking Soda
1/4 Teaspoon Salt

1/4 Cup Chilled Dairy-Free Margarine
1/4 Cup Flaked, Sweetened or Unsweetened Coconut
1/4 Cup Semi-Sweet Chocolate Chips
1 Teaspoon Vanilla Extract
5 to 6 Tablespoons Plain Milk Alternative of Choice
Turbinado Sugar (Optional)

Preheat your oven to 400ºF (205ºC) and line a baking sheet with parchment paper or a non-stick baking mat. In a medium bowl, whisk together the flour, cocoa, sugar, baking powder, baking soda, and salt. Add the margarine and use your finger tips to rub the margarine into the flour mixture until it resembles coarse sand: A few larger pieces are just fine to leave in, but try to avoid including large lumps of unmixed margarine. Stir in the coconut and chocolate chips, as well as the vanilla. Add in the milk alternative 1 tablespoon at a time, wetting it just enough for everything to come together in one cohesive ball. The amount necessary will vary depending on humidity and elevation, so just trust your instincts. Divide the resulting dough into 4 equal pieces and place them on your prepared baking sheet. Sprinkle with additional sugar for an extra crunch on top, if desired. Bake for 16 to 19 minutes, until a toothpick comes clean out of the center of each scone. Let the scones cool on the baking sheet for 5 minutes before removing them to a wire rack.

Some Store-Bought Recommendations for Breakfast:
There are many great brands on the market, but the following recommendations only include products that I purchase with some regularity or that a colleague highly recommended. For full lists of non-dairy, packaged foods and brands, see the product lists available on www.godairyfree.org.

Barbara's Bakery® (www.barbarasbakery.com, (866) 972-6879) ~ cold cereal
This is a great brand of all-natural cereals that has hit the mainstream. I am a big fan of their Shredded Oats cereal line, while my colleague Hannah can't get enough of the Puffins®.

Bob's Red Mill® (www.bobsredmill.com, (503) 654-3215) ~ hot cereal, pancake and waffle mixes
Bob's is truly a one-stop shop for grains and mixes. I enjoyed their organic whole grain pancake and waffle mixes (high fiber and 7-Grain), but they offer many other pancake mix varieties, including a gluten-free option that gets the seal of approval for taste and value. Bob's also offers a wide range of all-natural hot cereals.

Cherrybrook Kitchen® (www.cherrybrookkitchen.com, (978) 974-0200) ~ pancake and waffle mixes
Cherrybrook's mixes are excellent when allergies are a top concern, as they are promoted as nut and dairy-free, and they are intended to be made without eggs. They offer both wheat-based and gluten-free mixes.

Enjoy Life® (www.enjoylifefoods.com, (847) 260-0300) ~ granola
Enjoy Life is the main gluten-free, nut-free granola game in town, and it really is pretty good. This is an excellent option for multiple food allergies and intolerances, but you don't have to be gluten-free to enjoy it.

Golden Temple (www.goldentemple.com, (800) 964-4832) ~ cold cereal and granola
The company behind Golden Temple produces Peace Cereals®/Granolas and Golden Temple Bulk Granola. I am pretty sure the end product for most of the varieties is the same (one packaged nicely, one in bulk), so we tended to purchase the bulk bags of their granola, which is also available in the bulk bins of many natural food stores.

Nature's Path Organic (www.naturespath.com, (888) 808-9505) ~ cold/hot cereal, granola, and frozen waffles
Nature's Path has an enormous range of non-dairy cereals (both hot and cold), many of which are also gluten-free and organic. Back in my pre-home baked granola days, my husband easily inhaled a box of their Optimum™ Power cereal within three days. I liked their flaked cereals, which tended to be lower in sugar than most brands. I try to stick to homemade waffles, but do admit that their organic brand of frozen waffles is tasty and virtuous. Moms should definitely look into their Envirokidz™ line of cereals and frozen waffles.

Van's™ (www.vansintl.com, (323) 585-5581) ~ frozen waffles
Ingredient-wise, I actually prefer organic waffles by Nature's Path. However, from a price and availability perspective, it is hard to beat Van's. Not all of their waffles are dairy-free (and most are made on shared equipment), so use caution. However, they do offer organic, wheat-free, whole grain, and kid-friendly frozen waffles. One of my food allergy colleagues keeps these stocked for her little ones.

CHAPTER 19:
BAKING BREAD

Carrot or Zucchini-Pineapple Bread
Yields 10 to 12 Servings

I make this bread often, so I have tested it with eggs, applesauce, bananas, and yogurt. My husband likes it best with the banana, I like it best with the yogurt, and our friends like it best with applesauce. In other words, they all work great. The glaze makes this bread a deliciously sweet treat, but you can omit it when enjoying the loaf for breakfast.

Bread:
2 Cups All-Purpose (Plain) or Whole Wheat Pastry
   Flour
1 Teaspoon Ground Cinnamon
1/4 Teaspoon Ground Allspice
1 Teaspoon Baking Powder
1 Teaspoon Baking Soda
1/2 Teaspoon Salt
3/4 Cup Light Brown Sugar, Firmly Packed
1/2 Cup Grapeseed or Vegetable Oil or Dairy-Free
   Margarine, Softened

1 Cup Grated Zucchini or Carrot
1 8-Ounce Can Crushed Pineapple with Juice (do not
   drain!)
2 Eggs, 1/2 Cup Unsweetened Applesauce or Mashed
   Ripe Banana (about 1 medium), or 1/3 Cup Plain
   Dairy-Free Yogurt
1/2 Cup Chopped Raisins (omit if using zucchini)
1/2 Cup Chopped Pecans or Walnuts (optional)

Optional Glaze:
1 Tablespoon Pineapple Juice (from the crushed
   pineapple)
1/2 Cup Powdered / Confectioner's Sugar

1 Teaspoon Agave Nectar or Corn Syrup
1/4 Teaspoon Ground Cinnamon

Preheat your oven to 350ºF (175ºC) and grease the bottom of a 9x5-inch loaf pan. In a medium-sized bowl, sift together the flour, 1 teaspoon of cinnamon, allspice, baking powder, baking soda, and salt, and set aside. In a large mixing bowl, blend the brown sugar, oil or margarine, and eggs, yogurt, applesauce or banana until smooth and creamy. Reserve 1 tablespoon of the pineapple juice (if preparing the glaze). Stir in the rest of the pineapple with its juice and the carrot or zucchini. Add the flour mixture to your mixing bowl, and stir just to combine. Be careful not to over-mix, a few lumps are okay. Gently fold in the raisins and nuts, if using. Pour the batter into your prepared loaf pan. Bake for 45 to 55 minutes, or until a toothpick inserted in the center comes out clean. Allow the bread to cool for 10 minutes before removing it from the pan.

To make the glaze, combine the reserved 1 tablespoon of pineapple juice with the powdered sugar, agave or corn syrup, and 1/4 teaspoon of ground cinnamon. Mix until smooth, and spoon over the warm loaf. For an extra-moist loaf, poke holes in the top of the loaf before pouring on the glaze. Allow the bread to cool completely, wrap, and store in refrigerator.

Mini Loaf Option: Pour the batter into 4 mini-loaf tins and bake in a 350ºF (175ºC) oven for 25 to 30 minutes, or until a toothpick inserted in the center of a loaf comes out clean.

Multi-Purpose Muffins

Yields 12 Muffins

If you only have one muffin recipe on hand, this should be it. This simple formula will allow you to quickly churn out whatever flavor of fluffy pastry that your heart desires. See the Optional Add-Ins below for some possible variations.

2 Cups All-Purpose (Plain) or Whole Wheat Pastry Flour (or a combination of the two)
3/4 Cup Granulated Sugar
1 Tablespoon Baking Powder
1/2 Teaspoon Salt

1 Egg, 1/4 Cup Unsweetened Applesauce, or 3 Tablespoons Dairy-Free Yogurt
1 Cup Plain Milk Alternative of Choice
1/4 Cup Grapeseed or Vegetable Oil

Preheat your oven to 400ºF (205ºC) and grease 12 muffin cups or line them with cupcake liners. In a large bowl, sift together the flour, sugar, baking powder, and salt. Make a well in the center of your dry ingredients. In a glass measuring cup, beat the egg with a fork or add the applesauce or yogurt, and stir in the milk alternative and oil. Pour the liquid into the well of your dry mix. Gently stir the ingredients together, just until they are moistened. A few lumps are okay, you do not want to over-mix, as it will make the muffins tough. Distribute the batter between your prepared muffin cups. Bake for 20 to 24 minutes, or until the tops are golden and a toothpick inserted into the center of a muffin comes out clean. Allow the muffins to cool for 5 minutes in the cups, before removing them to a wire rack.

Optional Add-Ins:
~ Fold in 1 to 1-1/2 cups of your favorite fresh or frozen fruit just after you stir in the liquids. If using frozen fruit, such as blueberries, toss the fruit in a bit of the flour mixture before adding the liquids. This will help prevent the fruit from "bleeding" and sinking.
~ Fold in 1/2 to 3/4 cup of chopped nuts or chocolate chips just after you stir in the liquids.
~ Add 1 teaspoon of spice, such as cinnamon, ginger, etc. to the dry ingredients.
~ Add 1 teaspoon of extract (vanilla, almond, coconut, etc.) or zest (orange, lemon, lime) to the liquids.
~ Substitute light brown sugar or evaporated cane juice for some or all of the white sugar.
~ Substitute juice for some, or all, of the milk alternative.

Idea: Breakfast "Cupcakes"

Muffins by my standards are lower in sugar than cupcakes, and generally have some added ingredients (i.e. nuts, whole grain flours, fruit, or vegetables) to make them worthy (at least on occasion) of an early day meal. Yet, they still don't always have that staying power that my husband and I seem to require in the a.m. So as an added bonus, for both taste and nutrients, I often "frost" the muffins with some nut butter. I use a soft type of nut butter, such as almond, or warm the nut butter to ensure a spreadable consistency. It almost feels like I am sneaking a cupcake, but the lack of a sugar rush (and subsequent crash) reminds me that my indulgence was relatively wholesome.

Breakfast "Frosting" Options:
~ Dairy-Free Cream Cheese Alternative
~ Fruit Butter (apple, pumpkin, etc.)
~ 100% Fruit Jam
~ Nut or Seed Butter (almond, cashew, peanut, sunflower, etc.)

S'Mores Muffins

Yields 10 to 12 Muffins

Recipe adapted from the blog, VeggieGirl (veggiegirlvegan.blogspot.com) by Liz Stark - Anyone who knows Liz (aka VeggieGirl) is well aware of her fondness for calcium-packed carob, but these S'Mores work equally well with cocoa powder and chocolate chips. All of the ingredients below are typically dairy-free, but to keep the recipe vegan, Liz uses honey-free graham crackers (from Healthy Valley®, www.healthvalley.com) and gelatin-free marshmallows (from Sweet & Sara, www.sweetandsara.com, (718) 707-2808).

1-1/2 Cups Whole Wheat Flour
1/4 Cup Powdered / Confectioner's Sugar
1/4 Cup Carob or Cocoa Powder
1 Teaspoon Baking Soda
1 Cup Plain Milk Alternative of Choice

5 Tablespoons Unsweetened Applesauce
1 Teaspoon Vanilla Extract
1/4 Cup Carob Chips or Chocolate Chips
1/2 Cup Graham Crackers, Broken into Small Pieces
1/4 Cup Marshmallows, Chopped

Preheat your oven to 350ºF (175ºC) and grease 10 to 12 muffin cups or line them with cupcake liners. In a large bowl, combine the flour, powdered sugar, carob or cocoa powder, and baking soda, and mix well. In a separate bowl, combine the milk alternative, applesauce, vanilla, carob or chocolate chips, graham cracker pieces, and marshmallows, mixing well. Add the wet ingredients to the dry mixture, and stir just to combine. A few lumps are okay, you do not want to over-mix, as it will make the muffins tough. Distribute the batter between your prepared muffin cups, and bake for 15 to 18 minutes, or until a toothpick inserted in the center of a muffin comes out clean. Allow the muffins to cool for a few minutes in the cups, before removing them to a wire rack.

Maple Wheat Bran Muffins

Yields 12 Muffins

Most recipes for bran muffins call for white flour and loads of sugar. In my opinion, this defeats the purpose of the healthy bran. So I created this version, which is lighter on the sugar and made with whole wheat flour, but still wonderfully delicious according to my family.

1-1/4 Cups Plain Milk Alternative of Choice
1 Tablespoon Apple Cider Vinegar or White Vinegar
1 Cup Whole Wheat Flour
1 Teaspoon Ground Cinnamon
1-1/2 Teaspoon Baking Soda
1/2 Teaspoon Salt
1-1/3 Cups Wheat Bran

2 Tablespoons Ground Flaxseed
1/3 Cup Grapeseed or Vegetable Oil
1/3 Cup Pure Maple Syrup
1/4 Cup Lightly-Packed Brown Sugar or Evaporated Cane Juice
1 Teaspoon Vanilla Extract
2/3 Cup Raisins

Preheat your oven to 350ºF (175ºC) and grease 12 muffin cups or line them with cupcake liners. In a large mixing bowl, combine the milk alternative and apple cider vinegar. In a separate small bowl, sift together the flour, cinnamon, baking soda, and salt. Set aside. Stir the bran and flaxseed into your now soured milk alternative, and allow it to soak for a few minutes. Blend in the oil, maple syrup, brown sugar, and vanilla. Add the flour mixture, and stir just to combine. A few lumps are okay, you do not want to over-mix, as it will make the muffins tough. Gently fold in the raisins. Distribute the batter between your prepared muffin cups, and bake for 18 to 22 minutes, or until a toothpick inserted into the center of a muffin comes out clean. Allow the muffins to cool for a few minutes in the cups, before removing them to a wire rack.

Perfectly Pear Muffins

Yields 12 Muffins

These muffins got the seal of approval from my family for a rewarding breakfast treat. They use a bit less sugar than your average muffin, but make up for it with a light sugar topper and sweetened milk alternative. I use almond or rice milk to retain the delicate pear and cardamom flavors, but you can sub in your favorite milk alternative.

2 Cups All-Purpose (Plain) or Whole Wheat Pastry
    Flour (or a combination of the two)
1/2 Cup + 2 Teaspoons Granulated Sugar, Divided
1/2 Teaspoon Ground Cardamom
2 Teaspoons Baking Powder
1/2 Teaspoon Baking Soda (omit if using egg)
1/2 Teaspoon Salt

1 Cup + 2 Tablespoons Vanilla Almond or Rice Milk
1 Egg or 1/4 Cup Unsweetened Applesauce
1/4 Cup Grapeseed or Vegetable Oil
1 Teaspoon Vanilla Extract
1 Cup Peeled and Diced Pear (about 1 medium firm,
    but ripe pear)
1/2 Cup Walnuts (optional)

Preheat your oven to 350ºF (175ºC) and grease 12 muffin cups or line them with cupcake liners. In a large bowl, sift together the flour, sugar, cardamom, baking powder, baking soda (if using), and salt. Make a well in the center of your dry ingredients. In a glass measuring cup, whip the milk alternative, egg or applesauce, oil, and vanilla. Pour the liquid into the well of your dry mix. Gently stir the ingredients together, just until they are moistened. A few lumps are okay, you do not want to over-mix, as it will make the muffins tough. Fold in the diced pear and walnuts, if using. Distribute the batter between your prepared muffin cups. Sprinkle the muffin tops with the remaining 2 teaspoons of sugar. Bake the muffins for 18 to 22 minutes or until the tops just begin to take on a golden hue, and a toothpick inserted into the center of a muffin comes out clean. Allow the muffins to cool for a few minutes in the cups, before removing them to a wire rack.

<u>Apple Cinnamon Option</u>: Substitute 1 teaspoon cinnamon for the cardamom, 1/2 cup light brown sugar (firmly packed) or evaporated cane juice for the white sugar, and 1 cup peeled and diced apple for the pear.

Pumpkin Pecan Raisin Loaf

Yields 10 to 12 Servings

Recipe adapted from the blog, VeggieGirl (veggiegirlvegan.blogspot.com) by Liz Stark - Liz's famous pumpkin quick bread is the recipe that launched her VeggieGirl baking and blogging adventures. I can vouch for its deliciousness, as she actually shipped me an entire pumpkin loaf for a gift! Needless to say, we are still friends.

2 Cups Whole Wheat Pastry Flour
3 Tablespoons Evaporated Cane Juice or Light Brown
    Sugar, Firmly Packed
1 Teaspoon Ground Cinnamon
2 Teaspoons Baking Powder
1/2 Teaspoon Baking Soda

1 Cup Canned Pumpkin Puree
1 Cup Plain Milk Alternative of Choice
1/3 Cup Pure Maple Syrup
1/4 Cup Raw Pecans, Finely Chopped
1/3 Cup Raisins
1 Teaspoon Vanilla Extract

Preheat your oven to 350ºF (175ºC) and grease a 9x5-inch loaf pan. In a large bowl, combine the flour, sugar, cinnamon, baking powder, and baking soda. In a smaller bowl, mix together the pumpkin, milk alternative, maple syrup, pecans, raisins, and vanilla until fully combined. Add the wet mixture to the dry mixture waiting in your large bowl, stirring just to combine. Be careful not to over-mix, a few lumps are okay. Pour the batter into your prepared loaf pan and bake for 45 to 50 minutes, or until a toothpick inserted into the center of the loaf comes out clean.

Breakfast-Worthy Banana Bread

Yields 10 to 12 servings

Going out on a limb, I created a banana bread recipe that is completely void of added sugar of any kind, relying solely on the extra-ripe bananas for their natural sweetness. What resulted was a mildly sweet loaf of bread that my entire family adores. It is perfect for breakfast, and won't leave you face down on your keyboard by 10am. Feel free to make this bread the night before, allowing the banana flavor to infuse and giving the bread time to take on some moisture.

1/2 Cup Unsweetened Milk Alternative of Choice
2 Tablespoons Ground Flaxseed
2 Cups Whole Grain Spelt or Whole Wheat Flour
1 Teaspoon Ground Cinnamon
1/2 Teaspoon Ground Nutmeg
1-1/2 Teaspoons Baking Soda

1/4 Teaspoon Salt
1/4 Cup Grapeseed or Vegetable Oil
1 Teaspoon Vanilla Extract
3 to 4 Medium-Sized, Very (Very) Ripe Bananas,
     Mashed (about 1-1/2 to 2 cups mashed)*
1/2 Cup Nuts, Dried Fruit, or Other Add-ins (optional)

Preheat your oven to 350ºF (175ºC) and grease a 9x5-inch loaf pan. In a large mixing bowl combine the milk alternative and flaxseed and set aside. In a medium-sized bowl, sift together the flour, cinnamon, nutmeg, baking soda, and salt. Set aside. Returning to your mixing bowl, blend in the oil, vanilla, and bananas until well mixed. Stir in the dry ingredients by hand, being careful not to over-mix; a few lumps are okay. Gently fold in the nuts, fruit, or any other add-ins, if using. Spread the batter into your prepared loaf pan, and bake for 30 to 35 minutes, or until the top is browned and resilient to the touch. Allow the bread to cool in the pan for 10 to 15 minutes before removing it to a wire rack to cool completely.

* I prefer to use a full 2 cups of banana for the deepest flavor and a very moist bread, but using 1/2 cup less will allow the bread to rise a bit more.

Sinful Cinnamon Bread

Yields 10 to 12 Servings

Recipe adapted from the blog, Non-Dairy Queen (thenondairyqueen.blogspot.com) by Sarena Shasteen - When I mentioned this guide to Sarena, she promptly emailed this family favorite to share. Sarena's family prefers the gooey taste of this bread when prepared with the milk alternative alone, but if you would like a lighter loaf ... go with the buttermilk alternative.

1/4 Cup Grapeseed or Vegetable Oil
1-1/2 Cups Granulated Sugar
1 Egg or Flax "Egg" (1 tablespoon flax seeds, ground +
     3 tablespoons water)
1 Teaspoon Vanilla Extract
2 Cups All-Purpose (Plain) Flour

1 Teaspoon Ground Cinnamon
1 Teaspoon Baking Soda
1/2 Teaspoon Salt
1 Cup Plain Milk Alternative of Choice, Buttermilk
     Alternative (p130), or Dairy-Free Yogurt
Additional Cinnamon and Sugar for Sprinkling

Preheat your oven to 350ºF (175ºC) and grease a 9x5-inch loaf pan. Combine the oil, sugar, egg or flax "egg," and vanilla in a large bowl. In a separate bowl, combine the flour, cinnamon, baking soda, and salt. Gradually add the dry ingredients and the milk or buttermilk alternative (or yogurt) to the wet mixture, alternating between the two (ending with the flour) and gently stirring between each addition. Mix just until combined. Pour the batter into your prepared loaf pan, and sprinkle with a little cinnamon and sugar. Bake for 50 to 60 minutes, or until a toothpick inserted into the center of the loaf comes out clean. Allow the bread to cool for 15 minutes before removing it from the pan. The cinnamon and sugar topping makes a nice little crust on top.

Whole Wheat Bread

Yields 10 to 12 Servings

This was one of the first recipes I mastered when I turned to a dairy-free diet … after discovering that every loaf of wheat bread at my local grocer contained milk in some form! It makes fabulous sandwiches and breakfast toast, especially when cut nice and thick.

2-1/4 Teaspoons or 1 1/4-Ounce Package Active Dry Yeast

1/2 Cup Warm Water

3/4 Cup Warm Plain or Unsweetened Milk Alternative of Choice

2 Tablespoons Brown Sugar, Maple Syrup, or Sweetener or Choice

2 Tablespoons Grapeseed, Extra-Light Olive, or Vegetable Oil

1 Teaspoon Salt

1-1/2 Cups Whole-Wheat Flour

1/4 Cup 7-Grain Mix or Ground Flaxseed (optional)

1-3/4 to 2 cups Bread Flour, plus extra as needed

In a small bowl, sprinkle the yeast over the water and stir to dissolve. Let stand until foamy, about 5 to 10 minutes. In a large mixing bowl, combine the milk alternative, sweetener, oil, salt, and 1 cup of the whole-wheat flour, and mix until creamy. Add in the yeast mixture, the remaining 1/2 cup of whole wheat flour, and the 7-grain blend or flaxseed, if using, and mix well. Add the bread flour, 1/2 cup at a time, until the dough pulls away from the side of the bowl. Knead, and continue adding bread flour 1 Tablespoon at a time if the dough sticks, until smooth but slightly sticky when pressed, about 5 minutes. Lightly oil a large bowl, place the dough in the bowl and turn to lightly coat it with oil. Cover with a damp cloth and let it rise in a warm place until the dough had doubled in volume, about 1 to 1-1/2 hours.

Lightly grease a 9x5-inch or 8x5-inch loaf pan. Turn the dough out onto a lightly floured surface, and shape it into a long rectangle. Fold the rectangle like a letter, overlapping the short sides in the middle; press to flatten. Beginning at a narrow end, tightly roll up the dough into a thick log. Roll the log back and forth with your palms until it is the same length as the pan. Pinch the ends and the long seam to seal. Place the loaf seam side down, in your prepared loaf pan, tucking the end under to make a neat, snug fit. Cover with a damp cloth and allow the dough to rise again, until doubled in volume, about 1 hour.

When the dough is almost done rising, preheat your oven to 350ºF (175ºC). Bake for 35 to 40 minutes, or until the loaf is golden brown and pulls away from the sides of the pan. The time may vary slightly depending on the size of pan you are using. Remove the loaf from the pan and allow it to cool completely on a wire rack before cutting.

Optional Add-Ins: For a flavor variation, add raisins, dried blueberries, sunflower seeds, cinnamon, nutmeg, or savory flavors such as sun-dried tomatoes.

Perfect Peanut Butter Bread (Bread Machine-Friendly Recipe)

Yields 12 Servings

Recipe adapted from the blog, Have Cake Will Travel (www.havecakewilltravel.com) by Celine Steen - *I receive numerous requests for dairy-free bread machine recipes, and at last I have a place to direct people to. Celine gives a lot of love to her bread machine, as evidenced by the dozens of original bread recipes she has created and posted to her blog. According to Celine, "... this peanut butter bread is the one thing I could dine upon for the rest of my life without ever growing tired of it." Quite the testimonial, and for those who do not have a bread machine (like myself) she has included by-hand instructions.*

1 Cup + 1 Tablespoon Water

1/2 Cup Chunky Natural Peanut Butter

3 Tablespoons Light Brown Sugar, Firmly Packed

1 Teaspoon Salt (omit or reduce if using salted peanut butter)

2 Cups Whole Wheat or White Whole Wheat Flour

4 Teaspoons Vital Wheat Gluten

2 Teaspoons Active Dry Yeast or Bread Machine Yeast

1/2 Cup Semi-Sweet or Dark Chocolate Chips or Chunks (optional, switch to creamy peanut butter if using)

1 Cup Bread Flour

With the Machine:

Place all ingredients in your bread pan, following the manufacturer's instructions. Set it on DOUGH if you would like to bake it in the oven or BASIC if you want the machine to do all of the work. Keep in mind that the fat from the peanut butter may cause the crust to brown up a bit more. If you prefer a lighter crust set the machine to LIGHT CRUST if that setting is available.

Without the Machine:

In a large bowl, whisk together the water, peanut butter, sugar, and salt. Add the wheat flour, gluten, yeast, and chocolate chips, if using. Mix well. Gradually stir in the bread flour, working it with your hands when it gets too tough to stir with a spoon. Turn the dough out onto a lightly floured surface, and knead it until the dough is smooth and elastic, about 5 to 10 minutes. Don't worry if the dough is a little wet, it will work out. Shape the dough into a ball. Lightly oil a large bowl, place the dough in the bowl and turn to lightly coat it with oil. Cover with plastic wrap and let rise in a warm, draft-free place until the dough has doubled in volume, about 1 to 1-1/2 hours.

Grease an 8x5-inch loaf pan. Punch the dough down, and roll it out to about 11x16 inches. Roll it up like you would a Swiss roll, tightly and firmly. Pat it down on the sides and tops. Place the dough into your prepared loaf pan and press it down with your knuckles so that it covers the bottom surface. Cover with plastic wrap and let rise for another hour in the same warm, draft-free area. It will rise about 2 inches above the pan, like a mushroom, you'll see!

About 20 minutes before the dough is done rising, preheat your oven to 350ºF (175ºC). Remove the plastic wrap from the dough, and bake for 30 minutes or until an instant-read thermometer tells you your bread has reached at least 195ºF (90ºC) in its center. If you don't have an instant-read thermometer, tap the bottom of the bread to ensure it sounds hollow. Due to the peanut butter in the bread, it will have a tendency to brown a bit. To prevent this, you may want loosely tent the bread with foil part way through the baking. Remove the bread from the pan and let it cool completely before slicing.

Nut-Free Option: Substitute the peanut butter with tahini or sunflower butter.

Roll Option: You could also choose to go the sweet tooth way and roll the dough into 12 buns/rolls, throwing a little piece of dark chocolate in the center of each before the second rising. The rolls should only take about 10 to 15 minutes in a 350ºF (175ºC) oven.

Tender Squash Dinner Rolls

Yields 12 Dinner Rolls

Remember those buttery, soft, lightly sweet dinner rolls from the bakery? If so, then these rolls are bound to put a smile on your face. I prepared them for Thanksgiving one year, and my entire family couldn't stop raving. They have that soft, pull apart texture of bakery fresh bread. I like to use butternut squash (pre-cubed) in this recipe, but feel free to substitute canned pumpkin puree if it is more convenient. The fluffiness of these rolls will suffer with whole wheat flour, but you can substitute up to 1 cup of whole wheat flour for the all-purpose with only a minor change in density.

3/4 Cup Cubed Winter Squash (1/2 cup mashed)
3/4 Cup Plain Rice or Soymilk, Lukewarm
2-1/4 Teaspoons or 1 1/4-Ounce Package Active Dry
    Yeast

3 Cups All-Purpose (Plain) Flour, Divided
1/4 Cup Granulated Sugar
1 Teaspoon Salt
1/4 Cup Shortening

Boil or steam the squash until tender, roughly 15 minutes, and then mash it to a fairly smooth consistency. Set aside to cool. In a small bowl, dissolve the yeast in the warm milk alternative, and set aside for 5 minutes to proof. In a large mixing bowl, combine 2 cups of the flour, the sugar, and salt. Add the yeast mixture, shortening, and squash, mixing well. Add the remaining flour, 1/2 cup at a time, mixing well after each addition. When the dough has pulled together, turn it out onto a lightly floured surface and knead it until smooth and supple, about 5 minutes. Lightly oil a large bowl, place the dough in the bowl and turn to lightly coat it with oil. Cover with a damp cloth and let rise in a warm place until the dough has doubled in volume, about 1 hour.

Lightly grease a 9x13-inch baking dish. Divide the dough into twelve equal pieces and form each piece into rounds. Place the rounds in your prepared baking dish. Cover the dish with a damp cloth and allow the dough to rise again, until doubled in volume, about 30 minutes. When the dough is almost done rising, preheat your oven to 400º F (205º C). Bake the rolls for 10 to 15 minutes, or until the tops take on a golden hue.

Savory Sheesy Scones or Biscuits

Yields 8 Wedges or 10 Round Scones

I was privileged with some samples of Sheese® (www.buteisland.com, UK - 01700 505357), a cheese alternative from Scotland, just as it was hitting the United States. Unfortunately, while it tasted incredibly like real cheese, it just didn't want to melt atop my pizza. However, I noted that it did tend to "melt" on the stovetop or when combined with other ingredients. This made me wonder how it might do if I baked it in something rather than on top of it. And thus, these sheesy scones were born. Since melting is not the goal, most brands of vegan cheese should suit this recipe nicely.

1-1/2 Cups All-Purpose (Plain) Flour
1/2 Teaspoon Mustard Powder
1 Tablespoon Baking Powder
1/4 Teaspoon Salt

1/4 Cup Chilled Dairy-Free Margarine or Shortening
4 Ounces Cheddar or Cheshire Cheese Alternative,
    Grated
1/2 Cup Unsweetened Rice, Cashew, or Soymilk

Preheat your oven to 425ºF (220ºC). In a medium-sized bowl, sift together the flour, mustard powder, baking powder, and salt. Blend in the margarine or shortening with a fork or pastry blender until the mixture resembles fine crumbs. Stir in the grated cheese. Stir in the milk alternative to create smooth dough. If the mixture won't stay together, add a bit more milk alternative, one tablespoon at a time, as needed. Knead the scone mixture ever so lightly (just to bring the dough together) and roll or pat it on a lightly floured surface until it is about 1-1/2 inches thick. Using a 2-1/2-inch biscuit cutter cut the dough into rounds; transfer the rounds to a baking sheet. Alternately, you may pat the dough into a disk that is about 1-1/2 inches high, and cut it into 8 wedges. Bake the scones for 10 to 15 minutes, or until the tops are firm and golden.

Cheesy Potato-Onion Bread

Yields 4 Servings or 8 to 12 Slices

Recipe adapted from the blog, Diet, Dessert, and Dogs (dietdessertndogs.wordpress.com) by Ricki Heller - *Ricki is putting together a cookbook of the recipes she prepared in her popular Toronto Bakery in years prior. The book, to be entitled "Sweet Freedom," will encompass an array of desserts and baked goods that are free from dairy, eggs, refined sweeteners, and in many cases, wheat and gluten. Showing off the savory side of her baking skills, Ricki shared this deliciously cheesy bread, made purely for our dairy-free enjoyment.*

1 Tablespoon Ground Flaxseed	1/2 Teaspoon Salt
1 Teaspoon Grainy Dijon Mustard	1 Yukon Gold Potato, Grated (it need not be peeled)
1/2 to 2/3 Cup Plain Rice or Soymilk (as needed), Plus More for Brushing on the Bread	2 Tablespoons Nutritional Yeast Flakes
1-3/4 Cups Light Spelt Flour	5 Green Onions (white and light green part only), Finely Sliced
1/2 Teaspoon Smoked Paprika	1 to 2 Tablespoons Freshly Chopped Dill
2 Teaspoons Baking Powder	1 Small Roma Tomato, Chopped

Preheat your oven to 375ºF (190ºC), and lightly grease a cookie sheet or line it with a non-stick baking mat or parchment paper. In a glass measuring cup, stir together the flaxseed, mustard, and 1/2 cup of the soymilk. Set the soymilk aside while you prepare the other ingredients, or for at least 2 minutes. Sift the flour, paprika, baking powder, and salt into a medium-sized mixing bowl. Add the grated potato, nutritional yeast, onions, dill, and tomato and toss gently with your hands until all the vegetables are coated with flour and separated. Pour the wet mixture over the flour mixture and toss with a fork until everything comes together into slightly sticky dough. At this point, if the mixture is too dry, sprinkle with the remaining soymilk and toss again.

Transfer the dough to the cookie sheet and shape it into a domed round. If desired, score once or twice across the top with a sharp knife. Bake for 40 to 45 minutes, turning once after 20 minutes (at this point, you can also brush the top with additional soymilk for a more glossy crust, if desired). Bake until the top of the bread has a deep golden hue and the loaf has a slightly hollow sound when tapped on the bottom. Allow it to cool before devouring. This bread does freeze well.

Pizza Rolls

Yields 12 Rolls

Recipe adapted from the blog, Bittersweet (bittersweetblog.wordpress.com) by Hannah Kaminsky - *Hannah was a co-reviewer of Sheese® along with me and she simultaneously discovered the benefits of baking vegan "cheese" into food, rather than trying to force it to melt atop a pizza. However, she was not completely willing to give up the whole pizza theme. Feel free to add olives, mushrooms, onions or other "toppings" before rolling them up!*

1 Cup Plain Rice or Soymilk, Lukewarm
2-1/4 Teaspoons or 1 1/4-Ounce Package Active Dry
    Yeast
1 Cup All-Purpose (Plain) Flour
1 Cup Whole Wheat Pastry Flour
1 Teaspoon Granulated Sugar
1 Tablespoon Baking Powder

1/2 Teaspoon Salt
1/4 Cup Dairy-Free Margarine
1/3 Cup Pizza Sauce (store-bought or recipe on p208)
1/2 Teaspoon Garlic Powder
3 Ounces Mozzarella or Cheddar Cheese Alternative,
    Grated

Preheat your oven to 425ºF (220ºC). In a small bowl, dissolve the yeast in the warm milk alternative, and set aside for 5 minutes to proof. In a separate bowl, combine both flours, the sugar, baking powder, and salt. Blend in the margarine with a fork or pastry blender until the mixture resembles fine crumbs. Add the milk alternative mixture, and mix until it comes together to form a cohesive, but still rather moist, ball of dough.

Turn the dough out onto a well-floured surface, and with lightly-floured hands, pat it out into a rectangle measuring somewhere in the neighborhood of 13x8 inches. Being such loose dough, it won't play nicely with a rolling pin, so you just need to poke and prod it into shape with your hands. Once you achieve a satisfactory rectangle, spread the pizza sauce over it, going most of the way to the edges but leaving perhaps a centimeter uncovered all around. Sprinkle the garlic powder over it, followed by the grated cheese alternative. Try to cover the surface evenly with all of the above.

Gently roll the dough from the long side, moving with care and without stretching or pulling the dough. Once you have a nice log, cut 1-inch pieces with a sharp knife, using a sawing motion and as little downward pressure as you can muster to prevent the rolls from becoming completely smashed. Move the rolls to a baking sheet lined with parchment paper or a non-stick baking mat, spacing them out a bit and reshaping them if necessary. Bake for 13 to 17 minutes, or until golden brown. Enjoy warm or reheat in a toaster oven later.

Some Store-Bought Recommendations for Breads and Baking:
There are many great brands on the market, but the following recommendations only include products that I purchase with some regularity or that a colleague highly recommended. For full lists of non-dairy, packaged foods and brands, see the product lists available on www.godairyfree.org.

Bob's Red Mill® (www.bobsredmill.com, (503) 654-3215) ~ bread and muffin mixes (including gluten-free)
Bob's not only mills the grains for baking, they also package them into various bread mixes. Of special mention are their gluten-free whole grain and cinnamon raisin bread mixes, both of which got high marks from my most trusted GFCF taste tester.

Kinnikinnick (www.kinnikinnick.com, (780) 424-2900) ~ gluten-free baked goods
Kinnikinnick is a wonderful gluten-free company that makes a wide array of products, including popular premade loaves of bread and muffins. But, my favorite is their Kinni-Kwik Bread & Bun Mix. Keep in mind, I am not gluten-free, but the ability to whip up fluffy dinner rolls or a loaf of yeast-like bread by simply adding water and baking, is like a dream come true. Plus, I find them quite tasty. Not all of Kinnikinnick's products are dairy-free, but they readily offer allergen and ingredient information.

Pamela's Products™ (www.pamelasproducts.com, (707) 462-6605) ~ gluten-free cookies and cake mixes
I have been told that Pamela's Amazing Wheat-Free Bread Mix is the closest thing you can get to a regular slice of wheat breaad, while still maintaining a gluten-free / casein-free status. Plus, it is extremely easy to make, and quite versatile.

Roman Meal (www.romanmeal.com, (253) 475-0964) ~ bread products
As a native of the northwest, I grew up on Roman Meal bread, and even toured the factory as a tot. When my favorite milk allergy mom told me this is their bread of choice, I knew I had to include it in this guide. They now make many variations of whole grain bread, hot cereals, and snack bars, most of which are dairy-free (the butter wheat being an obvious exception). However, do keep an eye on the ingredient statements. Roman Meal breads are produced in 90 local area bakeries throughout the world, and they do warn that some of these bakeries may use whey. Strict vegans should be aware that honey is used liberally in the Roman Meal factory, which is still family owned and operated.

Rudi's Organic Bakery®(www.rudisbakery.com, (303) 447-0495) ~ bread products
Rudi's produces a very wide selection of bread products from their all-organic, certified kosher parve bakery. I like this brand because all of their products are dairy-free and egg-free, they are fairly priced for the higher quality, and their products are quite easy to locate. Rudi's products are sold in numerous natural food and mainstream grocers throughout the U.S. The core company for Rudi's is Charter Baking. They also own The Baker® (www.the-baker.com) and Vermont Bread Company (www.vermontbread.com) product lines, which I hear are also excellent quality options.

CHAPTER 20:
SIPS & SMOOTHIES

Idea: Smoothie Customization

Below are some ideas I use to customize home-blended smoothies to fit my current mood and/or nutritional needs.

<u>The Smoothie Base</u>: I am a big fan of using ripe bananas in smoothies for nutrition, texture, natural sweetness, and overall flavor. However, if you would like a different taste, feel free to replace each banana with 1/3 to 1/2 cup dairy-free yogurt (soy or coconut-based), 1/3 to 1/2 cup silken tofu or half an avocado plus a tablespoon of your favorite sweetener, or another rich fruit such as mango.

<u>Smoothie Add-ins</u>: Blended beverages are a great way to sneak a little extra nutrition into your diet, whether you are seeking vitamins, minerals, protein, healthy fats, or a flavor boost. Feel free to experiment with any of the following:

~ Protein Powder - See suggested dairy-free protein powders on p59.
~ Flax Seeds - I like to grind 1 tablespoon of flax seeds (per serving) in the spice grinder first, since the blender blades can sometimes miss a few of these little seeds.
~ Nuts / Nut Butters - Toss in 1 to 2 tablespoons of your favorite nut butter (almond, peanut, cashew, etc.) or up to 1/4 cup of raw, unsalted nuts per serving.
~ Greens - The mild flavor of leafy greens such as spinach and kale are virtually undetectable in smoothies. Toss a handful or two of leaves in per serving. If you are serving the smoothies to someone else, I recommend choosing berry, chocolate, or carob as your primary flavor; the darker color of these foods will mask the green nicely. They will be none the wiser, but definitely healthier for it.
~ Coconut - For a tropical vibe, I occasionally add 1 to 2 tablespoons of unsweetened, shredded coconut to fruit smoothies. For more of an infused flavor, I grind the coconut in my spice grinder before adding it to the blender.
~ Nutritive Oils - Coconut, hemp, and flaxseed oils are popular supplement oils. Rather than taking them in pill form, enjoy the richness that a tablespoon can add to your smoothie.
~ Natural Sweetener - When using ripe fruit in smoothies, additional sweetener is seldom required. However, feel free to add a bit of your favorite sweetener for some added indulgence, or if your base ingredients are a bit lacking in natural sugar. I highly recommend dates (1 to 2 per serving), agave nectar, honey, maple syrup, or a pinch of stevia (for sugar-free).

True Blue Smoothie

Yields 1 to 2 Servings

This is my go-to smoothie, and trust me on this one … don't omit the spinach. I don't care who you are serving it to, they will never know it is in there. The blueberries mask the green color, resulting in a beautiful purple beverage. As for the flavor … even the most adamant non-believers come back to me with surprise comments of delight. I never add sweetener, but feel free to add a bit if your fruit isn't very sweet.

1 Medium Very Ripe Banana, Broken into Chunks
1 Cup Frozen Blueberries (wild blueberries if possible)
1/2 to 1 Cup Plain or Vanilla Milk Alternative of Choice
1/4 Teaspoon Ground Cinnamon (optional)

1 Tablespoon Whole Flax Seeds (left whole or pre-ground in your spice grinder)
1/2 Cup Packed Fresh Baby Spinach Leaves
Sweetener, to Taste (optional)
1/2 Cup Ice (optional)

Toss the banana, blueberries, and 1/2 cup of the milk alternative into your blender, and process until smooth. Add the cinnamon (if using), flax seeds, and spinach, and blend until those little green specks vanish. Blend in more milk alternative until it reaches your desired consistency. If desired, blend in a handful of ice for a frostier treat.

Peachy Keen Almond Smoothie

Yields 2 Servings

I think of this smoothie as more of a snack or treat, which is why the serving size is a bit smaller. But don't be deceived, the almond butter makes it much more filling than it looks.

2 Cups Chopped Ripe Peaches (about 2 medium peaches), Frozen
2 Tablespoons Creamy Unsalted Almond Butter
3/4 to 1 Cup Unsweetened or Plain Almond Milk

1/2 Teaspoon Ground Cinnamon
Pinch Salt
2 Teaspoons Agave Nectar or Honey, or to Taste
3/4 Cup Ice (optional)

Blend the peaches, almond butter, and almond milk in your blender until smooth and creamy. You may need a little pulsing action to get it started. Add the cinnamon, salt, and agave or honey, and give it another quick blend. If desired, blend in some ice for a thicker, frostier treat.

Super C Smoothie

Yields 1 to 2 Servings

Enjoy the simplicity of this light and refreshing smoothie, which is naturally packed with vitamin C and potassium.

1 Medium Very Ripe Banana, Broken into Chunks
1 Cup Frozen Strawberries

1/2 Cup Orange Juice
1/2 Cup Ice (optional)

Toss the banana, strawberries, and orange juice into your blender, and process until smooth. If desired, blend in some ice for a thicker, frostier treat.

Mango Colada
Yields 2 Servings

For ease, I keep bags of frozen mango on hand, but even frozen mango has an "in-season." If the mango you are using isn't very sweet, feel free to add a teaspoon or two of your favorite sweetener (agave and honey go nicely with mango) to this smoothie.

8 Ounces (about 1-1/2 cups) Cubed Frozen Mango
1/2 Cup Canned Pineapple with Juice (I use crushed, grabbing a bit of the juice with the pineapple in my measuring cup)

1/2 Cup Regular Coconut Milk
1/2 to 1 Cup Water, Light Coconut Milk, or Plain Milk Alternative of Choice
2 Tablespoons Shredded Unsweetened Coconut

Combine the frozen mango, pineapple with juice, coconut milk, 1/2 cup of the water or milk alternative, and the coconut in your blender, and blend until smooth and creamy. Blend in additional water or milk alternative to your desired consistency.

Lower Fat Option: Replace the regular coconut milk with 1/3 to 1/2 cup plain coconut-based yogurt, and use water or rice milk for your blending liquid. The yogurt is a bit thicker, so you may need to add a little extra water or milk alternative to get the right consistency … but it is equally delicious!

Cheater's Instant Horchata
Yields 4 Servings

Horchata is a popular creamy, Latin American beverage that is often found in Mexican restaurants. Many traditional recipes rely on rice or almonds for the drink base, but in the U.S., milk is frequently used. I have made horchata from scratch, soaking and grinding the raw almonds and rice, and to be honest, I didn't like it as well as this simple beverage. Though not authentic by any means, this drink has a definite horchata vibe that is delicious and refreshing.

2 Cups Plain Almond or Rice Milk*
2 Cups Water
1 Cup Plain Dairy-Free Yogurt*

1/4 to 1/2 cup Granulated Sugar, Agave Nectar, or Honey, or to Taste
1 Teaspoon Vanilla Extract
1/8 to 1/4 Teaspoon Ground Cinnamon

Place the milk alternative, water, yogurt, 1/4 cup of the sweetener, vanilla, and cinnamon in your blender and give it a quick whirl. Traditional horchata is quite sweet, so feel free to blend in up to 1/4 cup of additional sweetener, or to your desired taste. Serve chilled over ice for a refreshing treat.

Mexican Chocolate Option: Who doesn't like chocolate? Blend in 2 to 4 tablespoons of cocoa powder depending on how strong your cravings are.

* I prefer to use plain (coconut-based) yogurt and plain milk alternative with pure vanilla extract added (the flavor is just a bit better to me), but feel free to "cheat" further by using vanilla yogurt or milk alternative. Just be sure to adjust the sugar accordingly as vanilla flavored products tend to contain more sweetener.

Chocolate Peanut Butter "Milk" Shake

Yields 1 Serving

This thick and rich shake is frequently requested in my household. Not only does it taste like a luscious dessert, but it also has a good amount of potassium and protein for a pre- or post-activity boost.

3/4 Cup Chocolate Milk Alternative of Choice
1 Medium Very Ripe Banana, Sliced and Frozen
1 to 2 Tablespoons Creamy Peanut Butter

2 to 3 Teaspoons Cocoa Powder
1/2 Cup Ice

Blend the milk alternative and frozen banana in your blender until smooth. Add the peanut butter and cocoa powder, adjusting the two flavors to your taste, and give it another blend. Add the ice and process until thick and creamy.

Chocolate Almond Option: For a more sophisticated shake, swap almond butter for the peanut butter, use chocolate almond milk, and add 1/4 teaspoon of cinnamon.

Minty Chocolate (or Carob) Shake

Yields 2 to 3 Servings

Avocado provides body to this simple recipe, without overwhelming the flavor. Plus, the addition of chocolate or carob masks the green color, and thus the secret ingredient. I prefer this recipe in shake form, but my friend found the pudding option (below) to be a bit addictive.

1 Small, Ripe Avocado (about 1/4 lb)
2 Cups Plain Soy, Rice, or Cashew Milk Alternative
1/4 Cup Carob or Cocoa Powder

1/4 Cup Agave Nectar, Honey, or Sweetener of Choice
1/8 to 1/4 Teaspoon Peppermint Extract
2 to 3 Cups Ice

In your blender, combine the avocado, milk alternative, carob or cocoa powder, sweetener, and peppermint. Blend in the ice to your desired texture and temperature.

Pudding Option: Follow the directions above, but use just 3/4 cup of milk alternative. If the mixture is too thick, thin with up to 1/4 cup of additional milk alternative. You should already have a nice pudding texture, but place it in a covered container and refrigerate for an hour or two for optimum taste.

Almost Vanilla "Milk" Shake

Yields 2 Servings

Vanilla frozen desserts are hard to mimic, but this vanilla-inspired shake is pretty tasty in its own right.

1/4 Cup Raw Cashews
1/3 Cup Regular Coconut Milk*
2/3 Cup Water*
1 Large Ripe Banana, Sliced and Frozen

1 Tablespoon Agave Nectar, Honey, or Granulated Sugar
3/4 Teaspoon Vanilla Extract
1 Cup Ice

If you have a spice grinder available, grind the cashews into a fine meal/powder. Place the coconut milk, water, cashews, frozen banana, sweetener, and vanilla in your blender, and blend until smooth and creamy. Blend in the ice.

* You may substitute the coconut milk and water with 1 cup of light coconut milk.

Thick & Spicy Pumpkin Pie Shake

Yields 2 to 3 Servings
This is about as healthy as pumpkin pie gets!

2 Medium to Large Very Ripe Bananas, Sliced and
    Frozen
1-1/2 Cups Plain or Vanilla Milk Alternative of Choice
1 Cup Canned Pumpkin Puree

2 to 4 Tablespoons Maple Syrup or Lightly Packed
    Brown Sugar
2-1/2 Teaspoons Pumpkin Pie Spice*
1 to 2 Cups Ice (optional)

Combine the bananas, milk alternative, pumpkin, 2 tablespoons of the sweetener, and spice in your blender, and blend until smooth and creamy. Blend in up to 2 tablespoons of additional sweetener to taste, and more milk alternative if you would like a thinner consistency. Blend in ice for a frostier experience.

* You may substitute the following ground spices for the pumpkin pie spice: 1 teaspoon cinnamon + 1/2 teaspoon ginger + 1/2 teaspoon nutmeg + 1/2 teaspoon allspice.

Coco-Nog

Yields 3 Cups
Recipe created by Hannah Kaminsky, author of My Sweet Vegan - There are a few brands of "soy nog" that pop on the market when the season rolls around, but this homemade version adds that extra dose of luxury. While it isn't very likely, if you have any leftover nog, give it a whirl in your ice cream maker for an instant frozen treat, or soak slices of crusty bread in it for a few minutes and pan-fry them to make decadent French toast.

1/2 Cup Macadamia Nuts
2 14-Ounce Cans Regular Coconut Milk
4 Whole Cloves
1 Cinnamon Stick
1/2 Cup Granulated Sugar

1/4 Cup Dark Brown Sugar, Firmly Packed
1/3 Cup Light or Dark Rum
1 Teaspoon Vanilla Extract
Pinch Salt
Freshly Grated Nutmeg

Bring about a cup of water to a boil and pour it over your macadamia nuts. Set aside to allow the nuts to soften a bit, which will make them easier to puree.* Place one can of coconut milk in the refrigerator for later. Pour the contents of the second can of coconut milk into a medium sauce pan, adding in the spices and both sugars. Gently heat the coconut milk over medium-low heat to dissolve the sugar, and allow it to simmer for about 10 minutes to let the spices infuse. Let the mixture cool completely before straining out the whole spices. Stir in the rum and vanilla.

Drain the water from the macadamia nuts, and thoroughly puree them in your blender or food processor with the coconut milk mixture. If the mixture still seems gritty, you may want to pass it a fine mesh strainer or a double layer of cheesecloth to strain. Take the chilled can of coconut milk out of the fridge, but do not shake it. Carefully open it and skim the thick cream off the top and put it into a chilled mixing bowl. Beat vigorously for a few minutes, until the coconut cream is somewhat whipped and fluffy. Fold the whipped coconut cream into the blended coconut mixture. Serve chilled and top with nutmeg.

* Alternately, you can grind the nuts in your spice grinder until they pass the powder stage and begin to clump.

Chocolate "Milk"

Yields 2 to 3 Dozen Servings (Though you don't have to make them all at once!)

This recipe actually does double-duty, as the syrup used to make the chocolate "milk" works well as a chocolate topping on "ice cream" or other desserts. The syrup is deep and dark; I prefer it with the lesser amount of sugar, but if you would like a sweeter sauce, feel free to up it a bit.

1 Cup Plain Milk Alternative of Choice   1 Tablespoon Chocolate Syrup, or to Taste (below)

Drizzle the chocolate syrup into your glass of "milk" while stirring. This syrup makes a very rich chocolaty flavor, so feel free to add a dash of additional sweetener for little ones, if desired.

Chocolate Syrup:
1-1/2 to 1-3/4 Cups Granulated Sugar   1 Cup Cold Water
1 Cup Sifted Cocoa Powder (sift then measure)   2 Teaspoons Vanilla Extract
Pinch Salt

Combine the sugar, cocoa, and salt in a large saucepan or pot. Gradually stir in the water, whisking until well combined and to remove any lumps. Set the pot over medium heat, while continuing to stir until the mixture comes to a boil. Allow it to boil for 3 minutes while stirring. Reduce the heat slightly if it threatens to boil over. Remove the syrup from the heat, and allow it to cool to room temperature. Strain the syrup through a fine mesh strainer or a double layer of cheesecloth to get a very smooth consistency. Stir in the vanilla. Store it in a covered container in the refrigerator, ready to report for duty whenever cravings strike.

"Milk" Chocolate Syrup Option: Use plain rice or almond milk alternative or light coconut milk in place of the water.

Carob "Milk" Option: Substitute half or all of the cocoa powder for carob powder.

Strawberry "Milk"

Yields 1 Serving

Strawberry syrup pales in comparison to this fresh strawberry beverage. Since the sweetness of this recipe could vary quite a bit, depending on the flavor of your strawberries and milk alternative, it is important to sweeten to taste.

1 Cup Unsweetened or Plain Milk Alternative of   1/4 Teaspoon Vanilla Extract
    Choice   2 to 4 Teaspoons Sugar, Agave Nectar, or Honey, or to
1/2 Cup Fresh or Frozen Strawberries   Taste

Combine the milk alternative, strawberries, and vanilla in your blender, and blend until smooth. Blend in the sweetener to taste. If desired, strain the "milk" through a fine mesh strainer or a double layer of cheesecloth to remove any lingering seeds.

Hot Double Chocolate

Yields 2 Servings

This rich beverage boasts a double dose of chocolate, and is perfect for those cold, damp evenings when you are chilled to the bone. To up the luxury one more notch, use light or regular coconut milk (or thinned regular coconut milk) in place of the milk alternative for a creamier base. This makes a sweet, dessert-like hot chocolate, so feel free to start with 2 tablespoons of sweetener, and add the remaining 2 tablespoons of sweetener only as desired.

2 Cups Plain Milk Alternative of Choice
2 Tablespoons Cocoa Powder
1/4 Cup Granulated Sugar, Agave Nectar, or
    Sweetener of Choice
2 Ounces Semi-Sweet Chocolate Chips or Bittersweet
    (Dark) Chocolate, Chopped

1/4 Teaspoon Vanilla Extract
Pinch Salt
Marshmallows (optional)
Whipped Coconut Cream (p253) (optional)

Place the milk alternative, cocoa, and sweetener in a medium-sized saucepan over medium heat. Allow it to come to a simmer as you whisk continuously, breaking up any clumps of cocoa. Add the chocolate and continue whisking until the chocolate is melted and the beverage is smooth. Whisk in the vanilla and salt while still simmering. Ladle into 2 mugs and top with marshmallows or coconut cream if desired.

Spiced Cocoa Option: In the first step, whisk in the following ground spices: 1/4 teaspoon cinnamon, 1/4 teaspoon cardamom, 1/4 teaspoon ginger, and a pinch of nutmeg.

Mocha Option: In the first step, whisk in 1 tablespoon of instant coffee.

Peppermint Option: Serve with a peppermint candy cane as a stir stick, stir in 1/4 to 1/2 teaspoon peppermint extract (to taste) with the vanilla extract, or (for adults only) stir in 2 ounces of peppermint schnapps after you remove the hot chocolate from the heat.

Carob Cocoa

Yields 2 Servings

This is a nice warm beverage variation for those seeking to cut caffeine, or who just like the taste of carob.

2 Cups Plain Milk Alternative of Choice
2 Tablespoons Carob Powder
4 Teaspoons Granulated Sugar, Agave Nectar, or
    Maple Syrup, or to Taste

1/2 Teaspoon Vanilla Extract
Pinch Salt
Marshmallows (optional)
Whipped Coconut Cream (p253) (optional)

In a small saucepan, whisk together the milk alternative, carob, sweetener, vanilla extract, and salt. Heat over medium-low heat until hot, but do not boil. Ladle into 2 mugs and top with marshmallows or coconut cream if desired.

Some Store-Bought Recommendations for Beverages:

There are many great brands on the market, but the following recommendations only include products that I purchase with some regularity or that a colleague highly recommended. For full lists of non-dairy, packaged foods and brands, see the product lists available on www.godairyfree.org.

Amazing Grass® SuperFood (www.amazinggrass.com, (415) 441-3326) ~ drink mixes
This is not a product that I had expected to fall in love with. I sampled quite a few "nutritional beverages" and while most were okay, they weren't something I looked forward to. Yet, when Amazing Grass hit my smoothies, I was delighted. I enjoy the Chocolate Superfood, using a scoop in place of the cocoa in my Chocolate Peanut Butter Shake (p164). As an added bonus, their SuperFood line is vegan, gluten-free, and soy-free, and they have a special Kidz SuperFood™.

Cabaret Brewed Chocolate® (www.brewedchocolate.com, (510) 219-1891) ~ hot beverage
This soothing beverage is a unique blend that exudes hints of hot chocolate, coffee, and tea, but in a more subdued environment that solely consists of brewed whole cocoa beans and organic evaporated cane juice (just a touch). While the small jar makes quite a few cups, this grown-up version of hot chocolate could easily get pricey since it is rather addictive.

Good Belly™ (www.goodbelly.com) ~ refrigerated beverages
This dairy-free, soy-free, wheat-free (it does contain barley and oats), all-natural, fruit juice-based beverage is a flavorsome way to get some of those beneficial bacteria (aka probiotics). In terms of taste and texture, it is like a cross between fruit juice and a smoothie, and it comes in a variety of unique fruity flavors that both my husband and I really enjoyed. The only catch is that it is sweetened with evaporated cane juice to get that perfect taste. I expect this drink to be a big hit with kids.

Odwalla® (www.odwalla.com, (800) 639-2552) ~ refrigerated beverages
It is hard to find nutritious options on the go, but Odwalla beverages and smoothies seem to appear in many convenient locations and in so many flavors. Our family favorite is the Mo' Beta®, a cheerful blend of OJ, peaches, and mango, but there are dozens of varieties to choose from. They also offer protein smoothie blends that are made with soymilk.

CHAPTER 21:
SNACKS & APPS

Instant Pudding

"How does one make instant pudding from the box without dairy?" If you have ever tried preparing instant pudding by just substituting milk alternative for the milk in the directions, then you likely ended up with a rather soupy pudding. To answer this question, I got to work in the kitchen and tested a variety of ways to whip up this snack/dessert, dairy-free style. I found many variations that worked, but for the record, my two favorites are the thickened cashew milk and the instant creamy mousse option at the end.

Start with:
1 3.9-Ounce Package Instant Pudding Mix (your flavor of choice)*

Then whisk in one of the following:
~ *Thickened Cashew Milk* – Grind 1/4 cup of cashews in your spice grinder until they begin to turn into a paste, about 1 minute. Place the cashew butter in your blender with 1 cup of cold water and blend until smooth, about 1 minute. Briefly blend in 1 additional cup of cold water. If you don't have a spice grinder, you can throw the cashews in your blender whole, with your water, but you will need to blend it for a minute or two longer. Pour the milk alternative through a fine mesh strainer, measuring out 2 cups. Whisk the 2 cups of thickened cashew milk alternative into your pudding mix, cover, and place it in your refrigerator. It will be soft set within five minutes, but you can chill it for longer if you prefer a firmer pudding.
~ *Light Coconut Milk* – Whisk in 2 cups of chilled light coconut milk or 1/2 cup of chilled regular coconut milk plus 1-1/2 cups of cold water. Cover, and place the pudding in your refrigerator. It will be soft set within five minutes, but you can chill it for longer if you prefer a firmer pudding.
~ *Unsweetened Milk Alternative* – Whisk in up to 1-1/2 cups of unsweetened milk alternative of choice, beginning with 1 cup and whisking in more 1/4 cup at a time until it reaches your desired consistency. Cover, and place the pudding in your refrigerator; it will be soft set within five minutes. It is important that you use unsweetened milk alternative since the reduced amount of liquid will cause the sugar from the mix to be more concentrated.
~ *Milk Alternative + Oil* – In a small saucepan, whisk 1-3/4 cups + 2 tablespoons of cold plain or unsweetened milk alternative of choice with the mix until smooth. Briefly heat the mixture over low heat, for just a minute or two, while whisking. Whisk in 1-1/2 tablespoons of coconut or palm oil until smooth. This version will need a couple of hours in the refrigerator to chill and set up.

Instant Creamy Mousse Option: Whisk the mix with 1 cup of regular coconut milk and 1 cup of cold water and allow it to chill for an hour or more for a rich and luxurious treat.

* You will find several flavors of the ever-so-popular Jell-O® brand instant pudding mixes that are made without milk ingredients, but a few do contain dairy, so be sure to check the label.

Pizza Fondue

Yields 4 to 6 Servings

This kid-friendly dip goes very well with crusty French bread, warm pita wedges, chicken fingers, or vegetables (such as lightly steamed cauliflower florets). It is also a great way to use vegan cheese alternatives, since some brands tend to be a bit stubborn when it comes to melting on their own.

1 15-Ounce or 2 8-Ounce Cans Plain Tomato Sauce
2 Slices Regular or Vegan Pepperoni, Diced (optional)
1/2 Teaspoon Dried Oregano
1/2 Teaspoon Dried Basil
1/4 Teaspoon Garlic Powder
Generous Pinch Crushed Red Pepper Flakes

1/4 Cup Unsweetened Soy, Rice, or Cashew Milk Alternative
3 Ounces (3/4 cup) Vegan Mozzarella or Cheddar Cheese Alternative, Shredded
2 Tablespoons Breadcrumbs of Choice (optional)
1/4 Cup Sliced Olives (optional)

Combine the tomato sauce, pepperoni (if using), oregano, basil, garlic powder, and red pepper in a small saucepan over medium-low heat, and bring it to a simmer. While that is simmering away, place the milk and cheese alternatives in a small skillet over medium heat. As the mixture begins to heat up, whisk continuously to break up any "cheese" shreds, cooking until most or all of the cheese melts to form a thick sauce. If you would like a heartier dip, add the breadcrumbs to the tomato sauce, and simmer for 2 to 3 minutes. Stir the cheese mixture into the tomato sauce until the two are well combined. Serve warm and top with sliced olives, if desired.

Five-Minute Nachos

Yields 4 Servings

These nachos were not only prepared in five minutes, but my husband and I also devoured every last chip in five minutes. This cheesy sauce also works well in other Mexican inspired recipes, including enchiladas.

1/4 Cup Raw Cashews
1 Cup Unsweetened Cashew, Rice, or Soymilk or Vegetable Broth
2 Tablespoons Olive, Grapeseed, or Vegetable Oil
2 Ounces Pimientos or Roasted Red Bell Peppers, Drained
2 Tablespoons Cornstarch or Arrowroot Powder
2 Tablespoons Nutritional Yeast Flakes

1 Tablespoon Lemon Juice
1/2 to 1 Teaspoon Salt
1 4-Ounce Can Diced Green Chilies, Drained (optional)
Tortilla Chips
Chopped Tomatoes (optional)
Chopped Avocado (optional)
Sliced Black Olives (optional)
Salsa (optional)

Grind the cashews in your spice grinder until they pass the powder stage, and just begin to clump, about 1 minute. Add the cashews, milk alternative or broth, oil, pimientos or bell peppers, arrowroot or cornstarch, nutritional yeast, lemon juice, and salt to your blender. Blend the mixture on high for 2 minutes, or until it is smooth. Place the liquid in a medium-sized saucepan over medium heat. Continue to cook and whisk the mixture until it reaches your desired consistency, about 5 minutes. Stir in the green chilies, if using. Place the tortilla chips on a serving platter and pour the nacho "cheese" sauce evenly over the top. If desired, top with chopped tomatoes, chopped avocados, and/or sliced black olives. Serve with a side dish of your favorite salsa.

Make it a Meal: Top the nachos with 1 15-ounce can of black beans (drained and rinsed), chopped and sautéed vegetables (I like zucchini and mushrooms), diced or shredded chicken, ground beef, or vegan mock beef crumbles. Roughly 3/4 to 1 lb of vegetables, meat, or mock meat should suffice.

Rich Eggplant Dip (aka Baba Ghanoush)

Yields 6 Servings

Hummus is nice, but eggplant takes it up a giant notch in my book. Serve this flavorful dip with French bread, pita wedges, or raw vegetables.

1 Large Ripe Eggplant (about 1-1/2 lbs)
1 Teaspoon Olive or Grapeseed Oil
2 Tablespoons Tahini, Plus More as Needed
2 Tablespoons Lemon Juice, Plus More as Needed
1 to 2 Garlic Cloves, Crushed or Minced

1/4 to 1/2 Teaspoon Ground Cumin
1/2 Teaspoon Salt, or to Taste
2 to 3 Teaspoons Extra-Virgin Olive Oil
1 Tablespoon Minced Fresh Parsley (optional)

Preheat your oven to 400ºF (205ºC). Cut the eggplant in half lengthwise. Drizzle the teaspoon of olive oil in a large baking dish, and place the eggplant cut sides down onto the oil, making sure the undersides of the eggplant are coated in the oil to avoid sticking. Bake for 30 to 40 minutes, or until the eggplant is very tender (the skin will be browned). Allow the eggplant to cool for a few minutes, and scoop the flesh out into a medium-sized bowl (you may be able to simply peel the skin off). Using a fork, hand mixer, food processor, or blender, mash the eggplant until it is relatively smooth but retains some of its texture.

Add the tahini, lemon juice, garlic, and cumin and mix well. Season with salt, then taste and add more tahini and/or lemon juice, if desired. Transfer the mixture to a serving bowl and spread with the back of a spoon to form a shallow well. Drizzle 2 to 3 teaspoons of extra-virgin olive oil into the well, and sprinkle with the parsley, if using.

Wine-n-Cheese Spread

Yields 1-1/2 Cups or 12 Servings

Recipe adapted from The Complete Idiot's Guide to Vegan Cooking by Chef Beverly Lynn Bennett - Beverly's newest book aims to "bring out the vegan chef and baker inside you" with over 200 recipes and an entire chapter devoted to making cheese and dairy alternatives. According to Beverly, "Wine and cheese are commonly paired together as an offering at parties and special events, which was the inspiration for this wine-flavored vegan cheese spread." She recommends using caution when selecting wine, as some wine makers will use animal-based agents, such as egg whites and casein to remove impurities. See p83 for resources to find dairy-free / vegan winemakers.

8 Ounces Firm or Extra-Firm Tofu
1 Garlic Clove
1/4 Cup Nutritional Yeast Flakes
2 Tablespoons Raw Tahini
1 Tablespoon Chickpea or Other Light Miso

1 Teaspoon Dijon Mustard
1/2 Teaspoon Paprika
1/2 Teaspoon Salt, or to Taste
2 Tablespoons or More Red Wine of Choice

Crumble the tofu into a food processor [or blender] using your fingers. Add the garlic and process for 1 minute. Add the nutritional yeast, tahini, miso, mustard, paprika, and salt, and process for 1 to 2 minutes or until completely smooth. Add the red wine and process 15 seconds longer. Taste and add additional salt or red wine as desired. Transfer the mixture to a small bowl. Serve with crackers, slices of bread, or fruit, or use as a spread for sandwiches. This spread can be stored in an airtight container in the refrigerator for up to 1 week.

Non-Alcoholic Option: Replace the wine with 2 tablespoons of lemon juice. You can also sprinkle finely chopped pecans or walnuts over the top of the spread, if desired.

Bryanna's Bagna Cauda (Hot Garlic Dip)

Yields 4 Servings or 2 Cups

Recipe adapted from *Nonna's Italian Kitchen* by Bryanna Clark Grogan - *As written by Bryanna, "Bagna cauda means 'hot bath.' It's a very old sauce from Piedmont, although it is eaten all over Italy now. It was popular as far back as the 16th century and today, as then, it makes a wonderful communal antipasto." Traditionally this recipe uses butter or cream, but Bryanna has actually improved the sauce to make it lower in fat, while maintaining its rich, creamy, and garlicky heritage. She recommends serving this dip with a platter of raw vegetables, such as bell peppers, cabbage wedges, celery, and fennel stalks or even cold cooked artichokes, lightly steamed vegetables, or some crusty bread.*

3/4 Cup Plain Almond, Rice, or Soymilk

6 Tablespoons (3 ounces) Extra-Firm Silken Tofu (can be a light version) or 3 Tablespoons Raw Cashews

6 Tablespoons Water

2 Tablespoons Soy, Chickpea, or Other Light Miso

1 "Chicken-style" Vegetarian Broth Cube (enough for 1 cup liquid), Crumbled or 1 Teaspoon Better than Bouillon No Chicken Broth Base

1/4 Cup Extra-Virgin Olive Oil

6 Garlic Cloves, Thinly-Sliced

Freshly Ground Black Pepper, to Taste

Combine the milk alternative, tofu or cashews, water, miso, and broth cube in your blender, and blend until very smooth. Set aside. In a small skillet, heat the olive oil over medium heat. Add the garlic and sauté it slowly until golden, but do not brown it. Remove the garlic [you can use it for another dish] and whisk in the blended mixture. Heat the sauce slowly and add black pepper to taste. Keep the sauce warm (like a fondue) in a heat-proof bowl over a small candle or other warming device.

Hazelnut Bagna Cauda Option: Use hazelnut (filbert) oil instead of the olive oil, and add 1/4 cup of ground, toasted hazelnuts or filberts. You will want to skin the hazelnuts before toasting them. To do this, bring 2 cups of water to boil in a saucepan and add the nuts. Blanch them for 3 to 4 minutes. Drain and rinse in a colander under cold running water; the skins will slide off. Once skinned, you can toast the hazelnuts in your oven, by spreading them evenly in a shallow pan, and baking them for 7 to 15 minutes in a 350°F (175ºC) oven, until they are golden brown. Check in often to stir them and to ensure that they do not burn. Alternately, you can toast them on the stove top, in a dry skillet over medium heat. Stir and shake them over the heat for about 4 minutes, or until the nuts begin to release there flavor.

Rawesome Nut Dip

Yields 1-3/4 Cups

Recipe adapted from Eat, Drink & Be Vegan *by Dreena Burton - In this versatile recipe, Dreena demonstrates her ability to transform simple, all-natural ingredients into flavorful, everyday dishes. According to Dreena, "This dip has a slight 'cheesy' taste, and is in fact a good cheese replacement [see the ideas following the recipe]. For a cheesier flavor, you can add 1 to 2 tablespoons of nutritional yeast, though nutritional yeast may not be considered 'raw'."*

1/2 Cup Raw Almonds
1/2 Cup Raw Pistachios
1/4 Cup Raw Walnuts
1/4 Cup Raw Pine Nuts (or more walnuts, see note)
1/2 Cup Red or Orange Bell Pepper, Chopped
3 to 3-1/2 Tablespoons Freshly Squeezed Lemon Juice
1 Very Small Garlic Clove, Sliced (may use a larger
    clove if desired)

1/2 Teaspoon Sea Salt
Freshly Ground Black Pepper, to Taste
4-1/2 to 6 Tablespoons Water, or More to Thin as
    Desired
1/2 Cup Fresh Basil Leaves
1 to 1-1/2 Teaspoon Fresh Thyme Leaves

In a food processor, combine the nuts, bell pepper, lemon juice (starting with 3 tablespoons), garlic, salt, pepper, and water (starting with 4-1/2 tablespoons), and puree until fairly smooth, scraping down the sides of the bowl several times. Add the basil and thyme, and puree again until well combined and to your desired smoothness. Add more lemon juice to taste and/or water to thin the dip, if desired.

Nut Note: You may change the proportions of nuts in this recipe or substitute with other nuts or seeds. Note that nuts differ in natural sweetness and bitterness; cashews, almonds, and pistachios have sweeter flavors, whereas walnuts and pine nuts have more savory and bitter tones. Since substitutions will affect the overall flavor, you may want to adjust the lemon juice or salt to taste. Truly raw almonds are hard to come by, but just make sure you are using nuts that are not roasted or salted.

How to Use: On her blog (vivelevegan.blogspot.com), Dreena offers a list of suggestions for how to use this recipe for much more than dipping:
~   Spread on bread/pitas with fresh vegetables for scrumptious sandwiches!
~   Layered in lasagna (dollop on one or two layers).
~   As a pizza base instead of tomato sauce. Spread on a whole-wheat (p207) or spelt crust (p208) then sprinkle on your toppings of choice.
~   As a baked potato topping. Either use raw, or mix with some of the potato flesh and re-bake for some super stuffed spuds!
~   Used as a filling for stuffing pastas like manicotti, giant shells, or ravioli.
~   Tossed into beans or spooned onto cooked grains.
~   As a soup garnish, especially for a lighter soup like tomato. Serve with a scoop of this dip.

Perfect Popcorn

Yields approximately 8 Cups (2 quarts)

3 Tablespoons Corn Oil or Other High Heat Oil (p113)   1/4 Teaspoon Salt, or to Taste (optional)
1/3 Cup Organic or Non-GMO Popcorn Kernels

Heat the oil in a large saucepan or pot over medium-high heat. Throw a few popcorn kernels into the pot and cover it. Once the kernels pop, your oil is hot enough to start. Add the rest of the popcorn kernels and the salt, if using. Cover, remove the pan from the heat and count 30 seconds. Return the pan to the heat. Once the popping begins, gently shake the pan by moving it back and forth over the burner. When the popping slows to more than 5 seconds between pops, remove it from the heat. Carefully remove the lid as some kernels may still pop and the steam is hot. Transfer the popcorn to a dish to serve.

Cheezy Popcorn

Yields 4 Cups

Recipe adapted from *The Ultimate Uncheese Cookbook* by Jo Stepaniak - *Impress everyone with a big bowl of this snack on your next movie night. Jo uses air-popped popcorn, but you can use the Perfect Popcorn recipe above.*

4 Cups Air-Popped Popcorn   1/2 Teaspoon Salt, or to Taste
Olive Oil Spray   1/2 Teaspoon Garlic Powder
1/3 Cup Nutritional Yeast Flakes   1/4 Teaspoon Onion Powder
1/2 to 1 Teaspoon Chili Powder or Curry Powder

Place the warm popcorn in a large bowl and mist it with olive oil. Toss gently and mist again. Repeat until all the kernels are lightly coated with the oil. Combine the remaining ingredients in a zipper-lock plastic bag. Seal the bag and shake until the seasonings are well mixed. Drop in the popcorn, a small amount at a time, seal the bag, and shake and turn the bag to coat the popcorn evenly. Continue to add a small amount of popcorn to the bag until all of the kernels are well coated. Store the popcorn in the zipper-lock bag. Gently shake again just before serving.

Caramel Corn

Yields 4 to 5 Cups

Recipe created by Hannah Kaminsky, author of *My Sweet Vegan*

4 to 5 Cups Popped Popcorn   1/4 Teaspoon Salt
1/3 Cup Granulated Sugar   1/8 Teaspoon Cream of Tartar
1/4 Cup Pure Maple Syrup, Agave Nectar, or Brown   1 Tablespoon Dairy-Free Margarine
   Rice Syrup   1/2 Teaspoon Baking Soda

Place the popped corn in a large mixing bowl with all un-popped kernels removed, and set aside. Lay a non-stick baking mat or sheet near the stove. In a medium-sized saucepan, combine the sugar, syrup or agave, salt, and cream of tartar. Bring it to a boil over medium heat and toss in the margarine, stirring until it melts. Clip on your candy thermometer and continue to cook the sugar syrup, stirring occasionally, until it reaches 250ºF (120ºC), or the firm ball stage. Turn off the heat, stir in the baking soda, and quickly pour the syrup over the popcorn, tossing to thoroughly coat. Spread the coated popcorn out on your non-stick mat and break up as many clumps as you can. Let cool and harden before storing the caramel corn in an air-tight container at room temperature.

Cheezy Quackers

Yields 30 to 60 Crackers

Recipe adapted from the blog, Have Cake Will Travel (www.havecakewilltravel.com) by Celine Steen - *The concept of homemade crackers never occurred to me until Celine came up with dairy-free cheesy crackers ... or quackers to be more specific. Yes, she even used mini duck-shaped cutters, but they will taste just as good cut into squares.*

1 Cup All-Purpose (Plain) or Whole Wheat Pastry
   Flour
1/3 Cup Nutritional Yeast Flakes
1 Teaspoon Sea Salt
1/2 Teaspoon Black Pepper, or to Taste

Generous 1/4 Cup Dairy-Free Margarine, 3
   Tablespoons Shortening, or 3 to 4 Tablespoons
   Oil (grapeseed, olive, or peanut will work well)
Up to 1/4 Cup Water

Place the flour, nutritional yeast, salt, pepper, and margarine, shortening, or oil in a large mixing bowl. Blend with a hand mixer until the mixture resembles coarse flour. Add the water little by little until the dough forms a ball. You probably won't need it all. If your dough isn't ready to be rolled out, place it in plastic wrap in the refrigerator to chill for 30 minutes or so.

Preheat your oven to 350ºF (175ºC) and line two baking sheets with parchment paper or non-stick baking mats. Roll your dough out on a clean surface to about 1/3 of an inch thick (this will yield "Goldfish" height crackers). Cut out shapes using the smallest cookie cutters you have. Re-roll the dough, and cutout shapes again, until there is no dough left. Place the crackers on your prepared baking sheets, and bake them for 15 to 17 minutes, or until the crackers are set and light golden on the bottom. Remove the crackers to a wire rack to cool. If you manage to keep them around for that long, they keep well in freezer/sandwich bags.

Wheat-Free Version: Follow the directions above, but use 1 cup plus 6 tablespoons of light spelt flour in place of the flour, use 1/4 cup of peanut oil (or other oil) for the fat, and use 4 to 6 tablespoons of water (however much is needed to make the dough manageable).

Chocolate Figs

Yields 4 Servings or 24 Bite-Sized Treats

I have experimented with several fig recipes, but I find that the simpler the better with this calcium-rich dried fruit. This recipe is equally delicious with white chocolate, should you happen to have a dairy-free variety on hand, or if you decide to make a batch from Hannah's recipe on p135. These are great for a decadent snack or for parties.

4 Ounces Semi-Sweet or Dark Chocolate, Chips or
   Chopped
24 Whole Dried Figs

1/2 Cup Finely Chopped Pistachios, Macadamia Nuts,
   or Your Favorite Nut (optional)

Line a baking sheet with wax paper, and place the nuts in a small bowl. Set both aside. Place the chocolate in a microwave-safe bowl and microwave it on HIGH in 30 second intervals (just 2 to 3 should suffice), stirring vigorously between intervals, until the chocolate has just melted and is smooth. Be careful not to overheat the chocolate, as it can scorch easily. If you prefer, you can melt the chocolate in a double broiler, stirring often, I am just a bit lazy. Dip a fig in the chocolate, then dip the bottom half in the chopped nuts, and place it onto a baking sheet lined with wax paper or a non-stick baking mat. Repeat this process with the remaining figs, chocolate, and nuts. Refrigerate for 20 to 30 minutes, or until the chocolate has hardened. Store them in an airtight container for up to one week.

Carob Fudgies

Yields 20 Bite-Sized Snacks

I am a true carob fan, so this is one snack I could easily enjoy as dessert and chocolate replacement. Though somewhat indulgent, these treats are packed with protein, "healthy" fats, and a good little dose of calcium per fudgie.

1/2 Cup Creamy Almond, Peanut, or Sunflower Butter
1/2 Cup Agave Nectar, Honey, or Light Corn Syrup
1/2 Cup Sifted Carob Powder (sift then measure)

1/2 Cup Sesame Seeds
1/4 Cup Unsweetened Shredded Coconut

In a small saucepan, combine the nut or seed butter and the sweetener. Stir over medium-low heat until the two are melted together, about 2 to 3 minutes. Remove from the heat, and gradually stir in the carob powder, followed by the sesame seeds, until everything is well combined. Place the carob mixture in the refrigerator for 10 to 15 minutes to set up. Place the coconut in a small dish. Remove the carob fudge from the refrigerator and using a spoon, scoop up some of the fudge. With your hands roll it into a 1-inch ball, and roll it in the coconut. Repeat with the remaining fudge. Store them in the refrigerator.

Trail Mix Carob Fudgie Option: Along with the sesame seeds, add 1/2 cup sunflower seeds and 1/2 cup chopped walnuts.

Chewy No-Bake Granola Bars

Yields 16 to 20 Bars

This is one of those recipes that literally took me a dozen times to perfect. After many failed attempts at baked granola bars, I realized that the chewy granola bar I was craving required no baking at all. My husband is addicted to these, so I often make a large batch, and store them in the refrigerator or freezer.

3 Cups Crispy Rice Cereal
2-1/4 Cups Quick-Cooking Oats
1/2 Cup Sliced Almonds
1/2 Cup Unsweetened Shredded Coconut
2/3 Cup Semi-Sweet Chocolate Chips (mini chips if available)

1/2 Cup Agave Nectar or Corn Syrup
1/4 Cup Light Brown Sugar, Firmly Packed
1 Cup Creamy Almond Butter or Peanut Butter
1-1/2 Teaspoons Vanilla Extract
1/2 Teaspoon Salt (omit if using salted nut butter)

Grease a 9x13-inch baking dish. Combine the cereal, oats, almonds, and coconut in a large bowl, and set aside. In a small saucepan, bring the agave or corn syrup and the brown sugar just to a boil over medium heat. Immediately remove from the heat and stir in the nut butter, vanilla, and salt. Gently stir this hot gooey mixture into your awaiting cereal mix until it is well incorporated. Let it sit and cool for about 2 minutes. Stir in the chocolate chips. Press the mixture firmly (as firm as you can manage!) into your prepared dish. Using a sheet of wax paper or a sandwich baggie around your hand while pressing will help to avoid sticking issues. Freeze the bars for 30 minutes.

Remove the granola from the freezer, and cut it into fourths lengthwise, and then cut each quarter into 4 to 5 longish granola bars. Store the bars in the refrigerator or freezer for an easy "anytime" snack.

Nut-Free Option: Replace the almonds with more oats, coconut, seeds, or chopped dried fruit and use sunflower butter in place of the nut butter. If coconut is also a problem, replace it with more oats, seeds, and/or dried fruit.

Fruity Frozen Yogurt Pops

Yields 4 Servings

This easy recipe has kid-friendly appeal, and offers a nice healthy treat on a hot day. I have been told that probiotics are preserved when frozen, so this is a cool way to enjoy the live active cultures in dairy-free yogurt.

1 Heaping Cup or 2 6-Ounce Containers Plain or Vanilla Dairy-Free Yogurt
1 Heaping Cup Fresh or Frozen Fruit (blueberries, strawberries, and peaches work well)

2 Tablespoons Agave Nectar, Honey, or Granulated Sugar
1 Teaspoon Lemon Juice (optional)

Place all of the ingredients into your blender, and blend to your desired consistency. Pour the mixture into 4 freezer pop molds. If you don't have freezer pop molds, fill 4 5-ounce paper cups with the yogurt mixture. Top the cups with foil and make a slit into the center of each and insert a wooden stick before freezing. Freeze for several hours, or until the yogurt pops are frozen solid.

Your Basic Vanilla Pudding

Yields 4 Servings

This easy pudding performs best with a milk alternative that has a little fat, such as soymilk, nut milk, or coconut milk (regular or light), but any milk alternative, including rice, will do in a pinch.

1/3 Cup Granulated Sugar
3 Tablespoons Cornstarch
1/4 Teaspoon Salt
2 Cups Cold Plain Milk Alternative (see intro)

1 Teaspoon Vanilla Extract
1 Tablespoon Dairy-free Margarine (optional)
Nutmeg (optional)

Combine the sugar, cornstarch, and salt in a medium-sized saucepan. Slowly add the milk alternative while whisking to eliminate any lumps. Once the mixture is smooth, place it over medium heat. Cook and stir until the mixture thickens enough to coat the back of a metal spoon, but do not allow it to boil. Remove from the heat, and stir in the vanilla and margarine, if using. Pour the pudding into four serving dishes, and sprinkle with a dash of nutmeg, if using. Chill for at least 2 hours before serving.

Instant Rice Pudding Option: After adding the margarine, stir in 2 cups of cooked brown or white rice. You may also stir in 1/2 teaspoon ground cinnamon and/or 1/2 cup of raisins, if desired. Chill as directed above.

Banana Pudding Parfait Option: Once the pudding has chilled and set, divide half of the pudding between four parfait glasses. Top the pudding with a few banana slices in each glass. Repeat the layers with the remaining half of the pudding, followed by another layer of banana slices. If desired, garnish or serve with vanilla wafers.

Custardy Option: Lightly beat 1 to 2 egg yolks. Before adding the vanilla, stir a small amount of the hot pudding into the egg yolks, and return it all to the pan. Cook and stir for 1 minute more before removing the pudding from the heat and stirring in the vanilla and margarine, if using.

More Menu Ideas: Quick Snacks

Of course, there are many other snack ideas which don't really require a recipe …

~ *Ants on a Log* - Go with black ants (raisins) on a peanut butter-filled celery log or red ants (dried cranberries) on an almond butter-filled celery log.

~ *Hummus with Pita Wedges* - Hummus is almost always dairy-free, whether store-bought or prepared at home, and it often comes in interesting flavor variations.

~ *Homemade Trail Mix* - Toss together your favorite nuts, seeds, dried fruit, and/or sweet treats, such as semi-sweet chocolate chips.

~ *Orange or Apple Wedges* - Sprinkle them with cinnamon (yes, the orange slices too) to bring out their naturally sweet flavor. If traveling, give the apples a quick squirt of lemon or pineapple juice to help prevent browning.

~ *Peanut Butter/Honey Dip* – Sweeten some peanut butter with honey or agave nectar to taste. Use it as a dip for apple slices or pretzels.

~ *Melon Wedges* - Fill them with a scoop of dairy-free yogurt.

~ *Cinnamon Nut Butter Spread* - Combine 2 tablespoons of your favorite nut butter with a few shakes of cinnamon, a dash of your favorite sweetener, and 2 tablespoons of raisins or other dried fruit. Use as a spread on plain rice cakes or whole grain toast.

~ *Edamame* - Boil these baby soybean pods in lightly salted water for 3 to 5 minutes, or until bright green. Sprinkle them with coarse sea salt, and enjoy popping the beans out as you eat them.

~ *Pumpkinseed Crunch* - Toast pumpkin seeds on a baking sheet coated with cooking spray. If desired, stir in seasonings, such as a teaspoon of olive oil, garlic powder, or mixed herbs.

~ *Oven Baked S'mores* - Split some graham crackers into halves, place one half of each on a baking sheet, and top with several mini-marshmallows (vegan or regular). Place the baking sheet in a 450ºF (230ºC) oven until toasty (just a few brief minutes). Remove and top the marshmallows with a couple squares of chocolate, followed by the other half of each graham cracker. Smash and enjoy.

~ *Tortilla Chips and Salsa or Guacamole* – This is my husband's go-to snack when the munchies hit. Most brands of plain or salted tortilla chips are dairy-free. Guacamole is typically dairy-free, but you should always check the labels for sour cream or other milk additives.

~ *Fruit Salad* - Toss together a seasonal blend of chopped fruit, for a nutritious and sweet snack. Feel free to defrost firm frozen fruits, such as mango or blueberries, for a flavor burst when fresh varieties are not in season.

~ *Banana "Ice Cream"* - Freeze banana slices and puree them in your food processor or blender until smooth. Viola, instant "ice cream!" If using a blender, you may need to let the bananas defrost for 10 minutes before pureeing, or add a touch of milk alternative or coconut milk to get things moving.

~ *Popcorn* - Make up a batch in an air popper or via the old-fashioned method (on the stove top), drizzle with a bit of oil or margarine, and sprinkle with salt, some nutritional yeast, and/or your seasonings of choice.

~ *Frozen Grapes* – Sometimes the simplest foods are the most rewarding. Grapes freeze wonderfully in baggies, and they make a perfect healthy snack on a hot summer day.

~ *Tortilla Roll-Ups* – Tortillas come in many sizes, shapes, and flavors (including brown rice and spelt for gluten-free and wheat-free, respectively). I like to grab a spinach flour tortilla and slather it with dairy-free "cream cheese" (homemade from p122 or store-bought), followed by some garlic and olive tapenade. I roll it up and slice it into rounds for a quick snack. Other roll-up fillings may include canned green chilies, sliced olives, sliced avocado or guacamole (in place of the "cream cheese"), deli meats, chopped walnuts or pecans, mayonnaise, lettuce, etc.

Some Store-Bought Recommendations for Snacks:
There are many great brands on the market, but the following recommendations only include products that I purchase with some regularity or that a colleague highly recommended. For full lists of non-dairy, packaged foods and brands, see the product lists available on www.godairyfree.org.

Arico Foods (www.aricofoods.com, (866) 98-ARICO) ~ chips and cookies snacks
There are several brands and generics of potato chips that will be perfectly suitable for dairy-free diets, but Arico's Cassava Chips are worth the occasional splurge in my opinion. All four flavors are free from dairy and gluten (this can be hard to find with the flavored chips varieties), and the taste and crunch are quite unique from your average chip.

Clif Bar® (www.clifbar.com, (800) 254-3227) ~ energy bars
For years we have been loyal Clif Bar customers, enjoying their original product line, in addition to their newer Clif Nectar™ and Clif Mojo™ bars. The Nectar bars have a simple "raw" base of dates and nuts, accompanied by some natural spices The Mojo bars are more trail mix in nature, covering those sweet and salty cravings nicely. The entire Clif line is dairy-free and vegan by ingredients, but they do run the risk of trace amounts of dairy due to manufacturing processes.

Eco-Planet™ (www.eco-planet.net, (310) 829-9050) ~ snack cookies and crackers
These are the most adorable and tasty snacks I could ever imagine giving to my nieces; okay, I might sneak a few for myself. Eco-Planet™ produces organic bite-sized crackers (including non-dairy cheddar!) and tasty morsels that liken themselves to animal cookies, but with a much better taste and a crispier crunch. Plus, these snacks come in eco-friendly shapes: windmills, winking suns, hybrid cars, and snapshots of the earth.

Emerald® (www.emeraldnuts.com) ~ nut and snack mixes
The glazed nuts from Emerald's border on dessert, but I have trouble resisting these bags whenever I spot them on sale at my local pharmacy. After all, how often do I find a bag of caramel-glazed pecans that is made without milk ingredients?

Envirokidz™ (www.naturespath.com, (888) 808-9505) ~ bar and cookie snacks
The Envirokidz™ line from Nature's Path offers Crispy Rice Bars in various kid-friendly flavors (though not all are dairy-free) in addition to some popular Animal Cookies.

Grandpa Po's (www.nutranuts.com, (323) 260-7457) ~ popcorn snacks
This simple mix of organic popcorn and soybeans, occasionally with a touch of salt or seasoning thrown in, is really quite addicting. This is another one I would be thrilled to stumble across on a road trip.

Kinnikinnick (www.kinnikinnick.com, (780) 424-2900) ~ animal crackers
For gluten-free animal crackers, look no further than Kinnikinnick. Actually, my gluten-loving sister and I could not stop inhaling these ourselves ... but, I have heard some rave kid reviews too.

Larabar® (www.larabar.com, (720) 945-1155) ~ energy bars
These are just about as pure as packaged energy bars get. They are made with unsweetened dried fruits, nuts and spices ... that's it. If you aren't a date fan, then they might not be to your liking, but overall the Larabar line is quite pleasing and popular. Plus, these raw bars are suitable for most special diets, aside from nut allergies.

Late July® (www.latejuly.com, (508) 362-5859) ~ cracker and cookie snack packs
Late July offers delicious Ritz-like crackers and Oreo™-like sandwich cookies that are organic, all-natural and made without milk ingredients. The crackers come as is, with a nice buttery taste, or with a layer of peanut butter sandwiched between (of course, stay away from their cheddar cheese filled sandwich crackers). The crackers, cracker sandwiches, and sandwich crème cookies are available in snack packs.

Lundberg (www.lundberg.com, (530) 882-4551) ~ rice products
As I type, nearly a dozen bags of Lundberg Rice Cakes are stashed in my pantry. I am utterly addicted to these slathered with nut butter or a homemade spread. They offer many flavors of rice cakes and rice chips (a few are not dairy-free), though I am still content with the plain, unsalted.

Peeled Snacks® (www.peeledsnacks.com, (646) 290-5313) ~ dried fruit snacks
I was convinced that dried fruit was dried fruit until I tasted the fruit and nut mixes from Peeled Snacks. They are void of additives and sugars (including the mango) and taste deliciously fresh. Even the nuts take freshness to a new level. I am hoping to see these in convenience stores soon.

Robert's American Gourmet® (www.robscape.com) ~ chips, crisps, and puffs
This company offers a variety of American-style snacks in an all-natural format, some dairy-free and vegan, some not. But their Tings®, which come in both baked and fried varieties, have a special place in the hearts of many. Like mellowed out Cheetohs®, Tings® have a puffy crisp and a cheesy vibe, but they are in fact dairy-free. Most of the Robscape product line is also gluten-free.

Toby's Family Foods (www.tobysfamilyfoods.com, (541) 689.8506) ~ creamy dip
Toby's Tofu Paté is a creamy, delightful, and insanely unique spread / dip that is unfortunately, hard to find. But … I always stock up when I do spot it in my local natural food store. It is great for parties, regular snacking, or as a bagel spread.

CHAPTER 22:
SOUP'S ON

Roasted Eggplant & Tomato Soup
Yields 4 to 6 Servings

The satiny finish of this delicate soup makes it perfect for impressing dinner guests or a light summer meal. The addition of coconut cream or nut crème really is optional, but it makes for a rich and comforting "crème of ..." experience. For a lighter indulgence, skip the crème, but top each bowl with a dollop of Sour Cashew Crème (p131).

2 Tablespoons Grapeseed or Olive oil, Divided (plus extra for greasing)
1 lb Tomatoes (about 3 medium), Halved
1 Medium Eggplant (1-1/4 to 1-1/2 lbs), Halved Lengthwise
6 Garlic Cloves, Peeled
1 Small Onion or 2 Large Shallots, Chopped

1 Tablespoon Chopped Fresh Thyme or Basil or 1 Teaspoon Dried
4 Cups Chicken or No-Chicken Broth
1/8 Teaspoon Crushed Red Pepper Flakes (optional)
1/2 Teaspoon Salt, or to Taste
1 Cup Nutty Crème (p128) or Regular Coconut Milk / Cream (optional)
Freshly Ground Black Pepper, to Taste (optional)

Preheat your oven to 400ºF (205ºC) and grease a large baking dish with oil. Place the tomatoes and eggplant halves cut side down in the baking dish, along with the garlic. Drizzle the vegetables and garlic with 1 tablespoon of the oil; ensure that everything is well-coated. Roast the vegetables in your preheated oven until they are very tender and the skins are brown in spots, about 40 to 45 minutes. Set aside to cool for a few minutes.

Heat the remaining 1 tablespoon of oil in a large pot over medium heat. Add the onions or shallots and sauté until tender and translucent, about 5 minutes. Add the thyme and sauté for just 30 seconds. Pour in the chicken broth, crushed red pepper (if using), and salt. At this point, you should be able to easily pinch off the skins of the tomatoes, and peel the pulp away from the eggplant shell. Add the eggplant and tomato pulp and the garlic cloves to your soup pot. Bring everything to a boil, reduce the heat to low, cover, and simmer for 5 to 10 minutes, allowing the flavors to meld. Using an immersion blender, puree the soup, or transfer it to your blender in batches (this will take 2 to 3 batches, depending on the capacity of your blender) and puree until smooth and creamy, about 2 to 3 minutes.

The eggplant and tomatoes have little seeds that may not be processed by your blender. If desired, after whirling, strain the soup back into your pot using a fine mesh strainer or a double layer of cheesecloth to create the smoothest consistency. Return the soup to the pot, stir in the nut crème or coconut milk/cream, if using. Give it a taste test, and season with additional salt and pepper, if desired.

Condensed "Cream" of Mushroom Soup

Yields 10-3/4 Ounces or the Equivalent to 1 Can of "The Original"

Here it is, one of the most requested dairy-free recipes on the planet. My engineer / at-home-chef husband and I dissected the ingredients on the original Campbell's can, calculated, tested, and finally came up with this version that we believe is as close as you can get without the MSG, "modified" ingredients, and secret spices used in their version. Amazingly, this mock recipe is fairly low in fat and takes just one pan and mere minutes to prepare.

1-1/4 Cups Cold Unsweetened Cashew, Rice, or
    Soymilk
2 Tablespoons All-Purpose (Plain) Flour or White Rice
    Flour
1 Tablespoon Cornstarch
1 Tablespoon Grapeseed, Canola, or Vegetable Oil

3/4 to 1 Teaspoon Salt
1/8 Teaspoon Onion Powder
Generous Pinch Garlic Powder
1/2 Cup Canned Mushrooms (pieces and stems),
    Drained

In a small saucepan, whisk together the cold milk alternative, flour, cornstarch, oil, 3/4 teaspoon of salt, onion powder, and garlic powder until smooth (or process the ingredients in your blender until smooth). Stir in the mushrooms. Place the soup over medium-low heat and whisk continuously until the mixture thickens significantly, about 10 minutes. Remember, you are looking for a very thick, condensed cream of mushroom soup consistency. Once complete, it will weigh out to roughly 10-3/4 ounces or 1-1/4 cups.

Use in recipes as you would the original. Alternately, prepare the soup by thinning with water (roughly 1 cup) over low heat, stirring continuously until it reaches your desired consistency and temperature.

Condensed "Cream" of Celery Option: Briefly sauté 1 cup of diced celery in 1 teaspoon of oil over medium-low heat, just 2 to 3 minutes. Add the celery to the original recipe in place of the mushrooms.

Light Vichyssoise (aka Potato-Leek Soup)

Yields 4 Servings

Who says you can't enjoy French cuisine without dairy? This year-round soup is delicious, whether served chilled, at room temperature, or heated. In my opinion, Yukon Gold potatoes are the best choice for their buttery taste, but feel free to substitute another white-skinned potato should they not be available.

4 Large Leeks (white part only), Thinly Sliced
1 Garlic Clove, Minced
3 Cups Vegetable Broth or Stock, Divided
1 lb Yukon Gold Potatoes, Peeled (optional) and
    Chopped into 1/2-Inch Chunks

2 Tablespoons Dairy-Free Margarine
Pinch Nutmeg
1/4 Teaspoon Salt, or to Taste
1/4 Teaspoon White Pepper
4 Chives or Green Onions (green part only), Chopped

Combine the leeks, garlic, and 1 cup of the broth or stock in a stockpot over medium-high heat. Bring the broth to a boil, reduce the heat to low, cover and cook until the leeks just begin to soften, about 6 to 8 minutes. Add the potatoes and the remaining 2 cups of broth, cover and cook until the potatoes are soft, about 20 minutes. Remove the soup from the heat, and stir in the margarine, nutmeg, salt, and pepper. Allow the soup to cool for a few minutes. Using an immersion blender, puree the soup until smooth, or transfer the soup to your blender in batches (this will take 2 to 3 batches, depending upon the capacity of your blender) and puree until smooth. This soup may be served immediately (hot), allowed to cool to room temperature, or chilled. To chill, cover and place in the refrigerator for at least 3 hours. To serve, top each bowl with the chopped chives or green onions.

Lightly Curried Cruciferous Soup

Yields 3 to 4 Servings

My husband dislikes the flavor of Indian curries and he really isn't a fan of cauliflower, but even he admitted that this was a subtler mix of spices, which seemed to work nicely with the creamy vegetable base. The fact that he went back for seconds solidified this one as a winner.

1 Tablespoon Olive Oil, Grapeseed Oil, or Dairy-Free Margarine

1/2 Cup Chopped Sweet Onion (about 1/2 small to medium)

1 to 2 Teaspoons Garam Masala, Store-Bought or Homemade (see below)

2 Garlic Cloves, Minced

4 Cups Chicken or Vegetable Broth

1/2 to 1 Teaspoon Salt, or to Taste

12 Ounces Cauliflower Florets (roughly 1 small head)

6 Ounces Broccoli Florets (roughly 1 medium crown)

1 Teaspoon Lemon Juice (optional)

Heat the oil or margarine in a large pot over medium-low heat. Add the onion and sauté for 5 minutes, or until it begins to soften. Add the garam masala and garlic and sauté everything for just 1 more minute. Stir in the broth, 1/2 teaspoon of the salt, and add the cauliflower and broccoli florets. Bring the soup to a boil, reduce the heat to medium-low, cover and allow the vegetables to simmer for 20 minutes, or until the cauliflower is quite tender. Using an immersion blender, puree the soup, or transfer it to your blender in batches (this will take 2 to 3 batches, depending on the capacity of your blender) and puree until smooth, about 2 to 3 minutes. Return the soup to the pot and stir in additional salt and lemon juice to taste, if desired.

Homemade Garam Masala:
Combine all of the following ingredients to make 2 teaspoons of Garam Masala:

1/4 Teaspoon Ground Cardamom

1/2 + 1/8 Teaspoon Ground Coriander

1/2 Teaspoon Ground Cumin

1/4 Teaspoon Ground Black Pepper

1/8 Teaspoon Ground Cloves

1/8 Teaspoon Ground Cinnamon

1/8 Teaspoon Ground Nutmeg

For a larger batch to keep on hand, the following will yield 1/3 cup of Garam Masala:

2 Teaspoons Ground Cardamom

5 Teaspoons Ground Coriander

4 Teaspoons Ground Cumin

2 Teaspoons Ground Black Pepper

1 Teaspoon Ground Cloves

1 Teaspoon Ground Cinnamon

1 Teaspoon Ground Nutmeg

Even Creamier Option: Reduce the broth by 1 cup. After blending the soup, return it to your pot and stir in 1 cup of unsweetened coconut, rice, or soymilk. Alternately, you can add a swirl of coconut cream or nutty crème (p128), or 1/2 to 1 cup of milk alternative to the recipe above after pureeing.

Potato Corn Chowder

Yields 4 Servings

Recipe adapted from the blog, Non-Dairy Queen (thenondairyqueen.blogspot.com) by Sarena Shasteen - *I can always count on Sarena for simple, nutritious, and comforting recipes. To keep this soup very low in fat, she uses Smart Balance™ Light (www.smartbalance.com, (201) 568-9300) for the margarine.*

2 Tablespoons Dairy-Free Margarine
1/2 Cup Chopped Onion (about 1/2 small to medium)
2 Tablespoons All-Purpose (Plain) Flour
3 Cups Plain or Unsweetened Rice, Almond, or
    Soymilk
2 Cups Diced Cooked Potatoes

1-1/2 Cups Frozen Corn
1-1/4 Teaspoon Dried Thyme
1 14.75-Ounce Can Cream-Style Corn
Salt, to Taste
Freshly Ground Black Pepper, to Taste

Melt the margarine in a large stockpot or Dutch oven over medium heat. Add the onion and sauté for 3 minutes, or until tender. Add the flour and cook for 1 minute, while stirring constantly. Gradually stir in the milk alternative, and add the potatoes, frozen corn, thyme, and cream-style corn. Bring the soup to a light boil while continuing to stir, and cook until it thickens a bit, about 5 minutes. Season the soup to taste with salt and pepper.

"Cream" of Asparagus Soup

Yields 6 to 8 Servings

When we lived in North Lake Tahoe there was a wonderful restaurant that we liked to visit on special occasions, Soule Domain. Every night, the chef prepared a soup that was served to every guest. It was always dairy-free and vegan, yet incredibly luxurious. One night, I asked the chef's secret. He said it was simple, "just boil some white rice in broth or water with your vegetable of choice, puree, and season to taste." He was right; it really is that simple ...

2 lbs Asparagus
2 Tablespoons Olive or Grapeseed Oil
2 Medium-Sized Onions, Chopped into 1/2-Inch
    Pieces (about 3 cups)
2 Garlic Cloves, Minced

2/3 Cup Uncooked White Basmati or Jasmine Rice
8 Cups Chicken, No Chicken, or Vegetable Broth
2 Sprigs Fresh Thyme or 1/2 Teaspoon Dried Thyme
1 Teaspoon Salt, or to Taste
Freshly Ground Black Pepper, to Taste

Trim the woody ends from the asparagus, and cut the remaining stalks into 1/2-inch pieces, reserving the tips. Set aside. Heat the oil in a large pot over medium heat. Add the onions and sauté for 5 minutes, or until soft and translucent. Add the garlic and sauté just 1 minute more. Stir in the asparagus pieces (but not the tips), rice, broth, thyme, and salt. Bring the soup to a boil, reduce the heat to low, cover and simmer for 25 to 30 minutes, or until the rice is very tender. If using thyme sprigs, remove them. Using an immersion blender, puree the soup, or transfer it to your blender in batches (this will take 3 to 4 batches, depending on the capacity of your blender) and puree until smooth and creamy, about 2 to 3 minutes. Return the soup to your pot, add the asparagus tips, and simmer for about 5 minutes, or until the asparagus tips are bright green and crisp tender. Season the soup with additional salt (if desired) and freshly ground pepper to taste.

"Cream" of Broccoli Option: Substitute 2 lbs of broccoli florets for the asparagus, reserving 1 cup of small florets to stir in at the end when you would be adding the asparagus tips.

Peanut Buttery African Stew

Yields 4 Servings

For years I was intrigued by the comforting sound of African stew. After perusing many recipe ideas, I finally got up the nerve to trial my own version. The result was this recipe of rich, peanut buttery deliciousness!

2 Tablespoons Peanut or Olive Oil
1 Cup Diced Onion (about 1 medium)
4 Garlic Cloves, Minced
1 Tablespoon Minced Fresh Ginger
1-1/2 lbs Sweet Potatoes (about 2 medium), Peeled
    and Cut into 3/4-Inch Chunks (about 4 cups)
1 lb Tomatoes, Diced
1/2 to 1 Teaspoon Minced Jalapeno Peppers,
    Deseeded

1 Cup Vegetable or Chicken Broth
1-1/2 Cups Water
1 Teaspoon Salt, or to Taste
3/4 lb Cauliflower Florets (about 6 cups)
1/4 Cup Creamy, Unsalted Peanut Butter
4 Cups Cooked Brown Rice, Couscous, or Quinoa
2 Cups Packed Baby Spinach Leaves
1 Small Lime, Cut into 4 Wedges

Heat the oil in a large pot over medium heat. Add the onion and sauté until tender and translucent, about 3 to 5 minutes. Add the garlic and ginger and sauté for another minute. Add the sweet potatoes, tomatoes, and jalapeno, and cook for 5 minutes. Add the broth, water and salt. Bring the stew to a boil, reduce the heat to medium-low, cover and simmer for 10 minutes. Add the cauliflower, cover, and cook 10 to 15 minutes more, or until the vegetables are tender. Remove about 1/2 cup of the liquid from the soup and whisk the peanut butter into it. Return the soup with the peanut butter to the pot, and continue to cook the stew for 5 minutes, uncovered, while stirring. It should thicken a bit. Spoon 1 cup of brown rice, couscous, or quinoa into each of four bowls. Top each bowl with 1/2 cup of fresh spinach leaves. Ladle the hot stew over top of the spinach, and serve each bowl with a lime wedge.

Quick & Creamy Bean Soup

Yields 4 Servings

I like to use pinto beans in this soup, due to the color they impart when cooked with the paprika and tomatoes, but black beans are equally tasty. If you are sensitive to salt, feel free to use low sodium broth and adjust the salt to taste after cooking, as the spices do help to flavor this soup quite a bit on their own.

2 Teaspoons Peanut, Olive, or Grapeseed Oil
1 Cup Chopped Onion (about 1 small to medium)
1 Small Jalapeno Pepper, Deseeded and Minced
2 to 4 Garlic Cloves, Minced
1-1/2 Teaspoons Ground Cumin
1 Teaspoon Dried Oregano
1/2 Teaspoon Paprika

2 Cups Vegetable Broth
1 14.5-Ounce Can Diced Tomatoes or 1 lb Tomatoes,
    Chopped
2 15-Ounce Cans Pinto or Black Beans, Drained and
    Rinsed
1 to 2 Teaspoons Lime Juice (optional)
1/4 to 1/2 Teaspoon Salt, or to Taste

Heat the oil in a large saucepan or pot over medium-low heat. Add the onions and sauté for about 5 minutes, or until they begin to soften. Add the jalapeno and garlic, and sauté for 1 minute. Add the cumin, oregano, and paprika, and sauté for 1 minute more. Slowly stir in the broth, and finally, add the tomatoes, beans, lime juice (if using), and 1/4 teaspoon of salt, if using. Bring the soup to a boil, reduce the heat to low, cover and simmer for 15 minutes. Using an immersion blender, puree the soup, or transfer it to your blender in batches (this will take 2 to 3 batches, depending on the capacity of your blender) and puree until smooth, about 2 to 3 minutes. Adjust the salt to taste, if desired.

Optional Garnish: Serve topped with a dollop of Sour Cashew Crème (p131), Silken "Sour Cream" (p131), chopped avocados, and/or crushed tortilla chips.

Spiced Autumn Soup

Yields 4 Servings

My good blogging friend Janelle, over at Talk of Tomatoes (www.talkoftomatoes.com), inspired this recipe. Using her Pumpkin Ginger Soup as a guide, I simplified the recipe for the time impaired, added some dairy-free touches, and voila, a rich and nutritious soup! This recipe provides a ton of beta carotene, or the "good" vitamin A. You can add up to 2 tablespoons of sweetener (Janelle used brown sugar) but I found the soup to be sweet enough as is.

1 Tablespoon Olive, Vegetable, or Grapeseed Oil
2/3 Cup Minced Onion (about 1 small)
2 to 4 Garlic Cloves, Minced
1/2 Teaspoon Ground Ginger
1/4 Teaspoon Ground Nutmeg
1/8 Teaspoon Ground Cloves
1/8 Teaspoon Ground Cardamom
3 Cups Vegetable Broth

1/4 Teaspoon Salt
8 Ounces Cubed Butternut Squash*
1 Cup Baby Carrots
2/3 Cup Canned Pumpkin Puree
1 Cup Plain or Unsweetened Milk Alternative of Choice
Freshly Ground Black Pepper, to Taste (optional)

Heat the oil in a large pot over medium-low heat. Add the onion and sauté for about 5 to 7 minutes, or until soft and translucent. Add the garlic, and continue to sauté for another minute. Add the ginger, nutmeg, cloves, and cardamom, and sauté for 1 minute more. Stir in the broth, salt, squash, and carrots, and bring everything to a boil. Reduce the heat, cover, and allow the soup to simmer until the vegetables are quite soft, about 15 to 20 minutes. Remove from the heat, and stir in the pumpkin. Using an immersion blender, puree the soup, or transfer it to your blender in batches (this will take 2 to 3 batches, depending on the capacity of your blender) and puree until smooth, about 2 to 3 minutes. Return the soup to your pot, stir in the milk alternative, and heat it to your desired temperature. Add some freshly ground pepper and additional salt to taste, if desired.

* Since butternut squash can be a pain to cut, I often purchase pre-cubed squash, which can be found in the refrigerated or freezer section of many grocers.

Cheesy Broccoli Soup

Yields 4 Servings

A craving for comfort food led me to create this rich and creamy soup for myself and my husband one lazy afternoon. He tends to shy away from the notion of cheesy dairy-free items, but this soup received two enthusiastic thumbs up. The taste is full of flavor, yet the cheesy notes are not overstated, perfect for timid dairy-free palates.

1/2 Cup (2.5 ounces) Raw Cashews	1 Tablespoon Tahini
4 Cups Water, Divided	2 Teaspoons Lemon Juice
1 Tablespoon Grapeseed, Olive, or Vegetable Oil	1/2 Teaspoon Paprika
1 Cup Chopped Onion (about 1 small to medium)	1/2 Teaspoon Mustard Powder
1 lb Cauliflower Florets (about 1 medium head)	1/4 Teaspoon Garlic Powder
6 Ounces Baby Carrots or about 3 Medium Carrots, Peeled and Sliced	1-1/2 to 2 Teaspoons Salt
	Freshly Ground Black Pepper, to Taste
5 Tablespoons Nutritional Yeast Flakes	1/2 lb Cooked Broccoli Florets (I prefer steamed)

Process the cashews in a spice grinder or food processor until they just begin to form a paste. Place the cashew powder/paste in your blender along with 1 cup of the water, and blend for 2 minutes. Set aside. Heat the oil in a large saucepan or stockpot over medium heat. Add the onion and sauté for about 5 minutes, or until slightly softened and translucent. Add the cauliflower, carrots, and the remaining 3 cups of water, and bring the mixture to a boil. Reduce the heat to medium-low, cover, and let the vegetables cook for 20 minutes, or until quite tender. Stir in the reserved cashew milk from your blender, nutritional yeast, tahini, lemon juice, paprika, mustard, garlic powder, salt, and pepper. Using an immersion blender, puree the soup, or transfer it to your blender in batches (this will take 2 to 3 batches, depending on the capacity of your blender) and puree until smooth, about 2 to 3 minutes. Return the soup to the pot. Break the broccoli florets into very small pieces or mash them with a fork. Stir the broccoli into the soup, and heat to your desired serving temperature.

More Menu Ideas: Old Stand-by Soups

To inspire your culinary ventures, these are soups for which many dairy-free (or easy to convert to dairy-free) recipes are available. I have divided my list of "frequently dairy-free" suggestions into two categories, those that can easily be made vegan and those that usually contain eggs, meat, or fish, and may be a bit more difficult to transform into vegetarian recipes.

Easily Vegetarian / Vegan:

~ Mushroom Barley	~ Thai Coconut	~ Vietnamese (Pho)
~ Gazpacho	~ Lentil	~ Mulligatawny
~ Ajo Blanco	~ Chili	~ Pasta E Fagioli (no Parmesan)
~ Vegetable	~ Split Pea	~ French Onion (hold the cheese)
~ Tomato	~ Tortilla	
~ Black Bean	~ Minestrone	

Almost Always Omnivorous:

~ Chicken Noodle	~ Egg Drop	~ Greek (Egg) Lemon Soup
~ Won Ton	~ Albondigas	~ Sopa de Ajo
~ Hot & Sour	~ Manhattan Clam Chowder	~ Bouillabaisse
~ Hamburger	~ Goulash	~ Cioppino
~ Italian Wedding (no Parmesan)	~ Borscht (hold the sour cream)	~ Beef Barley

Some Store-Bought Recommendations for Soup:

There are many great brands on the market, but the following recommendations only include products that I purchase with some regularity or that a colleague highly recommended. For full lists of non-dairy, packaged foods and brands, see the product lists available on www.godairyfree.org.

Amy's Kitchen (www.amys.com, (707) 568-4500) ~ canned soup and chili
My first discovery of the Amy's brand was via their canned chili. It quickly became a staple in my house, always on hand for throwing together last minute meals. As many will tell you, Amy's canned soups are also delicious, ranging from the creamy Organic Thai Coconut to the flavorful Organic Fire Roasted Southwestern Vegetable Soup. Amy's products are always vegetarian and many are dairy-free / vegan, in addition to gluten-free.

Imagine Foods (www.imaginefoods.com, (800) 434-4246) ~ ready to eat soup
Imagine sells an entire line of organic "creamy" soups, all of which are dairy-free, and pretty tasty. When on sale, I pick up an aseptic package or two of the Creamy Broccoli or Creamy Portobello soups, but they have many other varieties to choose from.

Pacific Foods (www.pacificfoods.com, (503) 692-9666) ~ ready to eat soup
Pacific sells loads of wonderfully organic soups that seem to go on sale with regularity. I enjoy their vegetable-based, creamy-style soups that are sold in aseptic packages, though only about half of them are dairy-free. They also have a line of organic canned soups, complete with organic beef and chicken, about half of which are also dairy-free, but at the time of writing, I had not yet sampled these.

CHAPTER 23:
SIMPLE SIDES & SALADS

Cheese-Free Scalloped Potatoes
Yields 6 Servings
While you could sprinkle some vegan "cheese" atop this dish, it really doesn't need it, it is deliciously rich as is. Also, this is a great make-ahead dish. Prepare it in the morning, and pop it in the oven an hour before dinner time.

4 Tablespoons Dairy-Free Margarine, Divided
2-1/2 lbs Potatoes (your choice), Thinly Sliced (peeled or unpeeled)
1 Large Onion (about 1/2 lb), Chopped
1/4 Cup All-Purpose (Plain) or Garbanzo/Chickpea Flour

1-3/4 Cups Vegetable or Chicken Broth
3 Tablespoons Vegan or Regular Mayonnaise
1/2 Teaspoon Salt, or to Taste
1/8 Teaspoon Black Pepper, or to Taste
Paprika for Sprinkling

Preheat your oven to 350°F (175ºC) and grease a 9x13-inch baking dish. Melt 1 tablespoon of the margarine in a saucepan over medium heat. Add the onions and sauté until they become slightly tender and translucent, about 5 minutes. Layer the potato slices and cooked onions in your prepared baking dish. Returning to your saucepan, melt the remaining 3 tablespoons of margarine and whisk in the flour until smooth. Gradually whisk in the broth. Add the mayonnaise, salt, and pepper, and continue to whisk and cook until the sauce gets a bit thick and bubbly. Pour the sauce evenly over the potatoes. Sprinkle the potatoes with a light dusting of paprika. Cover and bake for 1 hour.

Sweet Potato Apple Casserole
Yields 8 Servings
Recipe by Nicole Smith, author of Cody the Allergic Cow and founder of www.allergicchild.com - Nicole may be well known for her popular food allergy children's books and her helpful website, but first and foremost, Nicole is a mom, with a delicious recipe or two up her sleeve …

1 2-lb Can Sweet Potatoes, Sliced
1 Cup Pared Apples, Sliced 1/4-Inch Thick
3/4 Cup Pure Maple Syrup

1/4 Cup Dairy-Free Margarine, Melted
1 Teaspoon Salt

Preheat your oven to 350°F (175ºC) and grease an 8x12-inch or 9x13-inch baking dish. Arrange the potatoes in the bottom of your prepared baking dish, and layer the apples on top of them. Combine the syrup, margarine, and salt, and pour it over applies & potatoes. Cover and bake for 30 minutes. Uncover and bake for another 30 minutes.

Baked Cauliflower Au Gratin

Yields 8 Servings

Recipe adapted from Levana Cooks Dairy-Free! by Levana Kirschenbaum - I chose to feature this recipe as it nicely reflects Levana's style with an all-natural ingredient list, a touch of elegance mixed with comfort food appeal, and no fear of selectively using dairy alternatives where most appropriate. According to Levana, "This is a great French favorite and a wonderful way to dress up the unpretentious cauliflower and end up with a rustic yet elegant dish. For a more colorful presentation, use a combination of cauliflower and broccoli. For faster results, use 2-1/2 pounds frozen chopped cauliflower or a cauliflower-broccoli combination. This dish reheats very nicely, making it perfect for buffets."

2 Heads Cauliflower, Cut in Small Florets, Stems
  Trimmed and Sliced
3 Tablespoons Olive Oil
1 Medium Onion, Quartered
3 Shallots, Quartered
3 Tablespoons Flour of Choice

1 Cup Dry White Wine
1 Cup Plain Milk Alternative of Choice
Good Pinch Ground Nutmeg
Salt and Pepper, to Taste
1 Cup Grated VeganRella Cheddar Cheese
  Alternative*

Bring some water to a boil in a large pot. Add the cauliflower and cook until tender but still firm, about 5 minutes. Drain thoroughly, dry with paper towels, and set aside. Preheat your broiler. Heat the oil in a heavy skillet over medium heat. In a food processor, coarsely grind the onion and shallots, add them to your skillet, and sauté them until translucent. Lower the heat and add the flour. Cook, while continuously whisking, for 2 to 3 minutes, or until the flour mixture turns a light brown. Raise the heat again and add the wine and milk in a slow stream, whisking constantly to avoid lumps, until the mixture thickens, about 2 to 3 minutes. Add the nutmeg, salt, and pepper and stir until combined. Pour the vegetables in a greased 9x13-inch pan. Pour the sauce over them. Sprinkle the cheese over all. Place the pan under the broiler, about 6 inches away from the flame, for about 10 minutes, or until nicely colored and bubbly. Serve hot.

* This is the brand that Levana relies upon for best results, but you can substitute another brand of vegan "cheese."

Almost Traditional Green Bean Casserole

Yields 6 Servings

Just in case you don't have your own family recipe on hand, this is a dairy-free version of that oh-so-traditional, holiday green bean casserole.

1 Batch Condensed "Cream" of Mushroom Soup
  (p182)
1/2 Cup Unsweetened Cashew, Rice, or Soymilk
1 Teaspoon Soy Sauce or Wheat-Free Tamari
Freshly Ground Black Pepper, to Taste

4 Cups Green Beans (roughly 1 lb frozen green beans,
  2 14.5-ounce cans green beans, or 1-1/2 lbs
  fresh green beans, trimmed, washed, and
  cooked) or Broccoli Florets
1-1/3 Cups Canned French Fried Onions, Divided

Preheat your oven to 350°F (175ºC). In a medium-sized bowl, combine the condensed soup, milk alternative, soy sauce, and pepper. Add the green beans and half (2/3 cup) of the fried onions, and stir to coat. Place the mixture in a 1-1/2-quart casserole dish or a 9-inch round or square baking dish. Bake the casserole for 25 minutes. Give it a quick stir, and sprinkle the remaining onions on top. Bake for another 5 minutes.

Oven Roasted Potatoes

Yields 4 to 6 Servings

This recipe is an easy crowd pleaser, and a great solution to milk-rich side dishes at potlucks and family dinners. In fact, my grandma just requested that I bring a big batch of these potatoes to an upcoming birthday party.

2 lbs Potatoes (Yukon gold, white, or red), Cut into
  3/4-Inch Cubes
2 Tablespoons Olive Oil
2 Large Garlic Cloves, Minced
1/2 Teaspoon Dried Basil
1/2 Teaspoon Dried Oregano

1/2 Teaspoon Dried Parsley
1/2 Teaspoon Dried Thyme
1/2 Teaspoon Dried Dill Weed
1/4 to 1/2 Teaspoon Crushed Red Pepper Flakes
1/2 Teaspoon Salt

Preheat your oven to 450ºF (230ºC). Place the potatoes in a single layer in a large baking dish. Drizzle the olive oil and garlic over the potatoes and stir to coat. In a small dish, mix together the herbs, crushed red pepper, and salt. You may opt to give them a quick blend in your spice grinder for finer herbs, or simply shake them over top of your potatoes. Stir to ensure that the potatoes are evenly coated with the spices. Roast the potatoes for 25 to 35 minutes, checking in every 10 to 15 minutes to give them a quick stir, so that they evenly brown.

Spicy Sweet Oven Fries

Yields 2 to 4 Servings

One evening I got a hankering for seasoned French fries, but you can't always trust those restaurant fries to be dairy-free. So I decided to bake up my own fries with a nice flavorful seasoning. Admittedly, it is hard to get that crunchy exterior without a deep-fryer, but these are quite delicious and definitely French fry material.

1 lb Russet Potatoes
2 Teaspoons Olive, Peanut, or Grapeseed oil
1/2 Teaspoon Paprika
1/2 Teaspoon Mild Chili Powder (use a medium chili
  powder for a spicier potato)

1/2 Teaspoon Garlic Powder
1/2 Teaspoon Onion Powder
1/2 Teaspoon Salt
1/8 Teaspoon Crushed Red Pepper Flakes

Preheat your oven to 425ºF (220ºC). Slice the potatoes into rounds or French fry strips that are 1/4-inch thick and place them in a large bowl. Mix the oil, paprika, chili powder, garlic, onion, salt, and crushed red pepper together. Coat the potatoes with the oil/spice mixture and place them on a baking sheet. Bake the fries for 30 to 45 minutes, turning them every 15 minutes. The cooking time may vary depending on the thickness of your fries.

Sweet Potato Fries Option: Substitute sliced sweet potatoes for some or all of the russet potatoes. I like to do a half and half mix, but keep in mind that sweet potatoes will be much softer than the russets.

Traditional Mashed Potatoes

Yields 6 to 8 Servings

Family get-togethers and holidays are that much easier when the "staple" dishes can be easily made dairy-free.

6 Medium Russet Potatoes, Peeled and Cubed (about 3 lbs of cubed potatoes)
3/4 Cup Warm Unsweetened Rice, Oat, or Soymilk

6 to 8 Tablespoons Dairy-Free Margarine, Softened
1 to 1-1/2 Teaspoons Salt
Freshly Ground Black Pepper, to Taste

Place the potatoes in a large pot and cover them with water. Cover the pot and bring the water to a boil. Allow the potatoes to cook for 20 to 25 minutes, or until they are very tender. Drain well, and return the potatoes to the pot to help any remaining water evaporate. Add the milk alternative, margarine, salt, and pepper, and mash until the potatoes reach your desired consistency, adjusting the margarine, salt, and pepper to taste. For a coarser mash, use a fork. For a light and fluffy whipped consistency, use a hand held mixer.

Roasted Garlic Option: Preheat your oven to 400ºF (205ºC). Slice off the top of 1 head of garlic so the cloves are just peaking out. Brush the top with olive oil and wrap the garlic head in aluminum foil. Roast for 45 to 60 minutes, or until the tops of the cloves are golden brown and the individual cloves appear to have separated from the side walls of the head. Allow the garlic to cool and squeeze the bottom of the head to pop the garlic cloves out. Lightly mash the cloves and add them to the potatoes along with the milk alternative and margarine.

Leftover Mashed Potato Cakes: Make small patties out of the leftover potatoes, and dust them with flour (your choice of type). Place 2 to 4 tablespoons of high heat oil (p113) in a skillet with high sides, and fry the potato cakes over medium-high heat until they are browned on both sides. For cakes that hold together a bit better, you can optionally blend 1 egg or egg white into the leftover mashed potatoes.

Whipped Potatoes

Yields 6 Servings

Recipe adapted from What's To Eat? The Milk-Free, Egg-Free, Nut-Free Food Allergy Cookbook by Linda Coss - Linda comments, "Although this looks a lot like mashed potatoes, it tastes much different. The olive oil gives these whipped potatoes a rich, rustic flavor that I enjoy without any gravy."

1-1/2 lbs White Potatoes
3 Tablespoons Olive Oil
1 Teaspoon Bottled Minced Garlic

1 Teaspoon Seasoned Salt
Freshly Ground Black Pepper, to Taste

Peel the potatoes and slice them into 1/2-inch thick slices. Place them in a 3-quart stockpot and add enough water to just cover the potatoes. Cover the pot and bring the water to a boil over high heat. Reduce the heat to low and simmer, covered, for 20 minutes or until the potatoes feel soft when pierced with a fork. Drain. Place the potatoes back into the pot and add the remaining ingredients. Using an electric hand-held mixer beat the potatoes on high speed until light and fluffy. Serve hot.

Lively Lemon Stir-Fry

Yields 3 to 4 Servings

This calcium-rich side dish (packed with BOTH bok choy and broccoli) uses the tang of lemon rather than the sodium of soy for a flavor that is sweet, sour, and spicy all in one. Don't let the Asian-inspired "stir-fry" title fool you, as it will pair well with most main dishes. Since you will be stir frying over a relatively high heat, make sure all of your ingredients are prepared, measured, and next to the stove ready to go before beginning.

2 Tablespoons Peanut, Vegetable, or Other High Heat Oil (p113)
1 Medium Onion, Quartered and Thinly Sliced
4 Garlic Cloves, Minced
1 Tablespoon Grated or Minced Gingerroot
1/2 Teaspoon Salt

1/8 to 1/4 Teaspoon Crushed Red Pepper Flakes
1/2 lb Broccoli Florets
1 Large Bok Choy (about 1-1/2 lbs), Coarsely Chopped
2 Tablespoons Lemon Juice
2 Teaspoons Agave Nectar, Honey, or Granulated Sugar

Heat the oil in a large skillet or wok over medium-high heat. Add the onions, garlic, ginger, salt, and red pepper, and stir-fry for 2 minutes. Add the broccoli and bok choy, and stir-fry for 2 minutes. Finally, add the lemon juice and sweetener, and stir fry for another 2 to 3 minutes, or until the broccoli and bok choy are crisp tender.

Cumin-Spiked Rice and Peas

Yields 4 Servings

The process of cutting out dairy prompted me to discover new flavors through experimentation with spices. My husband and I soon discovered a mutual love of cumin, and thus this simple side dish was born. The use of toasted cumin seeds not only enhanced this basic rice, but it also got my husband to eat peas! Of course, frozen corn or mixed vegetables will also go nicely.

2-1/4 Cups Water
1-1/2 Cups White Jasmine or Basmati Rice
1 Teaspoon Grapeseed or Olive Oil
3/4 Teaspoon Salt
1 Tablespoon Cumin Seeds

1 Cup Frozen Peas, Defrosted
1 Tablespoon Dairy-Free Margarine or Good Quality Oil (such as extra-virgin olive oil)
1 Small Lemon, Cut into 4 Wedges

In a medium saucepan, bring the water to a boil. Add the rice, 1 teaspoon of oil, and salt, stir, and cover. Reduce the heat to low and cook for 20 to 30 minutes. Add up to 1/4 cup of water if the rice becomes dry before it is fully cooked. Meanwhile, in a small dry skillet, toast the cumin seeds (while stirring) over medium heat until fragrant, about 2 to 3 minutes. When the rice is done, stir in the cumin seeds, peas, and margarine or oil. Serve with the lemon wedges for seasoning to taste.

Brown Rice Option: Substitute long grain or jasmine brown rice for the white rice, and increase the water to 3 cups.

Spanish Baked Barley

Yields 4 Servings as a Meal or 6 to 8 Servings as a Side Dish

I love this recipe for its ease in preparation, and the ability to adjust the heat and taste based on our latest favorite salsa. For an extra dose of greens and calcium, I stir in 6 cups of thinly sliced curly kale (about 6 large leaves) during the last 10 minutes of cooking.

2 Tablespoons Olive Oil
1 Cup Pearl Barley (regular or quick cooking), Rinsed
1 Cup Chopped Onion (about 1 small to medium)
2 Garlic Cloves, Minced
3 Cups Vegetable or Chicken Broth

1 Cup Salsa (mild, medium, or hot, your choice)
1/2 Teaspoon Salt, or to Taste
Freshly Ground Black Pepper, to Taste
1 2.25-Ounce Can Sliced Olives

Preheat your oven to 350°F (175ºC). Heat the oil in a large skillet over medium heat. Add the barley, onion, and garlic and sauté until the onions begin to soften and the barley looks lightly toasted, about 5 to 7 minutes. Pour the mixture into a medium to large casserole dish, and stir in the broth, salsa, salt, and pepper. Cover and bake for 60 minutes if using quick cooking barley, 90 minutes if using regular pearl barley. If some liquid still remains after the time is up, uncover and bake for another 10 to 15 minutes, or until the remaining liquid cooks off. Stir in the sliced olives.

Make it a Meal: Stir in 1 15-ounce can of drained and rinsed pinto or black beans and/or 1 cup of cooked, diced chicken.

Creamy Wild Rice Salad

Yields 2 Servings

Recipe created by Hannah Kaminsky, author of My Sweet Vegan - While Hannah loves the creamy luxury of risotto, it typically contains cheese and can be time-consuming to make at home. Luckily, a serendipitous experiment at the dinner table led her to discover the wonderfully lustrous texture and flavor that hummus can provide without all of the fat and dairy. The leftovers are delicious when eaten cold the next day, packed into lunchboxes, or taken on picnics.

1/4 Cup Wild Rice
1/4 Cup Brown Basmati Rice
1/4 Teaspoon Salt, Plus Additional to Taste
1-1/2 Cups Vegetable Stock

1/2 Cup Regular or Garlic Hummus
1/2 Cup Chopped Celery
1/4 Teaspoon Ground Cumin

In a medium pot, combine both types of rice, the salt, and stock. Cover and bring the rice to a boil, reduce the heat to medium-low, and cook for 25 to 30 minutes, or until all of the liquid has been absorbed. Take the pot off the heat, and allow the rice to rest for 5 minutes, covered. Stir in the hummus, celery, and cumin. Sprinkle with additional salt to taste, if desired.

Greek Pasta Salad

Yields 8 Servings

The tofu in this recipe soaks up the flavors of the marinade to help replace the more traditional feta cheese.

1 lb Rotini or Fusilli Pasta (regular or gluten-free)
6 Tablespoons Olive Oil
6 Tablespoons Red or White Wine Vinegar
1/4 Cup Lemon Juice
2 Tablespoons Dried Oregano
4 Garlic Cloves, Minced
1/2 to 1 Teaspoon Salt, or to Taste
Freshly Ground Black Pepper, to Taste
8 Ounces Soft or Firm Tofu, Drained and Crumbled or Cut into 1/2-Inch Cubes

1 2.25-Ounce Can Sliced Olives, Drained
1 13.75-Ounce Can Artichoke Hearts Packed in Water, Drained and Quartered
1 Cup Garbanzo Beans (roughly half of a 15-ounce can)
1 Cup Chopped Onion (about 1 small to medium)
1 Bell Pepper (any color), Chopped
1/2 lb Tomatoes (any kind), Halved if Small or Cut into 1/2-Inch Chunks

Cook the pasta according to the package directions. While the pasta is cooking, combine the oil, vinegar, lemon juice, oregano, garlic, salt, and pepper in a large bowl with a lid. Add the tofu and toss to coat, allowing it to sit for a minute or two while you prepare the other ingredients. Once the pasta and remaining ingredients are ready, place them into the bowl and toss everything together to coat. Cover and refrigerate the salad for at least an hour, but preferably overnight. Preparing this dish 24 hours in advance will give the flavors time to meld. Check in to give it a stir every so often to ensure everything is well coated.

Seed "Cheese" and Tomato Salad

Yields 2 Servings

Recipe adapted from the website, The Healing Feast (www.thehealingfeast.com) by Janet L. Doane - *This simple, yet flavorful tomato salad uses Janet's sunflower seed "cheese" as the center of the flavor attention, though another nut or seed cheese should work equally well.*

2 Large Ripe Tomatoes
1 Green Onion
1 Cup Sunflower Seed "Cheese" (p121)

Salt (Celtic, Himalayan, etc.), to Taste
Freshly Ground Black Pepper
Dash Balsamic or Other Favorite Vinegar

Cut the tomatoes in half, and then cut the halves into 1/4-inch slices. Arrange the slices around the outside of 2 plates. Place 1/2 cup of the sunflower seed "cheese" inside each plate of tomatoes. Finely chop the green onion, and sprinkle it over the seed "cheese." Sprinkle a little salt and freshly ground pepper over the seed cheese, and top with a splash of your favorite vinegar.

Seven Minute Salsa Salad

Yields 2 to 4 Servings

Recipe by Gina Clowes, founder of www.allergymoms.com - Gina knows the importance of quick and easy dishes. With food allergy families, nearly every meal and snack must be prepared at home, so there is no time for complicated recipes. She was kind enough to share this reliable sample from her recipe collection. It can be served chilled or at room temperature with taco chips, as an appetizer or as a healthy side salad.

1 Lime
2 to 4 Tablespoons Olive Oil
1/4 to 1/2 Packet "Safe" Taco Seasoning (or 1/4 to
    1/2 batch of the recipe on p220)

Few Dashes "Red Hot" or Minced Jalapeño Pepper
1 15-Ounce Can Corn
1 15-Ounce Can Black Beans

Optional Add-Ins:
~   1/2 Cup Chopped Roasted or Fresh Red Pepper
~   1/2 Cup Chopped Fresh Tomato
~   1/2 Cup Cubed Cucumber
~   1/2 Cup Sliced Black Olives

~   1 Fresh Avocado, Diced (add just before serving)
~   1 Garlic Clove, Minced
~   2 Tablespoons Minced Green or Red Onion

Wash the lime and grate some of the zest. Roll it around on a clean, flat surface to make it easier to juice. Juice the lime and mix it with the olive oil, taco seasoning, and red hot or jalapeño. Drain and rinse the corn and black beans. Cut any other vegetables that you are using (excluding avocado) and toss the beans and vegetables together lightly with the dressing and a little of the lime zest. You will want to use more olive oil and possibly a second lime depending on how many optional vegetables you add in. Allow the salad to marinate for 1 hour. If using avocado, add it just prior to serving.

Carrot Cake Salad

Yields 4 Servings

This makes a quick and easy side dish or a refreshing breakfast. I do recommend coconut-based yogurt for this recipe, but soy-based will do in a pinch. If you don't have any yogurt on hand, just omit it for a nice, simple carrot salad.

1 6-Ounce Container Plain Dairy-Free Yogurt
1 Tablespoon Agave Nectar or Honey
1 Tablespoon Lemon Juice
1/4 Teaspoon Ground Cinnamon
1/8 Teaspoon Ground Nutmeg (optional)

Generous Pinch Salt
2 Cups Shredded Carrots (about 3 medium)
1/3 Cup Raisins
1/4 Cup Crushed Pineapple, Drained
1/4 Cup Chopped Pecans or Walnuts (optional)

In a medium-sized bowl, combine the yogurt, agave or honey, lemon juice, cinnamon, nutmeg (if using), and salt. Stir in the carrots, raisins, and pineapple. Cover and refrigerate for at least 15 minutes, or for a make-ahead salad, overnight. When ready to serve, sprinkle with the chopped nuts, if using.

CHAPTER 24:
FULL MEAL DEAL

Elegant Eggplant Cannelloni
Yields 3 to 4 Servings

My husband proclaimed this entrée to be "restaurant quality!" I was expecting it to taste good, but the luxurious results surprised us both. There is a little prep time involved, but really, this meal comes together rather quickly. I like to serve it with simple side dishes, such as rice and steamed vegetables or a nice green salad with some crusty bread.

1 Medium Eggplant (about 1-1/4 to 1-1/2 lbs)
Salt
Olive Oil for Brushing
1 Batch Organic Tomato Basil Sauce (p218) or 1 Jar
    Store-Bought Pasta Sauce

1 Batch Rich & Nutty Ricotta (p122)
2 Cups Spinach Leaves, Chopped*
Sliced or Chopped Olives (black, kalamata, or green)
    (optional)

Cut off the ends of the eggplant and cut it lengthwise, so that you end up with large, long slices that are quite thin, roughly 1/8 to 1/4-inch in thickness. Sprinkle the eggplant slices with some salt on one side, and allow them to sit for about 30 minutes, salt side up. While the eggplant is resting, this is a good time to throw the tomato sauce together (if using homemade) and blend up the Nutty Ricotta. When the Nutty Ricotta is prepared, stir the spinach into it and set aside.

Preheat your oven to 400ºF (205ºC). Using a paper towel or tea towel, wipe off any moisture that has surfaced on the eggplant along with the excess salt. Lightly brush each side of the eggplant slices with oil, and place them on a baking sheet. Broil the slices for about 3 to 4 minutes per side, watching carefully to ensure that they do not burn.

Pour about half of the tomato sauce in the bottom of a large casserole dish (9x13-inch will work). Divide the Nut Ricotta between the eggplant slices, placing about a tablespoon or two at one end of each slice. Roll the slices up beginning with the ricotta side, and place them seam side down in the sauce in your baking dish. Spread the remaining tomato sauce over the eggplant rolls, ensuring that they are relatively well coated. Cover and bake for 30 to 40 minutes. Top each serving with sliced or chopped olives, if desired.

* Whenever organic spinach is on sale, I freeze a big batch of the leaves. When it is time for this recipe, I measure out the 2 cups, and then crumble the frozen leaves with my fingers.

Lightly Herbed Pasta Alfredo

Yields 4 to 6 Servings

This is a lower fat version of the traditional pasta Alfredo, since it is prepared without any cheese or cream. I like this feature, because I can enjoy it as a light, stand-alone entrée in the summer, yet it still acts as a warm comfort food on chilly winter nights … especially when paired with white fish, chicken, or vegetarian "chicken" strips.

12 ounces Linguine or Pasta of Choice (regular or gluten-free)
1 lb Fresh Vegetables (zucchini, summer squash, broccoli, etc.), Sliced or Broken into Florets
2 Teaspoons Olive or Grapeseed Oil
1/4 Cup Minced Onion
2 to 3 Garlic Cloves, Minced
1 Teaspoon Dried Oregano
1/2 Teaspoon Dried Thyme or 1 Scant Tablespoon Fresh Thyme, Minced
1/4 Cup White Wine
1/4 Cup Dairy-Free Margarine
1/4 Cup All-Purpose (Plain) Flour or Flour of Choice
2 Cups Warm Unsweetened Rice, Cashew or Soymilk
3/4 Teaspoon Salt, or to Taste
1/4 to 1/2 Teaspoon White Pepper or Freshly Ground Black Pepper, or to Taste

Cook the pasta according to the package directions. Using a steamer basket, place the vegetables over boiling water to steam until they are crisp-tender. While those are cooking away, heat the oil in a large saucepan over medium-low heat. Add the onion and sauté for 3 minutes, or until translucent. Add the garlic, oregano, and thyme, and sauté for one minute more. Stir in the wine and margarine, cooking until the margarine has melted and the ingredients are well combined. Time to pull out the whisk! Slowly add in the flour while continuously whisking to form a smooth paste. Slowly whisk in the milk alternative, stirring and cooking until your desired consistency is reached. Season the sauce to taste with salt and pepper. In a large bowl, toss the pasta with the vegetables. Top with the sauce and toss lightly to coat.

Soy-Free Option: I do like the flavor and richness of margarine in this dish, but if you are unable to locate a soy-free margarine, then olive oil (even the extra-virgin kind) will work in a pinch.

French Bread Pizza

Yields 4 to 6 Servings

Recipe adapted from The Ultimate Uncheese Cookbook by Jo Stepaniak - Jo shows us how easy it is to make delicious vegan fast food with this recipe from her popular dairy-free cookbook. It is a very kid-friendly meal (though you may want to omit the cayenne), and by using gluten-free bread you can have a GFCF "pizza" on the table in minutes.

1 Loaf French Bread (regular or gluten-free), Cut in Half Widthwise and Lengthwise
8 Ounces Firm Tofu, Rinsed, Drained, and Crumbled
2 Tablespoons Unsalted Tomato Paste
2 Tablespoons Extra-Virgin Olive Oil
1 Tablespoon Reduced-Sodium Soy Sauce or Wheat-Free Tamari
1 Teaspoon Ground Fennel or Dried Basil
1 Teaspoon Dried Oregano
1 Teaspoon Crushed Garlic
1/8 to 1/4 Teaspoon Cayenne
Salt, to Taste
Freshly Ground Black Pepper, to Taste

Preheat your oven to 450ºF (230ºC). Place the bread, cut-sides up, on a dry baking sheet, pizza pan, or baking stone. Combine the tofu, tomato paste, olive oil, soy sauce, fennel or basil, oregano, garlic, and cayenne in a food processor, and blend into a smooth pâté. Season it with salt and pepper to taste and blend again. Spread the pâté evenly over the bread. Bake the pizza for 10 to 15 minutes, or until the pâté is hot and lightly browned, and the crust is crisp.

Creamy Pesto-Inspired Pasta

Yields 4 Servings

Once I discovered that pine nuts could be magically transformed into a rich cream with the simple whiz of a blender, it seemed only fitting that they should act as a base for a basil sauce. This sauce has a slightly rich, almost buttery feel.

1/2 Cup Pine Nuts, Plus Extra for Garnish
1 Cup Water
1-1/2 Tablespoons Cornstarch
1/4 Teaspoon Garlic Powder
3/4 to 1 Teaspoon Salt, or to Taste
2 to 4 Tablespoons (1/4 cup) Fresh Chopped Basil

1 5 or 6-Ounce Package Baby Spinach Leaves*
8 Ounces Angel Hair Pasta or Pasta of Choice (regular or gluten-free)
White Pepper or Freshly Ground Black Pepper, to Taste
Definitely Not Parmesan (p124) (optional)

Cook the pasta according to the package directions. While the pasta is cooking, whirl the pine nuts in your spice grinder or food processor until a paste forms. Combine the pine nuts, water, cornstarch, garlic powder, and salt in your blender, and blend on high until a smooth, creamy mixture forms. Strain the nut "cream" through a fine mesh strainer, into a medium-sized saucepan. Place the "cream" over medium-low heat, and cook while whisking often, until the sauce thickens to your desired consistency. Stir in the basil, and cook for just 1 minute more. Season the sauce to taste with pepper and/or additional salt, if desired. Drain the pasta, but do not rinse it. Return the pasta to its pan, and stir the spinach leaves into the hot noodles. Cover the pan allowing the spinach to steam for a few minutes. Add the sauce to your pasta and spinach, stirring to ensure that everything is well coated. Serve topped with Definitely Not Parmesan, and some extra pine nuts if desired. Serve with fresh steamed vegetables, chicken, or fish.

* This isn't a "hide the spinach" type of recipe, so if you are not spinach fans simply omit the greens or substitute with some sautéed mushrooms or fresh cherry tomatoes cut into halves.

Grilled "Cheese"

Yields 4 Sandwiches

Recipe adapted from the blog, Domestic Affair (domesticaffair.blogspot.com) by jae steele - This recipe launched my discovery of jae's work. jae shares, "I was pretty skeptical about the idea of a dairy-free version of this childhood favorite, but at first taste it became a staple in the first couple years I was vegan." She now has a delicious all-natural cookbook out, called Get it Ripe.

1/3 Cup Nutritional Yeast Flakes
1/4 Cup Flour of Choice (regular or gluten-free)
1 Garlic Clove, Crushed or Grated
1/4 Teaspoon Mustard Powder
1/2 Teaspoon Salt

Freshly Ground Black Pepper, to Taste
1/2 Cup Water
1 Tablespoon Olive Oil
Dairy-Free Margarine, For Spreading
8 Slices Whole Grain Bread (regular or gluten-free)

In a small saucepan, whisk together the nutritional yeast, flour, garlic, mustard, salt, pepper, and water. Place the mixture over low heat, and stir continuously. Once it gets pasty, add the oil, and a touch more water if necessary. Once the oil is incorporated, turn off the heat. Spread some margarine on one side of each slice of bread. Take four of the slices and slather the other half with the "cheese." Slap the other four pieces of bread on top of the cheesy ones, margarine side out. In a large skillet over medium heat, fry up the sandwiches until golden brown on each side. Slice the sandwiches in half and serve with ketchup and pickles.

Koushari

Yields 4 to 6 Servings

Recipe by Cynthia Mosher, chief editor and publisher of www.vegfamily.com - *This is one of Egypt's most popular national dishes and it just happens to be dairy-free, vegetarian, and flavorful. According to Cynthia, it pairs nicely with a green salad and crusty bread for a wonderful meal.*

2 Cups Cooked Short Grain Rice
1 Cup Cooked Elbow Macaroni
1 Cup Cooked Vermicelli Pasta
1/4 Cup Olive Oil, Plus Additional for Frying
1 Large Onion (about 1/2 lb), Chopped
1 to 2 Garlic Cloves, Chopped
1 Teaspoon Ground Cumin

1/2 Cup Brown Lentils, Rinsed
8 Ounces Tomato Sauce
Salt, to Taste
Freshly Ground Black Pepper, to Taste
1 Large Onion (about 1/2 lb), Thinly Sliced
1/2 Cup Cooked Chickpeas/Garbanzo Beans

The rice, macaroni, and vermicelli should be cooked simultaneously while the lentil sauce is being prepared, and kept warm until ready to assemble the dish. For the lentil sauce, heat the 1/4 cup of olive oil in a large saucepan over medium heat. Add the chopped onion and garlic, and sauté until tender, about 5 minutes. Stir in the cumin, allowing it to cook briefly in the oil. Add the rinsed lentils and sauté for 1 minute more. Stir in tomato sauce. Bring the mixture to a boil, reduce the heat to medium-low, and simmer until the lentils are tender, about 30 minutes. Add salt and pepper to taste. Fry the thinly sliced onion in enough olive oil to brown it. On a platter, place the cooked rice as the bottom layer, the macaroni as the next layer, followed by the vermicelli on top. Ladle the lentil sauce over top of all, and sprinkle with the chickpeas and fried onions to serve.

Pasta alla Puttanesca

Yields 4 Servings

Recipe adapted from *Vegan Fire & Spice* by Robin Robertson - *As much as I love spaghetti, it is easy to grow tired of this staple when following a dairy-free diet. Luckily, Robin came out with her flavorful cookbook of international cuisine, and included this almost traditional Italian recipe to breathe new life into pasta with red sauce. According to Robin, "This dish is named 'streetwalker style' because the sauce is simply too good to resist. The classic version contains anchovies but I think my interpretation is even more irresistible without them."*

2 Tablespoons Olive Oil
3 to 4 Garlic Cloves, Finely Chopped
1 28-Ounce Can Diced Tomatoes, Drained
1/2 Teaspoon Crushed Red Pepper Flakes
1/2 Teaspoon Dried Basil
1/2 Teaspoon Dried Oregano
Salt, to Taste
Freshly Ground Black Pepper, to Taste

1/2 Cup Imported Black Olives (such as kalamata), Halved and Pitted
1/2 Cup Imported Green Olives, Halved and Pitted
3 Tablespoon Capers, Drained and Rinsed
1/4 Cup Dry White Wine
1 lb Spaghetti or Other Pasta (regular or gluten-free)
3 Tablespoons Minced Fresh Parsley

In a saucepan, heat the olive oil over medium heat and add the garlic. When the garlic becomes fragrant, add the tomatoes, red pepper flakes, basil, oregano, and salt and pepper to taste. Bring the sauce to a boil, and then reduce the heat to low, stirring to help break up the tomatoes. Simmer for 20 minutes, stirring occasionally, until the tomatoes make a thick sauce. Add the olives, capers, and wine to the sauce and keep warm over low heat. Bring a pot of salted water to a boil. Add the spaghetti to the water and cook until it is al dente, about 10 minutes. Drain the pasta and transfer to a large serving bowl. Taste the sauce to adjust seasonings, pour it atop the pasta, and gently toss to combine. Serve immediately, sprinkled with minced parsley.

Very Veggie Lasagna

Yields 6 Servings

It was my personal mission to pack as many vegetables as possible into a single pan of lasagna, while still eliciting a meal of approval from my husband. This recipe easily passed the test, though he still prefers his veggie lasagna with some added ground beef.

12 Lasagna Noodles (regular or gluten-free)
2 Cups Spinach, Chopped
Dairy-Free Ricotta (1 batch Tofu Ricotta p123 or a
    double batch of Rich & Nutty Ricotta p122)*
1 Tablespoon Olive Oil
1 lb Zucchini, Diced
1 Red or Green Bell Pepper, Diced

8 Ounces Button or Cremini Mushrooms, Diced
1 Batch Elegant Pantry Marinara (p219) or 1 Large Jar
    of Store-Bought Marinara
Vegan Parmesan Substitute (p123) or Definitely Not
    Parmesan (p124) (optional)
Chopped Olives (optional)

Preheat your oven to 350ºF (175ºC), and cook the noodles according to the directions on the package. While the pasta is cooking, stir the chopped spinach into the ricotta and set aside. Heat the oil in a large skillet over medium-low heat. Add the zucchini and bell peppers, and sauté for about 5 minutes. Add the mushrooms and sauté for another 5 minutes, or until the vegetables are tender. Drain any excess liquid, and stir in all but 1 cup of the pasta sauce. Allow the sauce to simmer until your noodles are ready.

Cover the bottom of a 9x13-inch pan with the reserved 1 cup of pasta sauce. Add a layer of three lasagna noodles. Cover the noodles with 1/2 of the ricotta mixture, then another layer of noodles. Cover with 1/2 of the vegetable pasta sauce, then another layer of three noodles. Cover with the remaining 1/2 of the ricotta mixture, followed by the last layer of lasagna noodles and the last of the pasta sauce. Make sure the sauce covers the noodles completely. Bake the lasagna uncovered for 30 to 35 minutes. Remove from oven and let stand 5 to 10 minutes before cutting and serving. Serve topped with one of the parmesan substitutes or chopped olives, if desired.

More Cheez, Please: For a cheesier punch, top each of the ricotta layers with 2 Tablespoons of vegan parmesan, increase the nutritional yeast in the tofu ricotta to 1/4 cup, sprinkle shredded vegan cheddar or mozzarella atop each layer of ricotta, or top the lasagna with shredded vegan cheddar or mozzarella during the final 15 minutes of baking. At this lower temperature you may not see a good "melt" with any faux cheese sprinkled on top, so when the lasagna is almost done, turn the oven to broil. Broil the lasagna for about 5 minutes, or until the faux cheese becomes melty and begins to bubble.

Meaty Option: For a meat or faux meat lasagna, cook 1 lb of lean ground beef, turkey, or vegan mock beef crumbles and add it to the marinara sauce prior to layering the lasagna.

* I typically use the tofu ricotta for a more authentic lasagna feel, but the nutty ricotta will create a richer and more luxurious dish.

Lasagna with Eggplant, Portobello Mushrooms, and Fresh Tomatoes

Yields 8 Servings

Recipe adapted from *The Whole Foods Allergy Cookbook* by Cybele Pascal - *In her cookbook, Cybele produces a wide variety of food allergy-friendly dishes, from Fennel-Crusted Pork Tenderloin to a Chicken Pot Pie with Biscuit Crust. But like me, she has a love of vegetables, and includes numerous dishes incorporating these healthy gems, such as this one. Cybele states, "I created this lovely lasagna to use up fresh tomatoes from my neighbor, and was thrilled to discover that I liked it just as much as the high-fat version from the old days. You may substitute other vegetables if you wish, but I find that meatier vegetables such as eggplant and Portobello mushrooms add depth to the dish, which is more necessary when cooking without cheese. Ideally, you should make this the night before to really let it set."*

1 Medium Eggplant, Peeled and Sliced into 1/4-Inch Rounds
8 Ounces Rice Lasagna Noodles (or wheat, spelt, or corn/quinoa)
2 Cups Hot Unsweetened Rice or Oat Milk Alternative
1/4 Cup + 3 to 4 Tablespoons Olive Oil, Divided
1/4 Cup + 2 Tablespoons Rice or Oat Flour [or flour of choice]
Pinch Ground Nutmeg
1 Bay Leaf
Freshly Ground Black Pepper, to Taste

2 Large Portobello Mushrooms, Sliced into 1/4-Inch Strips
12 Shiitake or White Mushrooms, Sliced
3 Ripe Medium Tomatoes, Deseeded and Sliced into Thin Rounds (really important to drain as much as possible)
4 Cups Red Sauce [homemade marinara (p219) or store-bought]
20 Basil Leaves
Brown Rice Bread Crumbs, Cornflake Crumbs, or Other Bread Crumbs of Choice
Salt, to Taste

Preheat your oven to 350ºF (175ºC). Cook the sliced eggplant in your microwave for about 2 minutes, until just tender. Set aside. Cook the lasagna according to the directions on the box.

While the pasta is cooking, make a cream sauce. Start by warming your rice or oat milk. Then heat 1/4 cup of the olive oil in a saucepan over medium heat, stir in rice or oat flour, and cook 2 minutes, stirring continuously. Don't burn. Add the heated rice or oat milk slowly, while stirring. Add a pinch of nutmeg and the bay leaf. Bring it to a simmer and then reduce the heat to low. Thicken, while stirring, for 10 minutes or so. When the cream sauce has thickened, remove it from the heat, and grind in a few turns of fresh pepper.

Put about 1 tablespoon of olive oil in the bottom of a lasagna pan. Cover the bottom of the pan with half of the eggplant. Cover the eggplant with half of both types of mushrooms, followed by sliced tomatoes. Cover the vegetables with 1-1/2 cups of the red sauce. Spread out 10 of the basil leaves. Drizzle with half of the cream sauce. Cover with a layer of lasagna noodles. Sprinkle about 1 tablespoon of olive oil over the noodles. Layer the remaining vegetables, another 1-1/2 cups of the red sauce, 10 basil leaves, and the remaining cream sauce. Top with lasagna noodles. Spread the final cup of red sauce over top [to cover the noodles], sprinkle with the bread crumbs, and drizzle with a little more olive oil. Bake uncovered about 1 hour. Remove from your oven and let cool completely before serving, ideally overnight in the refrigerator; otherwise, just let it come to room temperature to set, or you'll have a soupy mess. Cut into portions with a sharp serrated knife.

Mushroom & Sage Stuffed Bell Peppers

Yields 6 Servings

Whenever I find a good deal on organic green bell peppers, I make this dish. They tend to be a bit "meatier" than conventional peppers, making for a very filling vegetarian dish. Sage gives the rice and lentils a delicious stuffing vibe in my opinion. Nonetheless, if sage is a bit too woodsy for your tastes, feel free to substitute basil or oregano or add the sage earlier in the recipe (to the lentils and rice with the salt and garlic powder) for a more subdued flavor.

1-1/2 Cups Long Grain or Jasmine Brown Rice
3/4 Cup Brown Lentils
4 Cups Mushroom (preferred) or Vegetable Broth
3 Tablespoon Olive Oil, Divided
1/2 Teaspoon Garlic Powder
1 Teaspoon Salt
Freshly Ground Black Pepper, to Taste

1 Teaspoon Dried Sage
1 to 2 Cups Packed Baby Spinach Leaves (optional)
8 Ounces Chopped Mushrooms
6 Medium to Large Bell Peppers (green, red, or yellow), Tops and Seeds Removed
Diced Garlic or Jalapeno Stuffed Green Olives or Definitely Not Parmesan (p124) (optional)

In Your Rice Cooker: Combine the rice, lentils, broth, 1 tablespoon of olive oil, garlic, salt, and pepper in your rice cooker, and turn it on.

On the Stove Top: Add the ingredients listed in the rice cooker directions plus 1/2 cup of water to a medium-sized saucepan. Bring the rice to a boil, cover, and reduce the heat to low. Allow the rice and lentils to simmer for about 40 to 45 minutes, or until all of the water is absorbed.

Preheat your oven to 350ºF (175ºC). Combine the rice and lentil mixture with the sage, spinach (if using), and mushrooms. Stuff the bell peppers with the rice mixture (go ahead and pack it in there), place the peppers in a large baking dish, and drizzle each pepper with 1 teaspoon of olive oil. Bake for 30 to 40 minutes, or until the peppers become soft. To serve, top each pepper with 1 to 2 teaspoons of diced green olives or parmesan alternative, if using.

Portobello-Ricotta Ravioli

Yields 6 to 8 Servings

There are few dairy foods that I miss these days, but I do have fond memories of a frozen food item, of all things. Our local grocery store kept stock of these simple, but delicious Portobello mushroom raviolis that we would boil up whenever we didn't feel like cooking. They weren't rich with dairy, but they did unfortunately harbor some cheese. One day I decided it was time to recreate them, in dairy-free fashion. I usually serve them topped with a marinara or tomato sauce (p119), a drizzle of olive oil and some parmesan substitute (p123 or p124) or a light white sauce (p216).

1 Tablespoon Olive or Grapeseed Oil
1/2 Cup Diced Onion (about 1/2 medium)
4 Garlic Cloves, Minced
2 Cups Diced White Button or Cremini Mushrooms

2 Cups Diced Portobello Mushrooms
1 Batch Tofu Ricotta (p123)
Wonton, Egg Roll, or Gyoza Wrappers*

Heat the oil in a large skillet over medium-low heat. Add the onions and sauté until translucent, about 5 minutes. Add the garlic and sauté for 1 minute longer. Add the mushrooms and sauté until they are soft and have released most of their juices, about 5 minutes. Drain the mushroom mixture of any liquid that remains. Stir the mushrooms into the ricotta mixture.

Lay out the wonton or gyoza wrappers and add a small amount of the mushroom filling to the middle of one half of the wrapper. Err on the side of less filling to ensure a proper seal and minimize exploding raviolis during the boiling process. Tap your finger in a bowl of water, and lightly dampen the outer edge of the wrappers. You just want them moist enough to stick, but not saturated as it will cause the dough to thin. Fold the wrappers over to cover the filling, and squeeze out any excess air as you press to seal each side of the raviolis. Watch those fingernails when pressing the dough down, as it can be easy to poke holes in the wrappers. Repeat this process until all of the filling is used up.

Bring a large pot of water to boil, and add the raviolis in batches. You want to make sure they have plenty of room to move around, so that you don't end up with a large clump of raviolis. Boil them for 3 to 5 minutes or until the wrappers are tender, like noodles. Remove the raviolis with a slotted spoon, and continue to add batches until they are all cooked.

Freezing: Prior to cooking, these raviolis do freeze nicely. Space them out on a baking sheet (I usually do this as I make them) and flash freeze for about 1 hour. Flip the raviolis, and flash freeze them for another hour. Place the raviolis in a freezer bag, and keep frozen until ready to use. When ready to eat, pop the frozen raviolis in boiling water and cook as instructed above.

* If using wonton or gyoza wrappers, about 70 to 80 wrappers will suffice for this recipe. You will need less if using egg roll wrappers. For the best performance, I purchase egg roll wrappers and cut them into sixths (in half horizontally and in thirds vertically). Just a teaspoon of filling is needed for each and they seem to be easy to put together with minimal loss during boiling. If you are vegan or simply egg-free, choose your wrappers carefully, as some wonton and egg roll wrappers are made with egg.

Grilled Vegetable Strudel

Yields 4 to 6 Servings

Recipe adapted from the blog, Vegan Visitor (veganvisitor.wordpress.com), by Dayna McIsaac - *As a food photographer, Dayna creates dozens upon dozens of recipes, which she shares on her blog, but this is one of her favorites and it is always a hit with guests. Amazingly, many brands of puff pastry are dairy-free and vegan, so you should be able to find a suitable brand at your local grocer.*

1 Fennel Bulb
1 Medium Zucchini
1/2 Medium Red Onion
3 Tablespoons Balsamic Vinegar
1 Tablespoon Olive Oil
1 Tablespoon Vermouth (optional)
Freshly Ground Black Pepper, to Taste

1 Orange Bell Pepper
1 Sheet of Puff Pastry*
2 Garlic Cloves, Minced
1 Tablespoon Chopped Flat Leaf Parsley (optional)
Salt, to Taste
Roasted Red Pepper Purée (recipe below)

Heat your grill to medium. Remove the top fronds (reserving them) and base from the fennel, and slice it down the center. Remove the ends from the zucchini, and slice it lengthwise. Slice the onion into 1/4-inch rounds. In a medium-sized bowl, toss the fennel, zucchini and onion with the vinegar, oil, vermouth (if using), and pepper. Grill the vegetables, along with the bell pepper, turning regularly, until they have even grill marks and have softened. Place the pepper into a bowl and cover it with plastic wrap to steam. Once the pepper has cooled a bit, peel away the skin, and pull the stem from the pepper to remove the seeds.

Preheat your oven to 350ºF (175ºC). Roll out the puff pastry to a 10-inch square. Chop the vegetables roughly. Add the garlic, parsley (if using), and fennel fronds (reserving some for the Red Pepper Purée below), and add salt and pepper to taste if necessary. Spoon the grilled vegetable mixture into the center of the pastry, and evenly distribute it to form a line. Pull the first side of the pastry over the vegetables, and roll the pastry and vegetables over into the remaining pastry. Dot the end with water to seal. Flip the pastry so the seal is on the bottom. Transfer the strudel to a non-stick baking dish or sheet. Score the top. Bake the strudel on the center rack for 25 to 30 minutes or until it is golden and crisp. Serve with a drizzling of Roasted Red Pepper Purée (below).

Roasted Red Pepper Purée: This concentrated sauce adds a nice flavor boost and just the right amount of moisture to the strudel. It can also be enjoyed lightly drizzled atop pizza (p207).

2 Large Sweet Red Bell Peppers
4 Garlic Cloves, Minced (2 teaspoons)
1 Tablespoon Olive Oil
1 Teaspoon Fresh Lemon Juice
2 Teaspoons Chopped Flat Leaf Parsley

2 Teaspoons Chopped Chives
2 Teaspoons Chopped Fennel Fronds
1 Teaspoon Chopped Fresh Basil
Salt, to Taste
Pepper, to Taste

Over a medium flame, roast the peppers whole, turning regularly. Once done, they should be evenly blackened, not charred to a crisp. Transfer the hot peppers to a bowl and cover with plastic wrap to steam. Once they have had some time to cool, hold the peppers by the stem and peel away the skins. A clean tea towel may be used, but resist the urge to run them under water; you will lose so much great flavor. Pull away the stem and slice the peppers lengthwise to remove the membrane and seeds. Place the peppers into your food processor and pulse until smooth. Add the garlic, oil, juice, and herbs, and continue to pulse to a sauce-like consistency. Season the puree to taste with salt and pepper, as needed. It is most flavorful when served at room temperature.

Thai Chick-Un Pizza

Yields 2 to 3 Servings (10-inch/25-centimeter pizza) or 4 to 6 Servings (12-inch/30-centimeter pizza)
Recipe adapted from *Eat, Drink & Be Vegan* by Dreena Burton - *When I asked Dreena what her favorite recipes were from her latest cookbook, this pizza appeared on the top of her list (Though, as someone who owns her cookbook, I am really not sure how she could even narrow the list down!). Dreena suggests serving this pizza with a salad of "cooling vegetables," including celery, cucumber, tomatoes, and jicama.*

2/3 Cup Natural Creamy Peanut Butter
1/3 Cup Ketchup
2 Tablespoons Rice Vinegar
2 Tablespoons Tamari, Regular or Wheat-Free [or soy sauce]
2 Large Garlic Cloves, Quartered
1-1/2 Tablespoons Fresh Ginger, Chopped
1/4 Teaspoon Crushed Red Pepper Flakes, or to Taste
1/4 Cup Light Coconut Milk or Other Plain Milk Alternative of Choice
1 to 2 Tablespoons Water, or Additional Milk Alternative

1-1/2 to 2 Teaspoons Agave Nectar (optional)
1 (10 to 12-inch/25 to 30-centimeter) Pizza Shell*
1 Cup Cooked Chickpeas/Garbanzo Beans**
1 to 1-1/2 Cups Red Bell Pepper, Thinly Sliced (about 1 medium to large pepper)
3/4 Cup Fresh Pineapple, Chopped (may use canned pineapple chunks, drained)
1/2 Cup Green Onions, Sliced (or sweet red onions, very thinly sliced)
1/2 Cup Mung Bean Sprouts
Peanuts, Chopped (for garnish)
Fresh Cilantro Leaves (for garnish)

To prepare the peanut sauce, add the peanut butter, ketchup, rice vinegar, tamari, garlic, ginger, and red pepper flakes to your food processor [or blender] and puree until smooth, scraping down the sides of the bowl as needed. Add the coconut milk and puree again until smooth (add 1 to 2 tablespoons of water to thin if desired – the sauce should be thick enough to spread on your pizza and not runny). Taste test, and if you would like a touch of sweetness, add the agave nectar.

Preheat your oven to 425ºF (220ºC). If using a pizza stone, place it in the oven to preheat, or line a pizza pan with parchment paper. Spread the peanut sauce evenly on the pizza shell (refrigerate any leftover sauce). In a bowl, lightly flatten the chickpeas with a large spoon (or in palm of your hand), and distribute them evenly over the sauce. Distribute the bell pepper slices and pineapple evenly. Place the pizza on your pizza stone or pan and bake it for 17 to 20 minutes, sprinkling on the green onions for the last minute of cooking, until the crust is golden and the toppings have heated through. Serve sprinkled with the bean sprouts, and a handful of chopped peanuts and cilantro, if desired.

Wheat-Free or Gluten-Free Option: Use a non-wheat pizza shell [store-bought or recipe on p207 for gluten-free or p208 for spelt / wheat-free].

Kid-Friendly Tip: Reduce the ginger to 1/2 tablespoon, and omit the crushed red chili pepper flakes and perhaps the onions.

* Since this sauce is rich, the pizza shell should not be too thin.
** Mock chicken strips or vegetarian chicken ground round can be substituted for chickpeas.

Make Your Own Pizza

Yields 1 Pizza or 6 Servings

I don't think I am alone when I say that pizza was one of the hardest things for me to come to terms with on a dairy-free diet. Yet once I realized that cheese really isn't an integral factor in creating a delicious pizza, the sky was the limit. You may find some convenient frozen dough at your grocer, but dairy-free pizza crust can actually be difficult to come by. So, I have included three pizza crust recipes below (regular, wheat-free, and gluten-free), along with sauce ideas to help you to build your own masterpiece.

No Rise Pizza Crust:

This simple crust benefits with up to 30 minutes of "resting time," but realistically, you can pop it in once your oven has had time to heat up.

1 Cup Warm Water
2-1/4 Teaspoons or 1 1/4-Ounce Package Active Dry
   Yeast
1 Teaspoon Granulated Sugar or Sweetener of Choice
1 Tablespoon Olive or Grapeseed Oil

1-1/2 Cups All-Purpose (Plain) Flour
1 Cup Whole Wheat Flour or More All-Purpose Flour
1 Teaspoon Salt
1 Teaspoon Italian Herbs (optional)

In a large bowl, combine the warm water, yeast, and sugar. Allow it to sit and proof for 5 minutes. Stir in the oil, followed by the flours, salt, and herbs, if using. Mix well, kneading with your hands as needed to bring the dough together into a smooth ball of dough. Let the dough rest for 10 to 20 minutes while you prepare the toppings and preheat your oven to 450ºF (230ºC). Roll the dough out to your desired size and shape, and bake it for 5 minutes. Remove it from the oven, top with your desired toppings, and bake for another 10 minutes, or until the crust takes on a nice golden hue.

Gluten-Free Pizza Crust:

Recipe adapted from Cooking Free *by Carol Fenster - To get just the right texture, Carol uses a variety of flours and binders, but you can omit the gelatin in this recipe if preferred. Xanthan gum is a binder that is sold among the flours and in gluten-free grocery departments. It may appear expensive, but one bag lasts for quite some time.*

1 Tablespoon Active Dry Yeast
2/3 Cup Brown Rice Flour
1/2 Cup Tapioca Flour
2 Teaspoons Xanthan Gum
1 Teaspoon Unflavored Gelatin Powder (may omit)
1 Teaspoon Italian Seasoning
1/2 Teaspoon Granulated Sugar

1/2 Teaspoon Salt
2/3 Cup Warm (110ºF/43ºC) Plain or Unsweetened
   Milk Alternative of Choice
1 Teaspoon Olive Oil
1 Teaspoon Apple Cider Vinegar
Extra Rice Flour for Sprinkling

Preheat your oven to 425ºF (220ºC). In a medium-sized mixing bowl using regular beaters (not dough hooks), blend the yeast, flours, xanthan gum, gelatin powder (if using), Italian seasoning, sugar, and salt on low speed. Add the warm milk alternative, oil, and vinegar. Beat on high speed for 2 minutes. The dough will resemble soft bread dough. If the dough is too stiff, add warm water 1 tablespoon at a time. Put the mixture on a greased 12-inch pizza pan or baking sheet. Liberally sprinkle rice flour on the dough, and then press it into the pan, continuing to sprinkle the dough with flour to prevent it from sticking to your hands. Make the edges thicker to hold the toppings. Bake the pizza crust for 10 minutes. Remove it from the oven. Top the crust with sauce and your preferred toppings. Bake it for another 20 to 25 minutes or until the top is nicely browned.

Wheat-Free Spelt Pizza Crust:

While it may sound ultimately hearty, spelt has a pleasant flavor that both my husband and I almost prefer to wheat. This crust is a bit "breadier" than your average white or wheat pizza crust, but tasty nonetheless.

2-1/2 to 2-3/4 Cups Whole Spelt Flour, Divided
1 Tablespoon Active Dry or Fast Rising Yeast
1 Teaspoon Salt

1 Cup Hot Water
1/4 Cup Olive or Grapeseed Oil

In a large bowl, stir together 1-1/2 cups of the flour, the yeast, and salt. Combine the hot water and oil, and add them to your flour mixture. Stir well. Add 1 more cup of the flour, and combine. Continue to knead the dough until it comes together adding the remaining 1/4 cup of flour 1 tablespoon at a time, as needed. The dough should be very soft and supple, but not sticking to your hands. Let it rest for 10 minutes or so while you prepare your pizza toppings. Preheat your oven to 400ºF (205ºC). Press the dough into a greased pizza pan or shape it on a baking sheet. The dough tends to pull apart a bit as spelt has less gluten then wheat, so carefully press it into shape rather than pulling and stretching. Top the pizza with your toppings of choice, and bake it for 20 to 25 minutes, or until the crust is nicely browned.

Cooking Free Pizza Sauce:

Recipe adapted from *Cooking Free* by Carol Fenster - *My husband's favorite pizza is cheese-free, made with a regular pizza sauce (such as this one), and topped with pepperoni, mushrooms, and olives. I love cheese-free pizza with Canadian bacon / ham and pineapple plus a sprinkling of crushed red pepper flakes; something about it just works. For a vegan option, substitute mock "meats" or enjoy your favorite sautéed or roasted vegetables atop your pizza.*

1 8-Ounce Can Tomato Sauce
1-1/2 Teaspoons Granulated Sugar
1/2 Teaspoon Dried Oregano
1/2 Teaspoon Dried Basil

1/2 Teaspoon Crushed Dried Rosemary
1/2 Teaspoon Fennel Seeds
1/2 Teaspoon Salt
1/4 Teaspoon Garlic Powder

Combine all ingredients in a small saucepan, and bring to a boil over medium heat. Reduce the heat to low, and simmer for 15 minutes.

More Sauce Ideas:

~ *Béchamel* (p216)
~ *Pesto* (p219)
~ *Olive Oil and Garlic* - Top it with sun-dried tomatoes, artichoke hearts, and/or olives for a focaccia-style pizza
~ *Barbecue Sauce* - There is something comforting about barbecue chicken pizza.
~ *Peanut Sauce* (p221)
~ *Aioli* - I light drizzle of this rich, mayonnaise-like sauce goes a long ways.
~ *Roasted Red Pepper Puree* (p20) – Use it as a very light spread or as a drizzle.
~ *Cheesy Sauce* (p217) - Use less water when preparing it for a thicker "spread."
~ *Tofu Ricotta with Basil* (p123) - Spread the crust with a bit of olive oil and dot with dollops of the tofu ricotta.
~ *Vegan Cheese Alternative* - It usually shreds well, but vegan "cheese" can be stubborn when it comes to melting. Near the end of the baking time, broil the pizza to help the cheese alternative soften and become a bit bubbly.
~ *Bruschetta* - My husband's newest invention is a wheat crust topped with store-bought bruschetta, chopped bacon (cooked), garlic, and flavorful sliced olives.

Nutty Guacamole Enchiladas

Yields 4 Servings

Enchiladas sans cheese … it is true! The richness of the filling more than compensates for the dairy typically found in enchiladas. I love using whole grains whenever possible, but I must admit that whole wheat tortillas just don't meld well in enchiladas. For this recipe I recommend organic or non-GMO corn tortillas or white flour tortillas.

2 Medium, Ripe Avocados
1 to 1-1/2 Tablespoons Lime Juice
1/2 Cup Dairy-Free Sour Cream Alternative (store-bought or recipe on p131), Plus Extra for Serving
3 Green Onions, Thinly Sliced
1/4 Cup Parsley or Cilantro, Minced
1 Small Jalapeno, Deseeded and Minced

1 Garlic Clove, Minced
1/2 Teaspoon Ground Cumin
1/4 Teaspoon Salt
1 Cup (5 ounces) Raw Cashews, Finely Chopped
8 Corn or White Flour Tortillas (6 or 8-inch)
1 15-Ounce Jar Red Enchilada Sauce or the Recipe Below

Preheat your oven to 350ºF (175ºC). Mash the avocados together with the lime juice until relatively smooth; it is okay if a few small chunks remain. Add the sour cream alternative, green onions, parsley or cilantro, jalapeno, garlic, cumin, salt, and cashews and stir until everything is well combined. Pour a shallow layer of enchilada sauce (just enough to cover) in a large baking dish (7x11-inch or 9x13-inch will work). Lay a tortilla in the enchilada sauce in the baking dish, and place some of the avocado-cashew mixture along one side of the tortilla. Roll it up and place the enchilada to one side of the baking dish. Repeat with the remaining tortillas and avocado-cashew mixture. Pour the enchilada sauce over the enchiladas to cover, making sure they are well coated. Cover and bake the enchiladas for 30 minutes. Serve each enchilada topped with a dollop of sour cream alternative.

Meaty option: Before rolling the tortillas up, top the filling with cooked, chopped or shredded chicken or mock chicken strips cut into chunks. About 1 cup of meat or faux meat will suffice, but you may need 2 to 4 extra tortillas, since the filling will go a bit further.

Red Enchilada Sauce: This recipe yields a generous amount of enchilada sauce, so you may have just a bit more than you need for the recipe above.

3 Tablespoons Vegetable or Grapeseed Oil
3 Tablespoons Cornstarch or Arrowroot Powder
2 Tablespoons Chili Powder (mild, medium, or hot, depending upon your tastes)*
1 Teaspoon Ground Cumin
2 Cups Vegetable or Chicken Broth

1/2 Cup Plain Tomato Sauce (such as Hunt's)
2 Teaspoons Granulated Sugar or Sweetener or Choice
1 Teaspoon Dried Oregano
1/2 Teaspoon Salt

Heat the oil in a medium-sized saucepan over medium heat. Add the cornstarch or arrowroot and cook for 1 minute, while whisking to remove any lumps. Add the chili powder and cumin, and continue to whisk and cook the sauce for 1 more minute. Gradually stir in the broth, whisking to eliminate any lumps. Stir in the tomato sauce, sugar, oregano, and salt. Reduce the heat to medium-low and simmer (do not boil) for about 5 to 10 minutes (no need to stir continuously, just check in every minute or two to whisk), or until the sauce thickens just a bit. It will thicken further when baking your enchiladas, so do not cook it for too long.

My family likes spice at the warm heat level rather than flame throwing. Thus, I use 1 tablespoon of mild and 1 tablespoon of medium chili powder in this recipe. For our tastes, this still has a spicy kick.

Karina's Sweet Potato & Black Bean Enchiladas

Yields 4 Servings

Recipe adapted from the blog, *Karina's Kitchen* (glutenfreegoddess.blogspot.com) by Karina Allrich - *Karina's list of food allergies is one of the longest I have seen, but what she does with the foods she can eat is pure magic. Her blog is a true delight for the senses. This dish is one of Karina's most popular. She notes, "...for company I prefer to nestle these babies into individual gratin dishes. It makes for a prettier presentation. And the chile sauce can be mild or hot. However you like it. Both are tasty."*

Quickie Green Chile Sauce:

1 Tablespoon Arrowroot Powder [or Cornstarch]

1 Generous Cup Chopped Roasted Green Chilies (hot or mild, canned or frozen), Thawed

1 Cup Vegetable Broth

2 to 3 Garlic Cloves, Minced

Ground Cumin or Chili Powder, to Taste

Enchiladas:

1 15-Ounce Can Black Beans, Rinsed and Drained

3 to 4 Garlic Cloves, Minced

Juice of 1 Lime

2 Heaping Cups Cooked Sweet Potatoes, Smashed a Bit, but Chunky*

2 or More Tablespoons Chopped Roasted Green Chilies (canned are fine)

1/4 Teaspoon Ground Cumin

1/4 Teaspoon Chili or Curry Powder (mild or spicy)

Salt, to Taste

Freshly Ground Black Pepper, to Taste

2 to 4 Tablespoons Vegetable Oil

8 Corn Tortillas

Monterey Jack, Mozzarella, or Cheddar Vegan Cheese Alternative, Shredded (optional)

Preheat your oven to 350ºF (175ºC). Make your Quickie Green Chile Sauce by dissolving the arrowroot in a little bit of water and combining it with the green chilies, broth, garlic, and cumin or chili powder in a saucepan over medium-high heat. Bring the mixture to a high simmer, and continue simmering until thickened. Pour about 1/4 cup of the Quickie Green Chile Sauce into the bottom of 9x13-inch or 8x12-inch baking dish and set aside.

Meanwhile, for the filling, place the black beans, garlic, and lime juice in a mixing bowl and toss to coat. In a separate bowl combine the lightly smashed sweet potatoes with the green chilies, cumin, and chili or curry powder. Season the potatoes with salt and pepper to taste. Grab a skillet and heat a bit of the oil. Lightly cook the corn tortillas to soften them - one at a time - as you stuff each one.

Lay the first hot tortilla in the sauced baking dish; wet it with the sauce. Spoon an eighth of the sweet potato mixture down the center of the tortilla. Top with an eighth of the black beans. Wrap and roll the tortilla to the end of the baking dish. Repeat this process with the remaining tortillas. Top with the rest of the Quickie Green Chile Sauce. Sprinkle the shredded vegan cheese alternative atop the enchiladas, if using. Bake for 20 to 25 minutes, or until the enchilada sauce is hot and bubbling around the edges. Serve with a crisp green salad spiked with Mandarin oranges or halved grapes.

* Karina cubes the potatoes, and then softens them just a little with a potato masher.

Chinese Five-Spice Noodles

Yields 4 Servings

This dish has a subtle flavor and a gentle warm heat, making it a perfect comfort food for both warm and cool days. For those salt cravings, serve with soy sauce or wheat-free tamari, but add it modestly; just a splash or two goes a long way. Feel free to change up the vegetables; red bell peppers and snow peas also work nicely.

8 Ounces Wide Rice Noodles / Sticks (similar to linguine in width)
1/2 Cup Orange Juice
1 Teaspoon Orange Zest
2 Tablespoons Soy Sauce or Wheat-Free Tamari
2 Teaspoons Agave Nectar or Honey
1 Teaspoon Chinese Five-Spice Powder
1/4 Teaspoon Crushed Red Pepper Flakes

1/4 Teaspoon Salt
1 Tablespoon Peanut or Olive Oil
1 Medium Onion, Cut into Thin Wedges
1 Cup Thinly Sliced Carrots
12 Ounces Portobello, Cremini, or Button Mushrooms, Thickly Sliced
2 to 4 Garlic Cloves, Thinly Sliced or Minced
4 Cups Small Broccoli Florets (about 1/2 lb)

Cook the noodles according to the package directions, but be sure not to overcook them; al dente is fine. Drain (but do not rinse) the noodles and cover to keep them warm. While the pasta is cooking, combine the orange juice, zest, soy sauce, agave or honey, five-spice powder, crushed red pepper, and salt in a small dish. Set aside. Heat the oil in a large skillet over medium heat. Add the onions and carrots, and stir-fry for about 4 minutes. Add the mushrooms and garlic, and sauté the vegetables for 1 minute more. Add the broccoli, cover and cook for 2 to 4 minutes or until the vegetables are crisp-tender. Add the reserved sauce and cooked noodles, and continue to cook while stirring continuously for about 2 minutes, allowing the flavors to meld.

Meaty Option: The flavors of this dish work quite well with pork or chicken. Thinly slice about 1/2 lb of meat, and sauté it in 1 tablespoon of oil until cooked through, but still tender. Add the meat with the sauce and noodles, tossing to coat. To keep it vegetarian, add about 1/2 lb of mock chicken strips, cut into bite-sized pieces.

Lentil Curry in a Hurry

Yields 4 Servings

I apologize for the cheesy name, but this really is a quick and easy dish with a mild, yet slightly spicy flavor to appease kids and spouses alike. My curry hating husband devoured every last lentil, stating, "I do like curry sometimes." For him, I use just 1-1/2 teaspoons of curry powder, but feel free to use 2 teaspoons if you have a curry-loving household.

1 Cup Red Lentils
2 Teaspoons Olive, Peanut, or Grapeseed Oil
1/2 Cup Chopped Onion (about 1/2 medium)
2 Cups Water
1-1/2 to 2 Teaspoons Curry Powder

1 Teaspoon Mild or Medium Chili Powder
1/2 Teaspoon Mustard Powder
1/2 Teaspoon Salt
1/2 Cup Regular or Light Coconut Milk
4 Cups Cooked White or Brown Rice

Rinse the lentils in cold water until the water runs clear, checking to remove any stones that may have slipped in. Set aside. Heat the oil in a medium-sized saucepan over medium heat. Add the onion and sauté until tender and translucent, about 3 to 5 minutes. Add the water, lentils, and the curry, chili, and mustard powders. Stir to combine, and bring the mixture to a simmer. Cover, reduce the heat to medium-low, and let the lentils cook for 10 to 15 minutes, or until they are tender. Stir in the salt and coconut milk, and allow the lentils to simmer for a few minutes more. Divide the rice between 4 plates, and top with the lentil curry.

Optional Add-Ins: Dice 1 medium tomato or mash 1 small banana and stir it in with the coconut milk.

Pineapple Teriyaki Bowl

Yields 4 Servings

One of my favorite meals is the humble rice bowl. You may choose to use leftover rice and vegetables, or cook some up in 15 minutes using a rice cooker with steamer basket. This simple dish also goes well with baked tofu, leftover chicken, or a basic white fish, or you can omit the starch and use the sauce as a flavorful marinade.

1 14-Ounce Can Crushed or Chunk Pineapple in Juice
1/2 Cup + 2 Tablespoons Soy Sauce or Wheat-Free
    Tamari
2 Tablespoons Mirin or White Wine*
1 to 2 Teaspoons Sesame Oil
1/2 Cup Light or Dark Brown Sugar, Lightly Packed
2 Teaspoons Cornstarch or Arrowroot Powder

1/2 Teaspoon Garlic Powder or 4 Garlic Cloves
1/4 Teaspoon Ground Ginger or 1 Tablespoon
    Chopped Ginger
1/2 Teaspoon Crushed Red Pepper Flakes, or to Taste
4 Cups Cooked Brown or White Rice
2 lbs Steamed Vegetables (broccoli, cauliflower,
    carrots, snow peas, etc.)

Toss the pineapple with juice (do not drain it), soy sauce, mirin or wine, sesame oil, sugar, cornstarch or arrowroot, garlic, ginger, and red pepper (if using) into your blender, and give it a quick puree. Pour the sauce into a medium saucepan, and simmer it over medium-low heat for 10 minutes, or until it thickens to your desired consistency. Divide the rice between four bowls, top with the steamed vegetables, and ladle some sauce over top of the vegetables.

*Mirin is a Japanese rice wine that contains a good dose of sweetness. I have used both mirin and white wine in this recipe with good success; the white wine is just a bit less sweet.

Almond Buttery Stir Fry

Yields 4 Servings

Almond butter, blackstrap molasses, broccoli, and tofu are all good sources of calcium. Combined into this quick and easy dish, they are also quite delicious!

1/2 Cup Creamy Almond Butter
1/2 Cup Hot Water (plus more as needed)
1/4 Cup Apple Cider Vinegar or Rice Vinegar
5 Tablespoons Soy Sauce or Wheat-Free Tamari,
    Divided
2 Tablespoons Blackstrap Molasses (honey or regular
    molasses will work in a pinch)
1/4 to 1/2 Teaspoon Crushed Red Pepper Flakes
1 lb Firm or Extra-Firm Tofu, Well Drained
2 Tablespoons Peanut or Olive Oil

1 Large Onion (about 1/2 lb), Cut into 3/4-Inch
    Wedges
1 Tablespoon Minced Ginger
4 Large Garlic Cloves, Minced
12 Ounces Broccoli Florets
1 Red Bell Pepper Cut into 3/4-Inch Wedges or Slices
3 to 4 Cups Cooked Quinoa or Brown Rice
1/2 Cup Almond Slices or Chopped Cashews
    (optional)
1 Small Lime, Cut into 4 Wedges

In medium-sized bowl, whisk together the almond butter and hot water. Stir in the vinegar, 2 tablespoons of the soy sauce, molasses, and crushed red pepper until all ingredients are well incorporated. Set aside. Cube the tofu, place it in a bowl, and drizzle with 1 tablespoon of the soy sauce to marinate. Stir to combine and set aside. Heat the oil in a large skillet over medium heat. Add the onion and sauté for 2 minutes. Add the ginger and garlic, and sauté for 1 minute more. Add the broccoli, bell pepper, and the remaining 2 tablespoons of soy sauce. Sauté until the broccoli and bell pepper are crisp-tender, about 4 to 5 minutes. Add the tofu and sauté for 2 minutes, or until the tofu is heated through. Remove the skillet from the heat, and stir in the reserved almond butter sauce. If it thickens too much, thin with additional water, 1 tablespoon at a time, until it reaches your desired consistency. Serve over the cooked quinoa or rice. Garnish with sliced or chopped nuts, if desired. Serve with lime wedges for seasoning to taste.

Sesame Soba Noodles with Calcium-Rich Kale

Yields 6 Servings

It is so easy to incorporate calcium and nutrient-rich vegetables into flavorful stir-fry and noodle dishes. You can substitute the kale with spinach or chard, but they do not provide as much usable calcium as kale.

12 Ounces Udon, Soba, or Spaghetti Noodles
1 Large Bunch Kale (1 to 1-1/2 lbs)
2 Tablespoons White or Black Sesame Seeds
1 Tablespoon Peanut or Other High Heat Oil (p113)
1 Tablespoon Minced Fresh Ginger

3 Tablespoons Soy Sauce or Wheat-Free Tamari, Divided
2 Tablespoons Sesame Oil
4 Tablespoons Water, or as Needed
1 Green Onion, Thinly Sliced (optional)

Prepare the noodles according to the package directions. While the pasta is cooking, cut the thickest stem portions away from the kale, and slice the remaining leaves into strips. Set aside. Place the sesame seeds in a large skillet over medium heat. Stir or shake the sesame seeds until they darken slightly (be careful not to burn them!) and become fragrant. Remove the seeds from the pan and set aside. Add the 1 tablespoon of peanut oil to your skillet, and warm it over medium heat. Add the ginger and sauté for 1 minute. Turn the heat up to medium-high, and add the kale and 1 tablespoon of the soy sauce. Stir fry the greens until they are wilted but still slightly crunchy, about 3 minutes. As the kale cooks, you can add water 1 tablespoon at a time, but only as needed. If you end up with excess liquid once the kale is cooked, drain it. Add the cooked pasta to the kale, along with the remaining 2 tablespoons of soy sauce, sesame oil, and sesame seeds. Toss to combine. Serve topped with green onions if desired.

Optional Add-Ins: I enjoy this as a very light meal on summer evenings, or when my appetite isn't quite so large, but you can add baked tofu slices, tempeh, more vegetables (bean sprouts, broccoli, bell peppers, etc.), pork, or chicken for a more sizable entrée.

Gluten-Free: You can easily make this meal gluten-free by using the wheat-free tamari and your favorite gluten-free noodles. I do recommend seeking out the 100% buckwheat soba noodles by Eden Foods (www.edenfoods.com, (517) 456-7424) as a special treat if you get the chance; they are wheat/gluten-free.

More Menu Ideas: Reliably Dairy-Free Meals

The following is a list of additional meal ideas, which are traditionally dairy-free or easy to find without dairy. Before you scour the list to combat my dairy-free claims, remember that this is just an inspirational list. While some recipes may add a cheese or cream twist, in general, these are dinners that you should be able to enjoy fully without dairy.

~ *Spaghetti* - I never tire of this staple, which can be dressed up in so many ways.

~ *Seasoned Meat / Meat Alternatives* - Try jerk, Cajun, Italian, orange, pepper, barbecue, or mustard seasonings.

~ *Kebabs* - Marinate vegetables, fish, and/or meat in a light dairy-free Italian dressing or in your favorite blend of herbs and spices, skewer them and grill or roast until cooked to perfection.

~ *Burger* - Traditional beef, chicken, buffalo, turkey, veggie, Portobello (just one big meaty mushroom), or eggplant (thick slices) grilled up and slapped between two slices of bread, hold the cheese.

~ *Sandwiches* - Enjoy a cold sub for summer (cold cut, grilled vegetables, etc.) or a toasted version in the winter.

~ *Chicken Marsala* - Enjoy the wine and mushroom sauce, but be sure to use olive oil rather than butter.

~ *Stew* - Beef, potatoes, vegetables, or whatever is to your liking.

~ *Ratatouille* - Though this French comfort food is usually served as a side dish, it makes a hearty main meal when accompanied by some bread or rice.

~ *Roasted Spaghetti Squash* - Once roasted, the flesh of this jumbo squash is easily scraped out with a fork to make a wonderful "noodle" stand-in that goes well with pesto or other light sauces.

~ *Spanish Rice* - When I was young, my mom made a "pantry" Spanish rice that was spiked with bacon (or turkey bacon), which I couldn't get enough of.

~ *Taco Night* - Place small flour or corn tortillas out with cooked ground beef (or vegan crumbles), chicken or fish, and an assortment of toppers, including beans, chopped avocado, guacamole, sour cream alternative (store-bought or recipe on p131), chopped olives, salsa, hot sauce, corn, tomatoes, sliced cabbage, and/or lettuce.

~ *Fajitas / Burritos / Wraps*

~ *Tamales*

~ *Jambalaya*

~ *Empanadas* - Traditional Argentine empanadas are made with beef, flavorful olives, eggs, and onions, but you can swap the meat and eggs for vegetables in this dinner-worthy pastry.

~ *Chile Verde*

~ *Paella* - You will often find this dish served with a mix of seafood, but you can enjoy the flavors vegetarian-style; the key is in the saffron.

~ *Fried Rice*

~ *Stir Fries* - The humble Chinese stir fry can be dressed up with so many flavors and is a brilliant way to stash those vegetables. Check your local grocer for jars of hoisin, kung pao, teriyaki, sweet and sour, or black bean sauce. They are usually dairy-free and should have quick and simple meal instructions on the label.

~ *Chinese Chicken Salad*

~ *Asian Buns, Dumplings, or Gyozas*

~ *Homemade Sushi* - No need to scour the stores for sushi-grade fish. Cooked fish and vegetables are equally delicious when rolled up in sheets of nori with sticky rice, and this meal is amazingly quick and fun to assemble.

~ *Pad Thai* - Full of flavor, this dish is traditionally made with fish sauce and eggs, but vegans can substitute soy sauce and omit the eggs in most recipes, if desired.

~ *Thai Curry* - Green, Yellow, Red, Panang ... Thai curries are so amazingly flavorful and simple because the pastes come in ready made cans at Asian food markets (cheapest options) or in small jars at traditional grocery stores. Just add coconut milk, the vegetables, and your favorite protein, and your meal is on the table.

~ *Aloo Dishes* - Dry Indian curry type recipes such as Aloo Phujia, Aloo Matar, Aloo Gobi, and Samosas are often dairy-free or easily adaptable.

~ *Falafel* - My favorite falafel recipe is a baked version from *The Whole Foods Allergy Cookbook*, but dairy-free falafel recipes abound.

Some Store-Bought Recommendations:

There are many great brands on the market, but the following recommendations only include products that I purchase with some regularity or that a colleague highly recommended. For full lists of non-dairy, packaged foods and brands, see the product lists available on www.godairyfree.org.

Amy's Kitchen (www.amys.com, (707) 568-4500) ~ frozen entrées
If you need some quick frozen entrées stashed in the freezer, then there is no better than Amy's organic products. Okay, so this is my personal opinion, but I know dozens of people who would agree. I have yet to have a bad meal from Amy's, and I have sampled their dairy-free pizzas, dinner pies, bowls, and their burritos (which are a quick, lower-priced option). Plus, since the Amy's brand is now mainstream, it does tend to go on sale for stocking up. Amy's is a vegetarian company (including no eggs), and they have a large range of vegan/dairy-free products. However, they do have some cheesy items, so be sure to read the labels.

Ian's® (www.amys.com, (707) 568-4500) ~ frozen entrées
Specifically designed for kids, Ian's frozen entrées are free from refined sugars, illegible ingredients, and hormones or antibiotics. Plus, they offer a special allergen-free line that is made without wheat, gluten, dairy, eggs, nuts, or soy. Thus far, we have kid-verified (two enthusiastic thumbs up) their gluten-free and casein-free chicken fingers meal, French bread pizza, and French toast sticks, but there are many more selections to go.

Namaste Foods (www.namastefoods.com, (866) 258-949) ~ pasta mixes
Namaste is best known for their gluten-free, food allergy-friendly baking mixes, but I love their pasta mixes. With names like Say Cheez and Pasta Pisavera, really, it is hard not to feel like a kid experimenting in the kitchen. These mixes (free from dairy, gluten, corn, soy, potato, nuts, and tree nuts) act as an easy base to a quick and tasty meal.

CHAPTER 25:
FEELIN' SAUCY

Bryanna's Béchamel or White Sauce

Yields 2 Cups or 8 Servings

Recipe adapted from Nonna's Italian Kitchen by Bryanna Clark Grogan - Bryanna offers numerous suggestions for this versatile white sauce, "It can be used as an all-purpose white sauce in all of your cooking, and as a topping for Greek dishes, such as vegetarian moussaka, and even as a substitute for melted cheese in many casseroles. In Italy, this type of sauce is used on lasagna rather than the heavy melted cheeses in American-style lasagna."

1 Cup Unsweetened Rice, Almond, or Soymilk
1/2 Cup Extra-Firm Silken Tofu or Regular Medium-
   Firm Tofu, Crumbled
1/2 Cup Water
1 "Chicken-style" Vegetarian Broth Cube (enough for
   1 cup liquid), Crumbled or 1 Teaspoon Better
   than Bouillon No Chicken Broth Base

1/2 Teaspoon Salt
2 Tablespoons Dairy-Free Margarine or Extra-Virgin
   Olive Oil
1 to 1/2-3 Tablespoons All-Purpose Flour (depending
   on thickness desired)
Pinch Freshly Grated Nutmeg
Pinch White Pepper

Place the milk alternative, tofu, water, broth cube, and salt in your blender, and blend until very smooth. Set aside. Melt the margarine in a medium, heavy saucepan and whisk in the flour. Whisk it over medium-high heat for a few minutes, but remove it from heat before it starts to change color (you want a white "roux"). Scrape this into your blender (where the tofu mixture awaits) and blend for a few seconds, then pour the entire mixture back into your saucepan. Stir over medium-high heat until it thickens and boils; turn the heat down and simmer on low for a few minutes. Whisk in the nutmeg and pepper.

Microwave Option: Melt the margarine in a large microwave-safe bowl or a 1 quart glass measuring cup on HIGH for 45 seconds. Whisk in the flour and microwave on HIGH for 2 minutes. Scrape this into the mixture in your blender, and blend briefly. Pour the mixture back into your measuring cup, and microwave on HIGH for 2 minutes. Whisk, and microwave for 2 more minutes. Whisk, and microwave for 2 more minutes. Whisk in the nutmeg and pepper.

Lower Fat Option: Leave out the margarine and simply cook the flour in a dry pan or microwave until it just starts to change color. You may also opt to use reduced fat tofu and soymilk.

Soy-Free Option: Omit the tofu; increase the milk alternative by 1/4 cup and add 1/4 cup raw cashews before blending. Since the cashews have a thickening effect, start with the lesser amount of flour. Also, use just 2 teaspoons of olive oil in place of the margarine.

Wheat-Free Option: Add the melted margarine or olive oil directly to the blended mixture, along with 1 to 4 tablespoons (depending on thickness desired) of white rice flour or mochiko flour (sweet/glutinous rice flour) instead of the wheat flour (omit the first cooking step). Sauces made with mochiko flour are excellent for freezing (for instance, if you freeze a prepared but not baked lasagna), because the sauce will not separate when thawed.

Mellow Cheesy Sauce

Yields 2 Cups or 8 Servings

This simple, kid-friendly "cheese" sauce has a pleasant flavor that goes well atop vegetables, rice, and baked potatoes. According to my husband, it is also wonderful with pasta for a quick macaroni & "cheese" (see below).

2 Cups Water
1/2 Cup Nutritional Yeast Flakes
1/2 Cup Cornstarch or Arrowroot Powder
1-1/4 to 1-1/2 Teaspoons Salt

1 Teaspoon Mustard Powder or Prepared Mustard
1/4 Cup Dairy-Free Margarine
1/2 Cup Unsweetened Rice, Cashew, or Soymilk

Combine the water, nutritional yeast, cornstarch or arrowroot, salt, and mustard in your blender, and give it a whirl for about 30 seconds. Melt the margarine in a medium-sized saucepan over medium-low heat. Pour in the mixture from your blender, and whisk until it begins to thicken, about 3 to 5 minutes. Slowly whisk in the milk alternative, and continue to cook, stirring constantly, until it reaches your desired consistency.

Soy-Free Option: Substitute olive or grapeseed oil for the margarine.

Macaroni & "Cheese" Option: Stir in 1 lb of cooked pasta (your choice, gluten-free or regular) for an easy stove top mac 'n cheez. I sometimes reduce the pasta to 3/4 lb (12 ounces) and add in steamed cauliflower and broccoli florets for a more complete meal that serves 4 to 6 people.

Orange Cheesy Sauce

Yields 2 Cups or 8 Servings

This cheerfully orange sauce offers that warm and fuzzy feeling of processed cheese, but with a much cleaner taste. It has a bit of a tang when compared to the mellow cheesy sauce, but not enough to call it sharp. I love this sauce stirred into pasta for an instant macaroni and "cheese" (see below), but I do believe it is multi-purpose and rather addictive.

1-3/4 Cups Water
1/4 Cup Olive or Grapeseed Oil
2 Teaspoons Lemon Juice
1/2 to 3/4 Cup Chopped Cooked (very soft) Carrots
1/4 Cup Nutritional Yeast Flakes

1/4 Cup Cornstarch or Arrowroot Powder or 1/3 Cup
    All-Purpose (Plain) Flour
2 Teaspoons Onion Powder
1-1/2 Teaspoons Salt
1 Cup Unsweetened Rice, Cashew, or Soymilk

Combine the water, oil, lemon juice, carrots, nutritional yeast, starch or flour, onion powder, and salt in your blender, and blend until all of the carrot bits have vanished and the mixture is smooth. For the smoothest results, pour the liquid through a fine mesh strainer (to remove any little carrot bits) as you pour it into a medium-sized saucepan over medium heat. Whisk continuously until it begins to thicken, about 3 to 5 minutes. Slowly whisk in the milk alternative, and continue to cook, stirring constantly, until it reaches your desired consistency.

Macaroni & "Cheese" Option: Stir in 1 lb of cooked pasta (your choice) for an easy stove top mac 'n cheez. I sometimes reduce the pasta to 3/4 lb (12 ounces) and add in steamed cauliflower and broccoli florets for a more complete meal that serves 4 to 6 people.

Powdered "Cheese" Mix

Yields 3 Cups or 24 Servings

Quite a while back, I ran into a bulk "cheese" mix recipe on the Internet. With a few changes, it quickly became a staple item in my pantry. It offers great versatility and is excellent to have on hand when those cheesy cravings strike.

1-1/2 Cups (7.5 ounces) Raw Cashews
1 Cup Nutritional Yeast Flakes
1/4 Cup Cornstarch or Arrowroot Powder
1-1/2 Tablespoons Garlic Powder

1-1/2 Tablespoons Onion Powder
3 to 4 Teaspoons Salt
3/4 Teaspoon Paprika
1/4 Teaspoon Black Pepper

Combine all of the ingredients in your blender or food processor, and blend until the nuts have been reduced to a very fine meal or powder. If your blender has trouble with nuts (as mine does), process the cashews and nutritional yeast together in your spice grinder. This may take 3 to 4 batches, but you should only need to blend each batch for 30 to 60 seconds. Combine the nuts and nutritional yeast with all remaining ingredients, making sure that everything is well incorporated. Place the mix in a container with tight fitting lid, and store it in the refrigerator. It should keep for several weeks.

To Prepare 4 Servings: In a small saucepan, whisk together 1/2 cup of the mix with 3/4 cup of cold water. Place the mixture over medium heat, and whisk continuously until it thickens, about 3 to 5 minutes. If it becomes too thick, add more water, 1 tablespoon at a time, until it reaches your desired consistency. For a slightly sharper flavor, whisk in 1/2 teaspoon of lemon juice.

Nacho Dip Option: When preparing, use 1/2 cup of your favorite salsa and 1/4 cup of water per 1/2 cup of mix. Add more water 1 tablespoon at a time until it reaches your desired consistency.

Nut-Free Option: Substitute sunflower seeds for the cashews, or a blend of sunflower and sesame seeds. The seeds are slightly bitter when compared to the sweetness of cashews, offering a different flavor.

Lower Fat Option: Technically, the above recipe only contains about 4g of fat per serving, but you can cut this in half and give the "cheese" a heartier flavor by omitting the arrowroot or cornstarch, reducing the cashews to 3/4 cup, and adding 3/4 cup rolled oats. Grind the oats (into a powder or flour) along with the cashews and nutritional yeast.

Fresh Organic Tomato Basil Sauce

Yields 1 Cup

This is one of those recipes that I love to make in the height of summer, when both tomatoes and basil are at their peak and a lighter sauce suits our mood. In my opinion, organic tomatoes further enhance the flavor, but conventional tomatoes will also work.

1 Tablespoons Olive or Grapeseed Oil
2 Large Garlic Cloves, Minced
1 lb Fresh Tomatoes, Diced (roma, cluster, or your
    favorite variety will work)

1/2 to 3/4 Teaspoon Salt
1/8 to 1/4 Teaspoon Freshly Ground Black Pepper
1/4 Cup Chopped Fresh Basil
Sliced or Chopped Olives, Black or Green (optional)

Heat the oil in a medium skillet over low heat. Add the garlic and sauté for just 1 to 2 minutes. Add the tomatoes, salt, and pepper to taste. Simmer on low for 20 to 30 minutes. Stir in the basil and cook for 2 to 3 minutes more. Add the olives, if desired.

Elegant Pantry Marinara

Yields approximately 5 Cups or 6 Servings

While you may think tomato sauce is safe territory for store-bought, it can often harbor milk, cream, cheese, or other milk based ingredients as I have accidentally found out on more than one occasion. Luckily, I have fallen in love with the wonderful flavors and simplicity of homemade tomato sauce. This recipe was originally thrown together to top the star entrée of the evening, eggplant raviolis. As it turned out, we hated the raviolis, but loved the sauce. It is a full-bodied tomato sauce that will hold its own with any Italian dish.

2 Tablespoons Grapeseed or Olive Oil
1 Cup Diced Onion (about 1 medium)
2 to 4 Garlic Cloves, Minced or 1 to 1-1/2 Teaspoons Crushed Garlic
1 Teaspoon Dried or 1 Tablespoon Fresh Thyme
1 Teaspoon Dried or 1 Tablespoon Fresh Oregano
Large Pinch Crushed Red Pepper Flakes

2 14.5-Ounce Cans Diced Tomatoes or 2 lbs Fresh Tomatoes, Diced
2 Tablespoons Tomato Paste
1 Cup Vegetable Broth
2 Teaspoons Agave Nectar or Sweetener of Choice
1 Tablespoon Balsamic Vinegar
1/2 Teaspoon Salt

Heat the oil in a large skillet over medium-low heat. Add the onion and sauté until it is soft and translucent, about 5 to 7 minutes. Add the garlic, thyme, oregano, and crushed red pepper, and sauté for another 3 minutes. Add the tomatoes, tomato paste, broth, sweetener, vinegar, and salt. Allow the sauce to simmer for 30 to 40 minutes, then remove it from the heat, allowing it to cool for 10 minutes. Place the sauce in your blender (this may take 2 batches) and pulse a few times. Return the sauce to your skillet, and keep it warm over low heat until needed. You should end up with a nice thick sauce, that is somewhat smooth, but with a hearty, chunky feel.

Sunflower Pesto

Yields 1 Cup or 4 to 6 Servings

Recipe adapted from What's To Eat? The Milk-Free, Egg-Free, Nut-Free Food Allergy Cookbook by Linda Coss - After months of weekly pesto dishes, my husband finally inquired what this pesto was made with. Knowing how frugal we both are, he couldn't imagine I was burning through bags of expensive pine nuts. With my cover blown, I revealed this secret recipe. True to Linda's claim, "this is as close to the taste of a traditional pesto that you can get without using nuts and cheese!"

1 Cup Packed Fresh Basil Leaves, Washed
1/2 Cup Raw Unsalted Sunflower Seeds*
1/2 Cup Olive Oil

2 Teaspoons Bottled Minced Garlic
1/2 Teaspoon Salt
Freshly Ground Black Pepper, to Taste

Place all ingredients in a food processor that has been fitted with a metal blade [or a blender]. Process approximately 2 minutes, until the basil leaves are finely chopped, the sunflower seeds are ground up, and the mixture has formed a thick sauce. Scrape down the sides of the food processor bowl and process for another 20 seconds.

Pasta Pesto Option: Toss the freshly made pesto with freshly cooked and drained pasta (about 12 ounces), and then serve immediately.

Available at Natural Foods stores. If allergic to nuts and/or peanuts, be sure to avoid roasted sunflower seeds, as most commercially available roasted sunflower seeds are roasted in peanut oil.

Flavorful Taco Seasoning

Yields 2-1/2 Tablespoons or the Equivalent of a 1/4-Ounce Packet of Store-Bought

My husband loves this seasoning in tacos, burritos, and fajitas. We use a mild chili powder, as we prefer to control the heat of our meals after the fact, with hot sauce or salsa to taste, but you can use a medium or hot one if you prefer.

1 Tablespoon Mild Chili Powder
1-1/2 Teaspoons Ground Cumin
1/2 Teaspoon Paprika
1/4 Teaspoon Garlic Powder
1/4 Teaspoon Onion Powder

1/4 Teaspoon Dried Oregano
1/8 to 1/4 Teaspoon Crushed Red Pepper Flakes
1 Teaspoon Salt
1/2 Teaspoon Freshly Ground Black Pepper (optional)

In a small bowl, stir all of the ingredients together. If not using immediately, store in an airtight container.

To Prepare: Add the full batch of this seasoning mix to 1 lb of almost cooked ground meat, cubed chicken, vegan "meat" crumbles, cubed tofu, or chopped vegetables. Finish cooking with the seasoning incorporated to help the flavors meld.

Cashew Gravy

Yields 2 Cups

Recipe adapted from Get it Ripe by jae steele - I was fortunate enough to be a recipe tester for jae's first cookbook. I love her focus on whole food ingredients, and was especially impressed by this gravy. While I am not usually a gravy fan, this one imparted an amazingly rich flavor on my meal. I use the full 3 tablespoons of soy sauce and skip the celery seeds to no ill effect.

1 Large or 2 Medium Garlic Cloves, Crushed or Grated
2 Tablespoons Olive Oil
1/2 Cup Cashews*, Ground or 1/4 Cup Cashew
    Paste/Butter
1/2 Teaspoon Celery Seeds (optional)

1-1/2 Cups Water
2 to 3 Tablespoons Soy Sauce or Wheat-Free Tamari
2 Tablespoons Arrowroot Powder or Cornstarch,
    Dissolved in an Additional 1/2 Cup Water
Freshly Ground Black Pepper, to Taste

Sauté the garlic in oil for just a few minutes in a medium saucepan or skillet over medium heat (don't let it get crispy!). Add the cashews, celery seeds (if using), water, and soy sauce or tamari. Turn up the heat. Stir in the starch mixture, and stir constantly until it all comes to a boil. Turn off the heat and grind in some pepper to taste. Serve over steamed or roasted vegetables or baked tofu. Use leftovers within 1 week.

* You can buy raw whole cashews and roast them for 5 minutes and then grind them for a more robust flavor.

Tahini Magic Sauce

Yields approximately 1 Cup or 2 to 3 Servings

Recipe adapted from www.meghantelpner.com, by Meghan Telpner - *Meghan is a certified nutritionist out of Ontario, who is always looking for ways to add healthy foods to her diet and those of her clients. She labeled this recipe as "magic" because it is jam packed with calcium. According to Meghan, no two foods have a higher concentration of calcium than tahini and parsley. Use this sauce for pasta, dipping, salads, or in Meghan's "Magic Rice Bowl" (below).*

1/2 Cup Tahini
1/3 Cup Finely Chopped Fresh Parsley
1 Garlic Clove, Minced
Juice of 1 Lemon

1/2 Cup Water, Plus More as Needed
Salt, to Taste
Freshly Ground Black Pepper, to Taste

In a small mixing bowl, combine the tahini, parsley, garlic, and lemon juice and mix thoroughly. Add 1/2 cup of water and mix. You may wish to add more or less water depending on how you want to use the sauce. Add salt and pepper to taste.

Magic Rice Bowl Option: For a quick and nutritious one-person meal, Meghan recommends layering 1 to 1-1/2 cups of cooked brown rice with 3/4 cup grated carrot, 3/4 cup fresh parsley, and 1/2 cup of the Tahini Magic Sauce.

Creamy Peanut Sauce

Yields 4 Servings

This recipe subs in beautifully for teriyaki sauce atop a rice or noodle bowl (p212) and pairs well with vibrant vegetables (think zucchini and colorful bell peppers), tofu, pork, or chicken. Plus, it can be prepared in just 5 minutes, and is extremely easy to customize to your tastes.

1/2 Cup Regular or Light Coconut Milk
1/4 Cup Creamy Unsalted Peanut Butter
2 Tablespoons Soy Sauce or Wheat-Free Tamari
1 Tablespoon Agave Nectar, Evaporated Cane Juice,
     Brown Sugar, or Sweetener of Choice
4 Teaspoons Rice Vinegar or Lime Juice

1/2 Teaspoon Ground Ginger*
1/2 Teaspoon Garlic Powder*
1/4 to 1/2 Teaspoon Crushed Red Pepper Flakes
2 Teaspoons Sesame Oil
2 Tablespoons Water (or more as needed)

Combine the coconut milk and peanut butter in a small saucepan over low heat, stirring continuously as the peanut butter melts. Add in the soy sauce, sweetener, vinegar or juice, ginger, garlic, and red pepper, and continue cooking and stirring for a few minutes more as the flavors meld. Add water to your desired consistency; it will thicken a bit as it cools. Turn off the heat and stir in the sesame oil.

* *I use ground spices for ease and a smoother sauce, but feel free to sauté 1-1/2 teaspoons each of crushed ginger and garlic in just a touch of oil for 2 to 3 minutes over low heat before adding the peanut butter and coconut milk.*

Spicy-Sweet Mustard Dressing

Yields 3/4 Cup

This recipe is a little bit of sweet, spicy, creamy, and tangy all drizzled together into one addictive salad dressing.

1/2 Cup Plain or Raspberry Dairy-Free Yogurt
2 Tablespoons Apple Cider Vinegar
1 Tablespoon Extra-Virgin Olive Oil
1 Tablespoon Dijon or Spicy Brown Mustard

2 Teaspoons Agave Nectar or Honey
1 Garlic Clove, Minced
1/2 Teaspoon Black Pepper
Generous Pinch Salt

Combine all ingredients in a small bowl, and whisk until smooth and creamy. Refrigerate for 1 hour before use to allow the flavors time to meld.

Japanese-Style Ginger Dressing

Yields 1-1/2 Cups

This light dressing reminds me of the small salads we receive at our favorite sushi restaurant before each meal. If your blender isn't very mighty (like mine) you may want to mince the onion, ginger, and garlic. Otherwise, just a quick chop will do before pureeing everything in your blender.

1/2 Cup Diced Onion (about 1/2 medium)
1/2 Cup Peanut or Vegetable Oil
1/3 Cup Rice Vinegar
1/2 Ounce Fresh Ginger, Sliced or 2 Tablespoons
   Minced Ginger
2 Tablespoons Ketchup
4 Teaspoons Soy Sauce or Wheat-Free Tamari

2 Teaspoons Agave Nectar, Honey, Light Brown Sugar,
   or Granulated Sugar
2 Teaspoons Lemon Juice
1 Teaspoon Sesame Oil
1 Garlic Clove, Sliced
1/4 to 1/2 Teaspoon Salt
Freshly Ground Black Pepper, to Taste (optional)

Combine the onion, peanut oil, rice vinegar, ginger, ketchup, soy sauce or tamari, sweetener, lemon juice, sesame oil, garlic, and 1/4 teaspoon of the salt in your blender, and blend for about 1 minute, or until all ingredients are well pureed. Give it a taste test and add more salt and freshly ground black pepper, if desired.

Taco Vinaigrette

Yields 1 Cup

Recipe adapted from Sophie-Safe Cooking by Emily Hendrix - This insanely simple salad dressing is sure to be a hit with both kids and adults, since it was created specifically for that purpose. All of Emily's recipes were designed with her food-allergic daughter's safety in mind, but they were also created for ease and enjoyment by her whole family. To meet with your family's tastes, you can adjust the spiciness of your end result by way of the chili powder, which can be purchased in mild, medium, or hot varieties.

1/2 Cup Oil of Choice
1/3 Cup Apple Cider Vinegar
1 Tablespoon Sugar
2 Teaspoons Chili Powder

1 Garlic Clove, Pressed
1/2 Teaspoon Salt
1/4 Teaspoon Black Pepper
1/2 Teaspoon Ground Cumin

Whisk all ingredients together. Serve atop green salads.

5-Star Ranch Dressing or Dip

Yields 1-1/3 Cups

While I do enjoy the lightness of vinaigrette, sometimes a thick and creamy ranch is the only way to go. Luckily, this delicious dairy-free ranch dressing or dip is just a blender-whirl away.

1/3 Cup Unsweetened Milk Alternative of Choice
1 Teaspoon Lemon Juice
1 Cup Mayonnaise (all-natural, organic, or vegan) or
    Dairy-Free Sour Cream Alternative (store-bought
    or recipe on p131)

2 Teaspoons Dried or Fresh Chopped Parsley
1/2 Teaspoon Garlic Powder
1/2 Teaspoon Onion Powder
1/8 to 1/4 Teaspoon Black pepper, or to Taste
1/8 Teaspoon Salt

In a small bowl, combine the milk alternative and lemon juice, and set it aside for 5 to 10 minutes. In the mean time, whisk together the remaining ingredients in a medium-sized bowl. Whisk the now soured milk alternative into the mayonnaise mixture until smooth. Add more milk alternative to thin if needed. Cover and refrigerate for at least 30 minutes before serving.

Quick Ranch Dip Option: Use the mayonnaise, but replace the milk alternative with dairy-free sour cream alternative (store-bought or recipe on p131).

Creamy Garlic Salad Dressing

Yields 1-1/3 Cups

Sunflower seeds provide thickening power to dressings when left to chill, and the added nutrition doesn't hurt either!

1/4 Cup Raw Sunflower Seeds
4 Ounces Firm Silken Tofu
1/4 Cup Water
1/4 Cup Lemon Juice
1 Tablespoon Agave Nectar, Honey, or Sweetener of
    Choice

1 Tablespoon Prepared Dijon or Yellow Mustard
2 Tablespoons Chopped Fresh Basil Leaves
3 Medium Garlic Cloves, Crushed
1/2 Teaspoon Salt, or to Taste
1/4 to 1/2 Teaspoon Black Pepper, or to Taste
2 Tablespoons Extra-Virgin Olive Oil

Process the sunflower seeds in your spice grinder until powdered. Combine the powdered sunflower seeds, tofu, water, lemon juice, sweetener, mustard, basil, garlic, salt, and pepper in your blender and process until smooth and creamy. With the motor running, slowly blend in the oil. This salad dressing will thicken a bit more as it chills. If it becomes too thick, feel free to add more water, 1 tablespoon at a time, until it reaches your desired consistency.

More Menu Ideas: Typically Dairy-Free Dressings

Dairy-free recipes abound for these simple salad dressings ... use caution though, as some store-bought brands or restaurant versions may using dairy ...

Thousand Island	Vinaigrettes	French
Honey Mustard	Oil & Vinegar	Sesame / Soy / Asian
Italian	Russian	Miso

Some Store-Bought Recommendations:
There are many great brands on the market, but the following recommendations only include products that I purchase with some regularity or that a colleague highly recommended. For full lists of non-dairy, packaged foods and brands, see the product lists available on www.godairyfree.org.

Amy's Kitchen (www.amys.com, (707) 568-4500) ~ pasta sauces
Yes, Amy's again … but this is not an everyday kind of recommendation. Their bottled pasta sauces are beyond an indulgence in taste and price. Amy's organic pasta sauces are packaged like homemade, taste like homemade, and unfortunately have the price tag of purchasing something homemade. But, if I spot them on sale, they are mine.

Annie's Naturals (www.anniesnaturals.com, 800-288-1089) ~ salad dressing and condiments
This is what I refer to as our old stand-by brand of salad dressing. Whenever I see Annie's dressings on sale, I pick up at least a few bottles of the organic selections (which always seem to be the same price as the non-organic – go figure). Annie's carries a wide range of dressings, many of which are dairy-free, making it fun to mix and match. The taste is good and reliable; we haven't found a flavor we didn't like yet. Amy Coccia, a good GFCF colleague and reviewer also raved about Annie's BBQ sauce.

Organicville® (www.organicvillefoods.com, (510) 655-1755) ~ salad dressing and condiments
If my budget allowed, I would load my cupboards with a year's supply of Organicville salad dressings and condiments. Other brands are good, but Organicville is simply the best. While they do offer a dairy-free ranch dressing (remarkable in its own right), it is impossible to ignore their other creative flavor offerings (such as Sundried Tomato & Garlic and Tarragon Dijon, just to name a couple of my favorites). They also produce organic ketchup and barbecue sauce, which are sweetened only with agave nectar, and definitely a notch above other brands in taste and sweetness. At the time of writing, the entire Organicville line was dairy-free and vegan.

Road's End Organics® (www.chreese.com, (805) 684-8500) ~ gravy and "cheese" mixes
Sarah, my favorite dairy-free mom, loves the Shiitake Mushroom Gravy Mix from Road's End so much that she has created recipes just to use it. You can ask her for the recipes via her blog, nowheymama.blogspot.com. She also recommends their most popular product, Chreese®, dairy-free "cheese" mixes. Because they come in powdered form in packets, the mixes have a long shelf-life, so even small stores are willing to carry them.

The Vegetarian Express (www.thevegetarianexpress.com, (734) 355-3593) ~ The ladies behind this business offer a full vegan product line that includes tasty gravy mixes and cheesy sprinkles, but what I like most are their seasoning blends. They offer a flavorful array of spice mixes for whipping up sauces and salad dressings in minutes, and making everyday meals come alive.

CHAPTER 26:
SWEET STUFF

Lemon Streusel Squares
Yields 16 Bars

A while back, I came across an intriguing recipe on the Internet for lemon streusel bars. While I do enjoy lemon bars, the concept of a brown sugar streusel sounded so much better. However, the recipe called for sweetened condensed milk. After some experimentation, I created a delicious sweetened condensed coconut milk (p127), which works perfectly in this recipe combination.

1 Batch Sweetened Condensed Coconut Milk (p127)
1/3 to 1/2 Cup Freshly Squeezed Lemon Juice*
2 Teaspoons Freshly Grated Lemon Zest
3/4 Cup Dairy-Free Margarine or Shortening, Softened

1 Cup Light Brown Sugar, Firmly Packed
2 Cups All-Purpose (Plain) or Whole Wheat Pastry Flour
1-1/2 Cups Rolled Oats
1/4 Teaspoon Salt

Preheat your oven to 350ºF (175ºC) and grease a 9-inch square or 7x11-inch baking dish.** In a medium-sized bowl, stir together the condensed coconut milk, lemon juice, and zest until well blended. Set aside. In a large mixing bowl, cream the margarine or shortening and the brown sugar. Add the flour and oats, and mix with a fork or pastry blender until the mixture resembles coarse crumbs. Reserve 2 cups of this streusel and press the remaining streusel into the bottom of your prepared baking dish. Spread the reserved lemon-coconut filling over the crust and sprinkle with the reserved streusel. Pat the streusel gently into the filling. Bake for 30 to 35 minutes, until the streusel is a light golden brown and slightly firm to the touch. Allow it to cool completely before cutting into bars. Yes, completely. My family actually preferred the bars chilled, so we stashed them in the refrigerator to enjoy whenever cravings struck.

Lemon Streusel Tartlets Option: For a fun presentation, pat the streusel base into 16 greased muffin cups (I recommend silicone cups for this). Divide the filling evenly between the muffin cups, and top each with the remaining streusel. Pat the streusel gently into the filling. Bake for 20 to 25 minutes, or until the tops are golden and they appear set. Allow the tartlets to cool in the cups for about 10 minutes, and pop out when ready.

My lemon-loving in-laws said "Bring on the lemon!" They loved the bars with a full 1/2 cup of lemon juice, proclaiming that even more would be good. My husband and my grandmother, however, like lemon in moderation. They preferred the bars with 1/3 cup lemon juice, which had a little less bite. I liked both. You choose which version works best for you.
***If you do not have one of the above sized baking dishes, use an 8-inch square baking dish, and cook the bars for 5 to 10 minutes longer.*

Bakery-Style Chocolate Chip Cookies

Yields 1-1/2 to 2 Dozen Cookies

Recipe created by Hannah Kaminsky, author of My Sweet Vegan - Unable to simply settle for ordinary chocolate chip cookies, Hannah created this scrumptious bakery-worthy version that holds its own in jumbo form. She uses bread flour in this recipe as it has higher protein content, making for a chewier cookie. While you can substitute all-purpose (plain) flour in a pinch, these cookies will have a better texture with bread flour.

1/2 Cup Dairy-Free Margarine
1/2 Cup Granulated Sugar
1/2 Cup Dark Brown Sugar, Firmly Packed
2 Tablespoons Whole Flax Seeds
3 Tablespoons Plain Milk Alternative of Choice
2 Tablespoons Plain Dairy-Free Yogurt
1/2 Teaspoon Vanilla Extract

1/2 Teaspoon Apple Cider Vinegar
2 Cups Bread Flour
1/2 Teaspoon Baking Powder
1/4 Teaspoon Baking Soda
3/4 Teaspoon Salt
1-1/2 Cups Semi-Sweet Chocolate Chips

Preheat your oven to 375ºF (190ºC) and line two baking sheets with parchment paper or non-stick baking mats. In a large mixing bowl, thoroughly cream the margarine and both sugars, until homogeneous and slightly fluffy. Grind the flax seeds to a fine powder in a coffee or spice grinder, and combine them with the milk alternative. Pour the flax mixture into the margarine and sugars, along with the yogurt, vanilla, and vinegar, and beat to combine. Sift in the flour, baking powder, baking soda, and salt, and mix until the flour has been completely integrated. Fold in the chocolate chips until they are evenly distributed throughout the dough. Scoop out about 1/4 cup of dough for each cookie, roll into balls with the palms of your hands, and flatten them slightly on your prepared pan. For best results, bake one sheet at a time for 10 to 12 minutes or until the edges are set and just beginning to turn golden brown. Let the cookies cool for about 15 minutes on the sheet before removing them to a wire rack to cool completely.

Chocolate Chip Cookies (Made with Oil)

Yields 3 to 4 Dozen Cookies

Since finding a suitable non-hydrogenated margarine was difficult in my early dairy-free years, and living without home-baked cookies was not an option, I decided to adventure making cookies with oil. The results were surprisingly successful, and have become a staple in my kitchen over the years. In fact, I have to act quickly when I take them out of the oven, before my husband attempts to tear the hot cookies right off the sheet!

2-1/2 Cups All-Purpose (Plain) Flour or Whole Wheat
   Pastry Flour
1 Teaspoon Baking Soda
1/2 Teaspoon Salt
1 Cup Light Brown Sugar, Firmly Packed
1/2 Cup Granulated Sugar
1/2 Cup Grapeseed, Coconut, or Extra-Light Olive Oil

1 to 2 Tablespoons Plain Milk Alternative of Choice
1 Teaspoon Vanilla Extract
2 Eggs or Scant 1/2 Cup (roughly 7 tablespoons) Plain
   Dairy-Free Yogurt
2 Tablespoons Ground Flaxseed (omit if using eggs)
1 Cup Semi-Sweet Chocolate Chips, or More if Desired

Preheat your oven to 375ºF (190ºC). In a medium-sized bowl, combine the flour, baking soda, and salt. Set aside. In a mixing bowl, blend the sugars, oil, milk alternative (add 1 tablespoon for a puffier cookie, 2 tablespoons for a slightly flatter, chewier cookie), and vanilla until creamy. Beat in the eggs or yogurt and flaxseed, until smooth. Gradually stir or beat in the reserved flour mixture until fully incorporated. Fold in the chocolate chips. Drop the dough by the large teaspoonful onto baking sheets (ungreased or lined with non-stick baking mats). Space the cookies a few inches apart, allowing room for them to spread. Bake until the cookies just begin to take on a light brown hue, about 10 to 12 minutes. Let them rest on the sheets for 2 minutes before removing them to a wire rack to cool completely.

Coffee House Cookies

Yields 1 Dozen Cookies

Recipe created by Hannah Kaminsky, author of My Sweet Vegan - Infused with a double-dose of caffeine, these lovely treats are perfect for any coffee-lover. This makes a petite batch, perfect for smaller households, but feel free to double the entire recipe if preparing it for a larger group.

1 Cup All-Purpose (Plain) Flour
1 Teaspoon Instant Coffee Powder
1/4 Teaspoon Cream of Tartar
1 Teaspoon Baking Powder
1/2 Teaspoon Baking Soda
1/4 Teaspoon Salt

1/2 Cup Dark Chocolate-Covered Espresso Beans
1/4 Cup Dark Brown Sugar, Firmly Packed
1/4 Cup Vegetable or Grapeseed Oil
1/4 Cup Light Agave Nectar or Corn Syrup
2 Teaspoons Vanilla Extract

Preheat your oven to 350ºF (175ºC). In a medium-sized bowl, sift together the flour, coffee powder, cream of tartar, baking powder, baking soda, and salt. Toss the coffee beans in the dry mix so that they're coated in flour, and set aside. Take out a mixing bowl, and combine the sugar, oil, agave, and vanilla until nicely emulsified. Pour this mixture into your dry ingredients, and stir carefully with a large spatula. I wouldn't recommend using a mixer to do this, because it is likely to power through those large coffee beans. Scoop relatively large balls of dough (slightly smaller than golf balls), roll them lightly in your palms, and flatten them on a baking sheet. Space them about 2 inches apart so that they have plenty of room to spread. Bake the cookies for 8 to 10 minutes, or until they are slightly golden around the edges. Don't worry if they are still very soft to the touch, as they will continue to bake outside of the oven. Let them sit on the sheet for at least 15 minutes in order to further firm up before removing them to a wire rack.

Soft and Chewy Oatmeal Cookies

Yields 5 Dozen Cookies

These cookies come out crispy on the outside, but wonderfully soft and doughy on the inside. Be careful not to cook them too long, as they will settle and flatten a bit as they cool.

2 Cups All-Purpose (Plain) or Whole Wheat Pastry
   Flour
3 Cups Quick-Cooking Oats
1 Teaspoon Ground Cinnamon
1 Teaspoon Baking Soda
1/2 Teaspoon Salt
1 Cup Dairy-Free Margarine, Softened

1/2 Cup Granulated Sugar
1 Cup Light Brown Sugar, Packed
6 Tablespoons Unsweetened Applesauce
2 Tablespoons Molasses
1 Teaspoon Vanilla Extract
1 Cup Raisins

Preheat your oven to 375ºF (190ºC). In a large bowl, combine the flour, oats, cinnamon, baking soda, and salt. Set aside. In a large mixing bowl, cream the margarine and sugars. Blend in the applesauce, molasses, and vanilla until creamy. Gradually stir or beat in the reserved flour mixture until fully incorporated. Fold in the raisins. Shape the dough into walnut-sized balls and place them on baking sheets (ungreased or lined with non-stick baking mats), spaced about 2 to 3 inches apart, allowing some room to spread. Bake for 8 to 10 minutes for soft and chewy cookies, or up to 12 minutes for crispy cookies. Let the cookies sit for 2 minutes before removing them to a wire rack to cool completely.

Oatmeal Chocolate Chip Option: Omit the cinnamon and use 1 cup of chocolate chips in place of the raisins.

Maple Spice Pumpkin Cookies

Yields 2 to 3 Dozen Cookies

When I was helping to test recipes for food allergy mom, Barb Nicoletti, these wonderfully soft pumpkin cookies came onto my radar. I made the slight addition of maple syrup and my latest cookie addiction was born!

Cookies:

2 Cups All-Purpose (Plain) Flour
1 Teaspoon Baking Powder
1 Teaspoon Baking Soda
1/2 Teaspoon Ground Cinnamon
1/4 Teaspoon Ground Nutmeg
1/2 Teaspoon Salt

1/2 Cup Shortening
1 Cup Pumpkin Puree
1 Cup Granulated Sugar
2 Tablespoons Maple Syrup
1 Teaspoon Vanilla Extract

Topping:

2 Teaspoons Granulated Sugar

1 Teaspoon Ground Cinnamon

Preheat your oven to 350ºF (175ºC). In a medium-sized bowl, combine the flour, baking powder, baking soda, 1/2 teaspoon cinnamon, nutmeg, and salt. Set aside. In a large mixing bowl, cream the shortening, pumpkin puree, 1 cup of sugar, maple syrup, and vanilla until light and fluffy. Slowly incorporate the flour mixture into the wet mixture. The dough will be rather sticky. You may want to chill it for 30 minutes to 1 hour to make it a bit more manageable. Drop the dough by the heaping tablespoonful onto baking sheets (ungreased or lined with non-stick baking mats).

For the topping, combine the 2 teaspoons of sugar and 1 teaspoon of cinnamon in a small dish, and sprinkle the mixture atop each ball of dough. Bake for 10 to 14 minutes, or until the tops take on a golden hue.

Super Yummy Ginger Cookies

Yields 2 Dozen Cookies

Recipe by Cynthia Mosher, chief editor and publisher of www.vegfamily.com *- Cynthia provided this recipe as a personal favorite and a healthier alternative to the typical refined flour cookie recipe.*

2 Cups Whole Wheat Flour
1 Teaspoon Ground Cinnamon
1/2 Teaspoon Ground Ginger
1/2 Teaspoon Ground Cloves
2 Teaspoons Baking Soda
1/2 Teaspoon Salt
3/4 Cup Coconut Oil

1 Cup Raw Turbinado Sugar, Plus Extra for Dipping
1/4 Cup Flax Goo (2 tablespoons ground flaxseed
   combined with 1/4 cup boiling water, and
   allowed to sit for 10 minutes)
1/4 Cup Molasses
2 Tablespoons Unsweetened Applesauce
2 Teaspoons Freshly Grated Ginger

Preheat your oven to 350ºF (175ºC). Sift together the flour, baking soda, cinnamon, ginger, cloves, and salt. In another bowl cream the coconut oil and 1 cup of sugar until soft. Blend in the flax goo, molasses, applesauce, and fresh ginger. Then add, a little at a time, the dry ingredients to this wet mix. Let the mix sit on the counter for about 5 to 10 minutes to let the flavors meld.

Form the dough into 1-inch balls, and dip just the tops into the turbinado sugar. Place each ball a few inches apart on an oiled baking sheet, sugared side up. Bake for 12 minutes; don't over cook or they will be hard when they cool. Let the cookies cool for just a few minutes on the sheet before transferring them to a wire rack.

Coconut Fudge Brownies

Yields 9 to 12 Brownies

This dessert is a house favorite, served alone or a la mode in traditional brownie sundae style. I prefer the brownies cooled, so that the chocolate chips re-solidify, but my husband likes them warm and gooey. For gluten-free connoisseurs, I have made this recipe many times with brown rice flour, and it also works well with GF flour blends.

3/4 Cup Flour of Choice
1/4 Cup Unsweetened Cocoa
1/4 Teaspoon Salt
1/4 Cup Grapeseed or Vegetable Oil or Shortening
1 Cup Granulated Sugar

2 Eggs (see note below regarding egg-free)
1-1/2 Teaspoons Vanilla Extract
1/2 Cup Unsweetened Flaked Coconut
1/3 to 1/2 Cup Semi-Sweet or Dark Chocolate Chips
1/4 Cup Chopped Walnuts (optional)

Preheat your oven to 350ºF (175ºC) and grease an 8-inch square baking dish. Sift the flour, cocoa, and salt together in a small bowl. Set aside. In a medium-sized mixing bowl, blend the oil or shortening, sugar, eggs, and vanilla until creamy. Slowly incorporate the reserved flour mixture into the wet mixture. Fold in the coconut. Spread the batter into your prepared pan. Sprinkle the chocolate chips and nuts (if using) over the top of the brownie mixture. Bake for 25 to 35 minutes, or until a toothpick inserted into the center of the brownies comes out clean. The brownies should be relatively firm to the touch.

Peanut Butter Brownie Option: Replace the coconut with 2 heaping tablespoons of peanut butter, or leave the coconut in for peanut butter coconut brownies.

Egg-Free / Vegan Option: See the Fudge Brownie Cookies recipe (below) for my egg-free spin-off from this recipe.

Fudge Brownie Cookies

Yields 2 Dozen Cookies

I was determined to keep my homemade brownies (above) fudgy while trying to create an egg-free option, rather than giving into the cakey versions that often result with vegan recipes. Unfortunately, failure after gooey failure nearly caused me to throw in the towel. But suddenly, I had an epiphany. Perhaps they were just being baked in the wrong form? And thus these cookies were born. Naturally delicious with no need for eggs at all, these cookies were devoured at a dinner party in mere minutes. Of course, I didn't mention the secret ingredient …

3/4 Cup All-Purpose (Plain) Flour or Whole Wheat
    Pastry Flour
1/4 Cup Cocoa Powder
1/2 Teaspoon Baking Soda
1/4 Teaspoon Salt

1 Cup Granulated Sugar
6 Tablespoons Grapeseed or Vegetable Oil
6 Tablespoons Mashed Ripe Avocado (2-3 avocados)
1-1/2 Teaspoons Vanilla Extract
1/2 Cup Semi-Sweet Chocolate Chips

Preheat your oven to 375ºF (190ºC). Sift the flour, cocoa powder, baking soda, and salt together into a small bowl. Set aside. In a medium-sized mixing bowl, blend the sugar, oil, avocado, and vanilla until the mixture is homogenous. Stir in the reserved flour mixture along with the chocolate chips. The dough will be rather stiff. Shape the dough into walnut-sided balls, flatten them just a touch with your palm, and place them a few inches apart on baking sheets (ungreased or lined with non-stick baking mats). Bake the cookies for 10 to 12 minutes, but no longer. They should have an external crust forming, but be soft in the center. The cookies will fall a bit as they cool. Let them rest on the sheets for 2 minutes before removing them to a wire rack to cool completely.

Coconut Fudge Cookie Option: Add 1/3 cup unsweetened flaked coconut to the flour mixture in the first step.

Raisindoras

Yields 12 Servings

Recipe adapted from *Allergen-Free Baking* by Jill Robbins – *According to Jill, "These are like chocolate-free brownies, with a taste similar to Hermits. They are fun to prepare, and make great school snacks!" Jill's baking business, HomeFree Treats (www.homefreetreats.com), and her cookbook focus on wheat-, dairy-, nut-, and egg-free sweets. To perfect their taste, many of her recipes use specialty flours, but if you do not have a problem with gluten or wheat, then feel free to substitute all-purpose, spelt, or wheat flour for the flours in this recipe.*

1 Cup Raisins
3/4 Cup Granulated Sugar
1/2 Cup Water
1 Teaspoon Ground Cinnamon
1/4 Teaspoon Ground Cloves
1/4 Teaspoon Ground Nutmeg
1/2 Teaspoon Salt

1 Teaspoon Baking Soda
1/3 Cup Safflower Oil
1/4 Cup Unsweetened Applesauce
2 Tablespoons Maple Syrup, Agave Nectar, or Honey
1 Cup Barley Flour
1/3 Cup Oat Flour
2 Tablespoons Sorghum Flour (or additional oat flour)

Put the raisins, sugar, water, cinnamon, cloves, nutmeg, and salt into a small pot. Stir and cover. Bring to a boil, uncover, and reduce the heat to medium-low. Gently boil the ingredients for 4 minutes, stirring occasionally. Remove from the heat. Gather any interested children to watch the next step! Add the baking soda, and watch the mixture immediately turn white and frothy. Stir briefly and cover. Let the mixture sit for 2 hours.

Five minutes before the 2 hours are up, preheat your oven to 325°F (165ºC), and grease and flour an 8-inch square baking dish. Add the oil, applesauce, and maple syrup, agave, or honey to the mixture in your pot, followed by the flours. Fold the ingredients in until they are just mixed. Spread the batter evenly into your prepared pan. Bake for 45 to 47 minutes. Let it cool in the pan on a cooling rack before slicing.

O'Henry Bars

Yields approximately 40 Bars

Recipe adapted from No Whey, Mama (nowheymama.blogspot.com), by Sarah Hatfield - *Sarah's version of this classic recipe caught my eye, since I used to love the peanut butter Oh Henry!® bars sold in Canada, which I never could find here in the states … and which, of course, are made with milk chocolate.*

2/3 Cup Dairy-Free Margarine, Softened
1 cup Light Brown Sugar, Firmly Packed
4 Cups Rolled or Quick Oats
1/2 Cup Light Corn Syrup or Agave Nectar

1 Tablespoon Vanilla Extract
1 Cup Semi-Sweet Chocolate Chips
2/3 Cups Chunky or Creamy Peanut Butter

Preheat your oven to 350ºF (175ºC). Cream the margarine and sugar together. Stir in the oats, syrup or agave, and vanilla until everything is well incorporated. Pat the mixture into a jelly roll pan or cookie sheet with high sides and bake for 15 minutes, or until the center is just barely firm. While still warm, sprinkle the bars with the chocolate chips and small spoonfuls of the peanut butter. Let stand 5 minutes while they melt a bit, and then spread the chocolate and peanut butter over the bars, swirling as you go to marbleize the two together. Allow it to cool completely, and then refrigerate for 15 minutes to set the topping. Cut into bars.

Nut-Free Option: If your school is a peanut-free zone, don't hesitate to substitute sunflower butter or a nut butter of your choosing for the peanut butter.

Pecan Pralines

Yields 2 to 3 Dozen Pralines

Recipe created by Hannah Kaminsky, author of My Sweet Vegan - This traditionally dairy-laden dessert is perfect for gift giving around the holidays, or when a sweet candy-like treat is in order.

1-1/2 Cups Granulated Sugar
1/2 Cup Dairy-Free Margarine
1/4 Cup Plain Soymilk
1/4 Cup Plain Soy Creamer or Coconut Milk
1 Tablespoon Light Corn Syrup
1/2 Teaspoon Apple Cider Vinegar

1/2 Teaspoon Baking Soda
Pinch Salt
1-1/2 Cups Pecan Halves
1 Teaspoon Vanilla Extract
1/2 Teaspoon Ground Cinnamon

First things first, it's very important to use a candy thermometer on a pot with tall sides for this one. Set that pot on your stove over medium heat with the thermometer attached in a stable place that it won't be in the way, and combine the sugar, margarine, soymilk, soy creamer or coconut milk, corn syrup, vinegar, baking soda, and salt in the pot. Once the margarine is melted and the sugar dissolved, it will begin to get frothy as it comes up in temperature and it is vital that you do not stop stirring! Continue agitating the mixture until it reaches 260ºF (127ºC), which is the hard ball stage. Kill the heat and stir in the nuts, extract, and cinnamon. Stir it for just 30 to 60 additional seconds, until it no longer looks quite as shiny. Working as quickly as possible (without creating a huge mess), drop large spoonfuls of the mixture onto a non-stick baking mat or piece of waxed paper. Let cool. Don't panic if it looks like your pot and utensils now look hopelessly encrusted in sugar - It will easily wash away after a good soak in hot water.

Peanut Butter "Truffles"

Yields approximately 2 Dozen "Truffles"

Casually elegant, these glorified peanut butter cups earned me rave reviews at a close friend's wedding. For party favors, we wrapped a few little treats up in tulle and placed one on each guest's plate. All night long, people I had never met approached me with recipe requests for "those incredible truffles." While I would love to gloat on my innovation and labor, the recipe is embarrassingly easy …

2 Cups Powdered / Confectioner's Sugar
3/4 Cup Smooth All Natural Peanut Butter
1/4 Cup Dairy-Free Margarine or Shortening,
    Softened

1/2 Teaspoon Vanilla Extract
1/4 Teaspoon Salt
6 Ounces Semi-Sweet or Dark Chocolate Chips
1/2 Teaspoon Shortening

Combine the sugar, peanut butter, margarine or shortening, vanilla, and salt in a medium-sized mixing bowl, and blend until smooth. Pinch off pieces of the peanut butter mixture and roll them into balls that are 1/2 to 1 inch in diameter. Since you won't be baking them, the thickness of the filling is really up to you. Place the peanut butter balls in a single layer on baking sheets lined with wax paper or non-stick baking mats (I flatten them slightly to keep them from rolling around), and freeze until they are firm, about 15 to 20 minutes. While those are chilling, Place the chocolate and 1/2 teaspoon of shortening in a microwave-safe bowl and microwave on HIGH in 30 second intervals (just 2 to 3 should suffice), stirring vigorously between intervals, until the chocolate has just melted and is smooth. Be careful not to overheat the chocolate, as it can scorch easily. Remove the peanut butter balls from the freezer, dunk them in the melted chocolate to coat, and return them to the baking sheets to dry. Place the truffles in the refrigerator or freezer to chill for 1 hour, or until the chocolate coating is firm. The truffles should keep in an airtight container in the refrigerator for up to 2 weeks.

Bittersweet Truffles

Yields 4 Dozen Truffles

Though luxurious, delicious truffles can be one of the simplest foods to prepare. Make sure you use a good quality chocolate; I like the big baker's dark bar from Scharffenberger's, which can often be found under generic labeling!

1 lb (16 ounces) Dark Chocolate, Coarsely Chopped
3/4 Cup (3.75 ounces) Raw Cashews
3/4 Cup Water

2 Tablespoons Liqueur or 1 to 2 Teaspoons Flavor Extract (optional)
Cocoa Powder, Finely Chopped Nuts, Powdered Sugar, or Coconut for Coating

Place the chocolate in a microwave-safe bowl and microwave it on HIGH in 30 second intervals (just 2 to 3 should suffice), stirring vigorously between intervals, until the chocolate has just melted and is smooth. Be careful not to overheat the chocolate, as it can scorch easily. Set aside to let the chocolate cool for a few minutes. If you have a spice grinder, use it to blend the nuts until they pass the powder stage and just begin to clump. Place the cashews or cashew paste and the water in your blender, and blend until smooth, about 1 to 2 minutes. If using a liqueur or extract, blend it in. Gently fold the resultant cashew crème into the melted chocolate until it is well combined. Cool the chocolate mixture in your refrigerator for 4 hours or until it is firm enough to handle. If it sets up too much, let it sit at room temperature to soften a bit. Scoop out balls of the chocolate mixture and roll them in your choice of coating or see the directions below for chocolate-dipped truffles. Store the truffles in the refrigerator until ready to devour.

Chocolate Coated Option: Melt 10 ounces of additional dark or semi-sweet chocolate with 1 teaspoon of shortening using the directions above. Dip the truffles in the chocolate and place them on baking sheets lined with wax paper or non-stick baking mats. Place the sheets in the refrigerator or freezer for 30 minutes to allow the chocolate to harden.

Nut-Free Option: Substitute 1 cup of coconut cream for the cashews and water. To get the thickest cream, allow two cans of coconut milk to chill and settle; no shaking! Skim off 1/2 cup of the thickest cream from the top of each can; use the remaining coconut milk in recipes as a light coconut milk.

Peanut Butter Chews

Yields 1 to 2 Dozen Treats

At the time of writing, Juventa Vezzani was in the process of creating and photographing recipes for her cookbook, The Milk Allergy Companion and Cookbook. She offered this candy-like recipe as a sneak preview of the work to come; it is actually one from her mother-in-law's collection, Janell Vezzani.

1 Cup Sugar
1 Cup Light Corn Syrup

1 12-Ounce Jar Extra-Crunchy Peanut Butter
6 Cups Corn Flakes

In a large saucepan, bring the sugar and corn syrup to a boil. Boil for 1 minute, stirring constantly. Remove from the heat, and add the peanut butter and corn flakes. Stir until everything is well coated. Drop the mixture by the spoonfuls onto waxed paper. Let cool. Serve with a tall glass of soymilk or rice milk!

Yellow Birthday Cake

Yields 10 to 12 Servings

There is something so rewarding about baking a birthday cake from scratch. The first time I baked this cake was for my Hawaiian food loving friend, Barb. For her, I prepared the pineapple upside down version below, but this versatile cake can be dressed up any way you like it.

1-1/4 Cups Buttermilk Alternative*
2-3/4 Cups All-Purpose (Plain) Flour
1-1/2 Teaspoons Baking Powder
1/2 Teaspoon Baking Soda
1/2 Teaspoon Salt

4 Eggs, Separated
3/4 Cup Dairy-Free Margarine (1-1/2 sticks), Softened**
2 Cups Granulated Sugar
2 Teaspoons Vanilla Extract

Preheat your oven to 350°F (175ºC) and grease and flour a 9x13-inch baking dish or two 9-inch round cake pans. Prepare the buttermilk alternative. Sift the flour, baking powder, baking soda, and salt into a medium-sized bowl and set aside. In a medium-sized mixing bowl, beat the egg whites with an electric mixer until stiff but not dry. Set aside.

In a separate mixing bowl, cream the margarine and sugar. Add the egg yolks and vanilla, and beat for 2 minutes, or until the mixture looks light and fluffy. Add about a third of the flour mixture to the mixing bowl, followed by a third of the buttermilk alternative, just mixing to combine (but not overbeating) after each addition. Continue this alternating pattern with the remaining flour and buttermilk alternative. Gently fold the stiff egg whites into the batter with a rubber spatula. Pour the batter into the prepared pan, spreading it with your spatula to even out the top. Bake for 35 minutes or until a toothpick inserted in the center comes out clean. Set the cakes on a rack to cool for 15 minutes, before turning them out of the pans to cool completely.

Egg-Free Option: Unfortunately, the egg yolks are what give this cake its yellow vibe, but for a vegan and egg-free birthday cake option, I have created the Simply Wonderful White Cake recipe that follows (p234).

Pineapple Upside Down Cake Option: Do not grease and flour your baking dish or cake pans. The following instructions are for the 9x13-inch baking dish, but divide the ingredients between your two cake pans if using. Coat the bottom of the baking dish with 6 tablespoons of melted dairy-free margarine. Sprinkle 1/2 cup of firmly packed light brown sugar atop the margarine. Optionally sprinkle 1/3 cup of shredded coconut (sweetened or unsweetened) atop this. Finally, spread 1-1/2 cups of well-drained (juice reserved) crushed pineapple atop all. When preparing the yellow cake use the reserved pineapple juice in place of the buttermilk alternative.

* To make the buttermilk alternative, place 1 tablespoon of white vinegar or lemon juice in a glass measuring cup. Add the plain milk alternative of your choice until it reaches 1-1/4 cups. Let it sit for a few minutes while you prepare the other ingredients.
** Margarine really adds to the flavor, density, and color to this cake, but in a pinch, you can substitute your favorite baking oil.

Simply Wonderful White Cake

Yields 10 to 12 Servings

For years, I have received recipe requests for a basic white cake, yet I didn't have any place to point people too. So I set out to create my own dairy-free white cake, and while I was at it, I went egg-free too! I like a cake that is sweet, but not too sweet, letting the frosting take center stage; but if you like your cake on the sweet side then you can increase the sugar to 1 cup. For a birthday cake, double the entire recipe to fit a 9x13-inch pan or two 8-inch round cake pans.

1-1/2 Cups All-Purpose (Plain) Flour
1 Teaspoon Baking Powder
1 Teaspoon Baking Soda
1/2 Teaspoon Salt
3/4 Cup Granulated Sugar

1/4 Cup Vegetable, Grapeseed, or Extra-Light Olive Oil
1 Tablespoon White Vinegar
1 Teaspoon Vanilla Extract
1 Cup Vanilla Rice or Almond Milk

Preheat your oven to 350ºF (175ºC) and grease an 8-inch square baking dish. In a medium-sized bowl, sift the flour, baking powder, baking soda, and salt together. In a large mixing bowl, combine the sugar, oil, vinegar, and vanilla. Stir in the rice or almond milk. Add the flour mixture and stir until the batter is smooth. Pour the batter into your prepared baking dish, and bake for 30 to 35 minutes, or until a toothpick inserted in the center comes out clean. Allow the cake to cool for 10 minutes before frosting.

Cupcake Option: Line a dozen muffins cups with cupcake liners. Divide the batter between the twelve liners and bake at 350ºF (175ºC) for 18 to 22 minutes or until a toothpick inserted in the center of a cupcake comes out clean.

Chocolate Wacky Cake

Yields 10 to 12 Servings

Needing virtually no introduction, various versions of this war-era pantry cake are prepared around the globe every day. Not only can it be prepared with inexpensive, common pantry items alone, but it is also an easy one to mix up by hand. For a birthday cake, double the entire recipe to fit a 9x13-inch pan or two 8-inch round cake pans.

1-1/2 Cups All-Purpose (Plain) Flour
1 Cup Granulated Sugar
1/4 Cup Cocoa Powder
1 Teaspoon Baking Soda
1/2 Teaspoon Salt

5 Tablespoons (scant 1/3 cup) Vegetable, Grapeseed, or Extra-Light Olive Oil
1 Tablespoon White Vinegar
1 Teaspoon Vanilla Extract
1 Cup Cold Water or Chocolate Milk Alternative of Choice

Preheat your oven to 350ºF (175ºC) and grease an 8-inch square baking dish. In a large bowl, sift the flour, sugar, cocoa, baking soda, and salt together. Make 3 small wells in the flour mixture, placing the oil in one well, the vinegar in the second, and the vanilla in the third. Pour the cold water or milk alternative over all, and stir until well combined. Pour the batter into your prepared baking dish, and bake for 30 to 35 minutes, or until a toothpick inserted into the center of the cake comes out clean. Allow the cake to cool for 10 minutes before frosting.

Cupcake Option: Line a dozen muffins cups with cupcake liners. Divide the batter between the twelve liners and bake at 350ºF (175ºC) for 18 to 22 minutes or until a toothpick inserted in the center of a cupcake comes out clean.

Chocolate-Orange Option: Replace the cold water with cold orange juice, and add 2 teaspoons of orange zest or 1/2 teaspoon of orange extract.

Rice Crispy Cake

Yields 10 to 12 Servings

Recipe adapted from the blog, Bittersweet (bittersweetblog.wordpress.com) by Hannah Kaminsky - I absolutely fell in love with Hannah's idea for this simple, kid-friendly cake. It is naturally free-from gluten, dairy, eggs, nuts, and peanuts (choose your crispy cereal wisely!) and can easily be made in advance. Hannah notes, "There is nothing fancy or sophisticated about this creation, no exotic flavors or ingredients, just sweet crunchy cereal stuck together with more sugar and topped off with a thick coat of vanilla "butter cream." You don't even need to heat up your oven for this one, a serious plus for all of those summer birthdays! Don't let these basic instructions stifle your creativity, either. Think different flavors - peanut butter crispy rice cereal with chocolate frosting, perhaps? The sky's the limit!"

Cake:

8 Cups Crispy Rice Cereal
1 Tablespoon Dairy-Free Margarine, Shortening, or
   Coconut Oil

1 Cup Light Corn Syrup or Agave Nectar
3/4 Cup Granulated Sugar
1 Teaspoon Vanilla Extract

Very Vanilla Frosting:

1 Cup Vegetable Shortening
3 Cups Powdered / Confectioner's Sugar

2 Tablespoons Vanilla Milk Alternative of Choice
2 Teaspoons Vanilla Extract

Begin by pouring half of the cereal into a very large bowl and set it aside, but keep it near the stove for easy access. Lightly grease two 8-inch round cake pans. Set a saucepan over medium heat and add in your margarine, shortening, or oil, heating until it has just melted. Pour in the corn syrup and sugar, stirring constantly until it bubbles up and becomes frothy. Reduce the heat slightly so that it's at a steady boil and cook for about 5 minutes. Turn off the stove and stir in the vanilla. Pour half of the sugar mixture over your waiting cereal, and carefully but quickly fold it in using a wide spatula. Add in the remaining cereal and sugar mixture, combining again until fully coated. Drop half of the sugared cereal into each pan, and press gently using the spatula so that it evenly fills both pans. Allow the layers to cool completely (you can refrigerate them to speed this up) before frosting. If you have difficulty removing the layers, simply dip the bottoms of the pans into boiling water (be careful of your fingers!) to slightly melt the sugar and loosen it from the sides.

To make the frosting, combine all of the ingredients in a mixing bowl and whip on high with a mixer for about 3 minutes or until creamy and fluffy. Decorate the cereal layers as desired, sandwiching a layer of frosting in between the two for stability.

Cookie Garnish Option: Cut vanilla or chocolate sandwich crème cookies in half, and press the cookie halves into the frosting around the sides of the cake (with the flat, cut edge of the cookie halves touching the serving platter). This will help to easily cover up any uneven frosting where the cake meets the plate. Also, you can press handfuls of colorful sprinkles into the frosting around the sides for a festive presentation.

Banana Crumb Coffee Cake

Yields 9 to 12 Servings

According to my husband, this cake could be sold at Starbucks. The first time I made it, the two of us polished off the entire pan within 24 hours. Since our waistlines don't need quite that much cake, I now make sure to bake it when there are more mouths around to feed. Nonetheless, if you are making this for a get together or a bigger household, double the entire recipe and bake it in a 9x13-inch pan.

Topping:

1/3 Cup Chopped Pecans, Walnuts, or Nuts of Choice
1/4 Cup Light Brown Sugar, Firmly Packed
2 to 3 Tablespoons All-Purpose (Plain) or Whole Wheat Pastry Flour

1/2 Teaspoon Ground Cinnamon
2 Tablespoons Cold Margarine or Shortening, Broken into Small Pieces

Cake:

1-1/2 Cups All-Purpose (Plain) Flour (or 1 cup all-purpose flour + 1/2 cup whole-wheat pastry flour)
1/2 Teaspoon Ground Cinnamon
1/4 Teaspoon Ground Nutmeg
1 Teaspoon Baking Powder
1/2 Teaspoon Baking Soda
1/4 Teaspoon Salt

1 Cup Ripe Mashed Banana (2 medium or 3 small)
1 Tablespoon Ground Flaxseed combined with 3 Tablespoons Pure Maple Syrup
1/4 Cup Coconut Oil or Dairy-Free Margarine, Softened
1/4 Cup Light Brown Sugar, Firmly Packed
1/4 Cup Granulated Sugar

Preheat your oven to 350ºF (175ºC) and grease an 8-inch square baking dish. For the topping, combine the pecans, brown sugar, 2 tablespoons of flour, and the cinnamon, in a medium-sized bowl. Add the margarine, and mix with a fork or pastry blender, until coarse crumbs form. If the mixture is too wet, add another tablespoon of flour. Set aside.

For the cake, sift together the flour, cinnamon, nutmeg, baking powder, baking soda, and salt, and briefly set aside. In a large mixing bowl, combine the banana, flax/maple mixture, margarine or oil, and the two sugars until creamy. Gently stir the reserved flour mixture into the wet mixture in your mixing bowl. Pour the batter into your prepared baking dish, it will be a bit thick, so you will want to use a spatula to evenly smooth it out. Sprinkle the reserved crumb topping over the cake, and bake it for 30 to 35 minutes, or until a toothpick inserted into the center of the cake comes out clean.

Nut-Free Option: Substitute the nuts in the topping with rolled or quick oats.

Sweet Apple Snackin' Cake

Yields 9 to 12 Servings

When testing a Cinnamon Applesauce Muffin recipe for a food allergy cookbook by colleague Barb Nicoletti, my penchant for experimentation got the best of me. The result was this wonderfully moist and tender cake. I use Granny Smith or Golden Delicious apples as they stay a bit firm when baked and offer a nice contrast to the sweetness.

1-2/3 Cups All-Purpose (Plain) Flour or Whole Wheat Pastry Flour
1 Teaspoon Ground Cinnamon
1/4 Teaspoon Ground Nutmeg
1 Teaspoon Baking Soda
1/4 Teaspoon Salt
1/2 Cup Shortening or Dairy-Free Margarine, Softened

3/4 Cup Unsweetened Applesauce
1/2 Cup Light Brown Sugar, Firmly Packed
1/2 Cup Granulated Sugar
1 Tablespoon White or Apple Cider Vinegar
1 to 2 Apples, Peeled, Cored, and Cut into 1/4 to 1/2-Inch Thick Slices or Chunks

Preheat your oven to 350ºF (175ºC) and grease an 8-inch square baking dish. In a medium-sized bowl, combine the flour, cinnamon, nutmeg, baking soda, and salt. Set aside. In a large mixing bowl, cream the shortening or margarine, applesauce, sugars, and vinegar. Slowly incorporate the flour mixture into the wet mixture in your mixing bowl; being careful not to over mix, a few small lumps are okay. Layer the bottom of the baking dish with the apple chunks/slices. Evenly spread the batter over top of the apples, and bake for 25 to 35 minutes or until the cake is firm to the touch, and a toothpick inserted into the center of the cake comes out clean.

Cookies & Cream Muffin-Cakes

Yields 12 Muffin-Cakes

Recipe adapted from the blog, VeggieGirl (veggiegirlvegan.blogspot.com) by Liz Stark - *According to Liz, her family was smitten with this three-treats-in-one baked good, stating "Aside from featuring an enticing combination of cookie-, muffin-, and cupcake-goodness, these muffin-cakes have a deliciously chocolate-y flavor, moist center, and a bit of crunchiness from the cookie on top."*

1 Cup Whole Wheat Flour
1/2 Cup All-Purpose (Plain) Flour
1/3 Cup Evaporated Cane Juice or Unrefined Sugar
1/4 Cup Cocoa Powder
1 Teaspoon Baking Soda
1/3 Cup Chocolate or Carob Chips

8 Chocolate Cream-Filled Sandwich Cookies, Crushed
1 Cup Plain Milk Alternative of Choice
5 Tablespoons Unsweetened Applesauce
1 Teaspoon Vanilla Extract
3 Additional Chocolate Cream-Filled Sandwich Cookies, Each One Broken into Quarters

Preheat your oven to 350ºF (175ºC) and line one dozen muffins cups with cupcake liners. In a large bowl, combine the flours, sugar, cocoa powder, baking soda, carob chips and crushed cookies, and mix well. In a small bowl, combine the milk alternative, applesauce, and vanilla, and mix well. Add the ingredients from the small bowl to the large bowl, and stir the mixture by hand, until fully combined. Pour the batter into your prepared muffin cups, and gently press a quarter-cookie segment on top of each muffin-cake. Bake for 22 to 25 minutes, or until a toothpick inserted in the center of a muffin-cake comes out clean.

Orange Chocolate Chunk Cupcakes

Yields 12 Cupcakes

Recipe created by Hannah Kaminsky, author of *My Sweet Vegan - Hannah takes the traditional flavor combination of orange and chocolate one step further, infusing them into this delicious dessert.*

1 Cup Orange Juice
1/2 Cup Granulated Sugar
1/3 Cup Vegetable or Grapeseed Oil
1/4 Teaspoon Vanilla Extract
1-1/2 Teaspoons Orange Zest

1-1/3 Cup All-Purpose (Plain) Flour
1/2 Teaspoon Baking Powder
1/2 Teaspoon Baking Soda
1/4 Teaspoon Salt
3 Ounces Dark Chocolate, Roughly Chopped

Preheat your oven to 350ºF (175ºC) and line a dozen muffin cups with cupcake papers. Whisk together the orange juice, sugar, oil, vanilla, and zest to combine, and set aside. In a separate bowl, sift together the flour, baking powder, baking soda, and salt, and stir well. Toss in the chocolate chunks to coat them with the flour, so that they don't just sink to the bottom of your cupcakes. Pour the wet ingredients into the dry, and stir just until combined. Divide the batter between your prepared muffin cups and bake for 15 to 20 minutes, or until a toothpick inserted into the center of a cupcake comes out clean. Frost the cupcakes with the Chocolate Ganache Frosting recipe (below), if desired.

Cake Option: Pour the batter into a lightly greased 8-inch round cake pan, and bake it for 20 to 25 minutes or until a toothpick inserted into the center of the cake comes out clean. You can double the recipe for a 2-layer cake.

Chocolate Ganache Frosting

Yields a Small Batch to Frost 12 Cupcakes

Recipe created by Hannah Kaminsky, author of *My Sweet Vegan – Hannah created this frosting to go with her Orange Chocolate Chunk Cupcakes (above), but it is quite versatile, and can be used with other cupcake recipes.*

6 Ounces Bittersweet (Dark) Chocolate
1/4 Cup Plain Soy Creamer or Light Coconut Milk

1/2 Cup Dairy-Free Margarine, Softened
1 Cup Powdered / Confectioner's Sugar

Melt the chocolate with the soy creamer (in the microwave in 30 second intervals or in a double broiler), stirring until completely combined and no lumps remain. Let it sit to cool for a couple of minutes, until roughly room temperature. Combine the chocolate with the margarine and sugar in a mixing bowl, and beat them on low speed for 1 minute. Turn your mixer up to high speed, and continue beating the frosting for about 5 minutes, or until light and fluffy.

Whipped Icing

Yields 2 to 2-1/2 cups (enough to frost an 8 or 9-inch double layer cake)
This deliciously addictive white icing is like a cross between rich frosting and fluffy whipped cream.

1 Cup Cold Plain Milk Alternative of Choice
1/4 Cup All-Purpose or White Rice Flour
1/2 Cup Dairy-free Margarine, Softened

1/2 Cup Shortening
1 Cup Granulated Sugar
1 Teaspoon Vanilla Extract

Whisk the cold milk alternative and flour together in a small saucepan until no lumps remain. Place the pan over medium heat, and cook, while whisking, until it reaches a pudding-like texture, about 3 to 5 minutes. Set aside. In a medium-sized mixing bowl, cream the margarine, shortening, and sugar for 3 to 4 minutes. Add the pudding-like mixture and the vanilla, and beat for 3 to 4 minutes or until the icing is nice and fluffy.

"Buttercream" Frosting

Yields approximately 3 Cups (more than enough to frost an 8 or 9-inch double layer cake)

1 Cup Dairy-Free Margarine, Softened
1 Teaspoon Vanilla Extract
Pinch Salt (optional)

3-1/2 to 4 Cups Powdered / Confectioner's Sugar
2 to 4 Tablespoons Plain Milk Alternative of Choice

In a large mixing bowl, cream the margarine. Beat in the vanilla and salt, if using. Add the powdered sugar 1 cup at a time, beating it on low speed until it is combined. Turn the mixer up to medium or high and whip the frosting for 2 minutes. Mix in the milk alternative as needed to reach your desired consistency.

Decorator's "Buttercream" Option: If the frosting is being used for decorating, replace 1/2 cup of the margarine with 1/2 cup shortening.

Soy-Free White Frosting Option: Use 1 cup of shortening in place of the margarine and optionally add 1 teaspoon of almond extract with the vanilla extract.

Chocolate "Buttercream" Option: Add 1/2 cup of cocoa powder with the powdered sugar.

"Cream Cheese" Frosting Option: Use just 1/2 cup of dairy-free margarine or shortening, but cream it with 1/2 cup of dairy-free cream cheese alternative. You can omit the milk alternative, but increase the vanilla to 2 teaspoons. For a cream cheesier taste, use up to 8 ounces (1 package) of cream cheese alternative.

Idea: Baking Box Cake Mixes

Birthday cakes are a big deal in the dairy-free world, especially when dealing with milk allergic or intolerant little ones. While I always prefer a cake baked from scratch, you still have some options when it comes to cake mixes. At the time of writing, there were a few brands with dairy-free flavors readily available:

~ *Cherrybrook Kitchen*® (www.cherrybrookkitchen.com, (978) 974-0200) - This is a good option for multiple food allergies, and they also have gluten-free mixes available. See the end of this chapter for company information.
~ *Dr. Oetker Organics* (www.oetker.ca, (905) 678-1311) - This is a Canadian brand, but it is sold internationally. You will recognize the box as "Organics."
~ *Duncan Hines*® (www.duncanhines.com, (800) 362-9834) - Not all versions will necessarily be dairy-free so check the ingredient label, but most are kosher parve and dairy-free. This is the easiest brand to find, but my least recommended since it is often filled with unsavory ingredients and additives.

As for preparation, most will have dairy-free instructions or close to dairy-free instructions. They may call for eggs, oil, and water in the simplest of scenarios. If they call for butter, use dairy-free margarine or oil. If they call for milk, use your favorite plain or unsweetened milk alternative. If you want to replace the eggs, use a scant 1/4 cup of applesauce or other fruit puree per egg. Of course, there are also a couple of shortcuts that are dairy-free, egg-free, vegan, and consequently, quite low in fat. Skip the directions entirely (no eggs, milk, water, butter, etc.), and combine the cake mix with one of the following:

~ 1 15-Ounce Can of Pumpkin Puree (this is great with white or spice cake mixes, but it even works with chocolate)
~ 1 12-Ounce Can Seltzer Water (feel free to use a flavored variety to go with your cake mix of choice)

Fudgy Chocolate Frosting

Yields 2-1/2 cups (enough to frost an 8 or 9-inch double layer cake)

This fudgy frosting made an entire two-tiered white birthday cake vanish in minutes!

2-1/2 Cups Powdered / Confectioner's Sugar
1/2 Cup Cocoa Powder
1/2 Cup Dairy-free Margarine, Softened

3 Tablespoons Agave Nectar or Honey
2 Tablespoons Water
1 Teaspoon Vanilla Extract

Sift together the powdered sugar and cocoa powder, and set aside. In a mixing bowl, cream the margarine, agave or honey, water, and vanilla using a hand mixer. Add the sugar and cocoa mixture, and beat at low speed until the ingredients are mostly incorporated. Increase the speed on your hand mixer to medium or high, and whip the frosting for 2 minutes, or until it is nice and fluffy.

Peanut Butter Fudge Frosting

Yields 2-1/2 cups (enough to frost an 8 or 9-inch double layer cake)

Recipe adapted from No Whey, Mama (nowheymama.blogspot.com), by Sarah Hatfield – For a peanut-free frosting, substitute your favorite nut or seed butter for the peanut butter.

1/2 Cup Creamy, Unsalted Peanut Butter (see intro)
1/4 Cup Dairy-Free Margarine, Softened
1/4 Cup Plain Milk Alternative of Choice

1 Teaspoon Vanilla Extract
Dash Salt
2 Cups Powdered / Confectioner's Sugar

Combine the peanut butter, margarine, milk alternative, vanilla, and salt in a mixing bowl, and cream with a hand mixer. Sift in the powdered sugar, and beat the frosting on low speed until the sugar is mostly incorporated. Increase the speed on your hand mixer to medium or high, and whip the frosting for 2 minutes, or until it is nice and fluffy.

Cashew Chai Frosting

Yields 2 Cups

This is a great make-ahead frosting as the spices meld and it thickens when allowed to chill overnight. Since it is made without shortening or margarine, it is denser than your average fluffy frosting, so I prefer it atop cookies, cupcakes or as a dessert-like spread on graham crackers.

1 Cup (5 ounces) Raw Cashews
1/4 Cup Plain Milk Alternative of Choice, Plus Extra as Needed
4 Teaspoons Grapeseed or Vegetable Oil
1/4 Teaspoon Vanilla Extract
3/4 Teaspoon Ground Cinnamon

1/4 Teaspoon Ground Nutmeg or Allspice
1/4 Teaspoon Ground Ginger
Generous Pinch Ground Cloves
Pinch Salt
2 Cups Powdered / Confectioner's Sugar

Grind the cashews in your spice grinder or food processor until they pass the powder stage and begin to clump into a paste. This may take a couple of batches if using a spice grinder. Place the cashew paste in a medium-sized mixing bowl and blend in the milk alternative, oil, and vanilla, followed by the spices and salt. Blend in the sugar, 1/2 cup at a time, until it is completely incorporated and the frosting is smooth. If it is too thick, add more milk alternative 1 tablespoon at a time until it reaches your desired consistency. If you have time, refrigerate the frosting for several hours or overnight. It will thicken a bit as it chills, so blend in additional milk alternative if needed.

Key Lime Mousse Pie

Yields 8 Servings

This thick and creamy pie has a flavor that is reminiscent of key lime pie, but with a much richer consistency. For a different presentation, this also makes a great layered dessert. Layer graham cracker or vanilla wafer cookie crumbs or chunks with the pie filling and whipped coconut cream (p253) in nice clear glasses.

1 Large Ripe Avocado
1 Batch (14 Ounces) Sweetened Condensed Coconut
 Milk (p127)

1/4 to 1/3 Cup Fresh Squeezed Lime or Key Lime Juice
1 Prepared Traditional or Vanilla Wafer Pie Crust*
Whipped Coconut Cream (p253) (optional)

Combine the avocado, condensed coconut milk, and juice in your blender, and blend until the mixture is completely smooth and creamy. Pour the filling into your prepared piecrust, and refrigerate for at least 2 hours. Top each slice with a dollop of whipped "cream" to serve.

* You can use a dairy-free store-bought or homemade pie crust. For homemade, I like to use the Chocolate Crust from the Pumpkin "Cheesecake" recipe below, substituting vanilla wafer cookie crumbs for the chocolate ones.

Pumpkin "Cheesecake"

Yields 8 to 10 Servings

Recipe created by Hannah Kaminsky, author of My Sweet Vegan - Switch things up a bit for the holidays or any day for that matter, and you won't be disappointed. This cheesecake has all the flavor and fun of pumpkin pie, but without the hassle of a traditional crust. If a chocolate crust doesn't strike a chord, substitute gingersnaps or lemon cookies.

Chocolate Crust:
2 Cups (8.5 Ounces) Chocolate Wafer Cookie Crumbs
 (regular or gluten-free)

6 Tablespoons Dairy-Free Margarine, Melted

Pumpkin "Cheese" Cake Filling:
2 8-Ounce Containers Dairy-Free "Cream Cheese"
1-1/4 Cups Pumpkin Puree
1/4 Cup Plain Soy Creamer or Coconut Milk (light or
 regular)
1 Teaspoon Vanilla Extract
1/3 Cup Dark Brown Sugar, Firmly Packed

1/4 Cup Granulated Sugar
1-1/2 Teaspoons Ground Cinnamon
1/2 Teaspoon Ground Ginger
1/4 Teaspoon Ground Allspice
Pinch Ground Nutmeg
1/2 Teaspoon Salt

Preheat your oven to 350ºF (175ºC) and lightly grease a 9-inch springform pan. Make sure that the cookie crumbs are very fine and even, almost to the point of being powdery. This may require a food processor or spice grinder, but you can also use a rolling pin to crush them inside a plastic bag. Move the crumbs into a small bowl, and mix in the melted margarine until all of the crumbs are moistened. Press the mixture firmly into the bottom of your prepared pan, and bake for 10 minutes until set. Set aside and lower the oven temperature down to 325ºF (160ºC) before proceeding.

To make the main body of the cheesecake, simply mix all of the filling ingredients in a large mixing bowl until smooth and homogeneous. Pour the filling on top of your baked crust; spread it out evenly, and smooth down the top with a spatula. Drop the pan on the counter a few times to release any air bubbles before moving it into the oven. Bake for about 45 to 50 minutes, although it won't seem the least bit done. It will be very loose and perhaps even bubbly around the sides, but let it cool completely and move it into your refrigerator. Once thoroughly chilled (after at least 4 hours), it should be solid, set, and easily sliceable.

Mini Icebox "Cheesecake"

Yields 2 to 4 Servings

Recipe adapted from *My Sweet Vegan* by Hannah Kaminsky - *Though this easy recipe can be enjoyed any time of year, its no-bake status is perfectly suited to summer, when the temperatures are just too hot to warrant turning on the oven. In terms of the cake's size, Hannah offers the following notes, "This is perfectly sized for an intimate party between a few close friends, but should you prefer a larger cake for a bigger party, double the recipe and use a 10-inch springform pan instead. It will be slightly taller than the small version, but I don't see any problem with bigger slices!"*

Graham Cracker Crust:

1 Cup Graham Cracker Crumbs [regular or gluten-free]

3 Tablespoons Dairy-Free Margarine

1 Tablespoon Brown Rice Syrup [or substitute corn syrup or more maple syrup]

1 Tablespoon Pure Maple Syrup

"Cheese" Cake Filling:

8 Ounces Dairy-Free "Cream Cheese"

1/3 Cup Granulated Sugar

1/4 Cup Plain Soy Creamer [or Light Coconut Milk]

2 Teaspoons Vanilla Extract

1/2 Teaspoon Lemon Juice

1/4 Cup Jam of Choice

Place the graham cracker crumbs in a medium-sized bowl. Melt the margarine and pour it over the crumbs, along with both syrups. Mix until all of the crumbs are moistened, and press the mixture firmly into a 6-inch round springform pan. Press the crust about 1 inch up the sides. Chill it in the freezer while you assemble the filling.

Blend the "cream cheese," sugar, soy creamer, vanilla, and lemon juice in a food processor or blender until the mixture is completely homogeneous. Remove the crust from the freezer, and pour the filling carefully inside. Cover the cake with plastic wrap, and return it to the freezer for at least 3 hours, or until firm. Top with your jam of choice before serving.

Chocolate Espresso Truffle Pie

Yields 8 Servings

Recipe adapted from the website, Everyday Dish (www.everydaydish.tv), by Julie Hasson - *When asked to demo a quick and easy decadent dessert, Julie whipped up this chocolaty creation. According to Julie, this pie never disappoints! You can view a demo of her making this pie (and many other recipes) on the Everyday Dish website.*

1-1/2 12.3-Ounce Boxes (about 18 ounces total) Silken Firm or Extra Firm Tofu (room temperature)

10 Ounces Dark Chocolate, Melted

1 Cup Powdered / Confectioner's Sugar

1/4 Cup Espresso, Strong Brewed Coffee, or Chocolate Soymilk

2 Teaspoons Vanilla Extract

1 Prepared 9-Inch Chocolate Cookie Crumb Crust (store-bought or recipe on p241)

Coarsely Crushed Chocolate Cream-Filled Sandwich Cookies (for garnish, regular or wheat-free)

Place the tofu in your blender, and blend until smooth. Add the melted chocolate, blending again until smooth. Add the powdered sugar, espresso, coffee, or soymilk, and vanilla, and blend until the mixture is smooth and fluffy. Spread the chocolate mixture into the pie shell and top with the crushed chocolate cookies. Refrigerate the pie for several hours or until it is firm enough to slice.

Virtuous Chocolate Mousse

Yields 4 Servings

Venturing out on that "chocolate is healthy" limb once again, this quick and easy dessert does seem to sway toward the nutritious side, while still fulfilling the need for a little indulgence. For an elegant presentation, layer it in parfait glasses with your favorite fresh berries.

1 12.3-Ounce Package Firm Silken Tofu
2 Medium-Sized, Ripe Bananas
8 Ounces Semi-Sweet Chocolate Chips

1 Teaspoon Vanilla Extract
Pinch Salt

Place the tofu and bananas in your blender, and process until smooth. In your microwave, heat the chocolate in 30-second intervals until it just melts, whisking vigorously between intervals. Pour the melted chocolate into your blender, along with the vanilla and salt. Blend until the mixture is smooth and creamy. Divide the mousse between 4 serving glasses, cover and chill in the refrigerator for at least 1 hour before serving.

Buttahscotch Dessert Pudding

Yields 4 to 6 Servings
Recipe created by Hannah Kaminsky, author of *My Sweet Vegan*

1/4 Cup Dairy-Free Margarine
1 Cup Dark Brown Sugar, Firmly Packed
3 Tablespoons Cornstarch

2 Cups Cold Plain Soymilk, Divided
1/2 Teaspoon Salt
1 Teaspoon Vanilla Extract

Place a medium saucepan over the stove and turn up the heat to medium. Melt the margarine before stirring in the brown sugar, cooking briefly until it is dissolved. Whisk the cornstarch with 1/4 cup of the soymilk, ensuring that no lumps remain. Quickly whisk the cornstarch mixture into your saucepan until it is completely incorporated and the mixture is smooth. Add in the remaining soymilk and the salt, whisking thoroughly to scrape up anything that might be left on the bottom of the pan, and cook until it comes to a boil. It should feel significantly thicker at this point. Cook for another minute before taking the mixture off the heat and whisking in the vanilla. Pour the liquid pudding into individual heat-safe cups. Place a piece of plastic wrap over the surface to prevent a skin from forming. Move the cups into your refrigerator, and let chill until set, about 4 hours.

White Chocolate Mousse

Yields 4 to 6 Servings
Recipe adapted from the blog, Bittersweet (bittersweetblog.wordpress.com) by Hannah Kaminsky - *According to Hannah, this deceptively rich dessert doubles as a topping for fresh berries, cupcakes, or hot chocolate.*

3 Ounces White Chocolate (a dairy-free store-bought version or the recipe on p135)

1 10-Ounce Container "Whippable" Soy, Oat, or Coconut Cream, Divided (p127-128)
3/4 Teaspoon Agar Powder

Melt the white chocolate with 2-1/2 ounces of the cream, stir vigorously until smooth, and let it cool for 10 minutes. With a mixer, whip the remaining cream for 3 to 4 minutes, until soft peaks form, and slowly stream in the melted chocolate on the side. It will liquefy a bit and appear to have gone awry, but do not panic. Sprinkle the agar on top, whisk to fully combine, and place the bowl in your refrigerator for 30 minutes. Once thoroughly chilled, whip it for 5 to 6 minutes until fluffy but firm. Serve, or pipe it into bowls and refrigerate for up to 6 more hours before serving.

Triple Chocolate Pudding

Yields 4 Servings or 3-1/2 Cups

Recipe adapted from the DVD, Everyday Dish (www.everydaydish.tv), by Julie Hasson - *Upping the indulgence factor of ordinary pudding, Julie infused it with a triple dose of chocolate. You can view a demo of Julie making this recipe on her DVD, which includes demos and corresponding vegan recipes from her, Dreena Burton, and Bryanna Clark Grogan.*

3/4 Cup Granulated Sugar
1/3 Cup Unsweetened Cocoa Powder
1/4 Cup + 2 Tablespoons Cornstarch
Pinch Salt

3 Cups Cold Chocolate Soymilk or Other Chocolate Milk Alternative
1/4 Cup Semi-Sweet Chocolate Chips
1 Teaspoon Vanilla Extract

In a large pot, whisk together the sugar, cocoa, cornstarch and salt. Add the soymilk, whisking until smooth. Bring the mixture to a boil over medium heat, whisking continuously. Lower the heat and simmer gently, whisking continuously, for 5 to 10 minutes or until the pudding is thick. Remove the saucepan from the heat and stir in the chocolate chips and vanilla. Serve the pudding warm, or scoop it into a bowl, press a piece of plastic wrap onto the surface of the pudding (to prevent a skin from forming), and refrigerate until ready to serve.

Glorified Rice

Yields 6 to 8 Servings

Recipe by Jennifer McCann, author of *Vegan Lunch Box* (www.veganlunchbox.com) - *This classic U.S. dish reached its height of popularity following the Great Depression, but the traditional recipes rely heavily upon whipped cream or heavy cream. As Jennifer's story goes, "I grew up eating sweet, fluffy Glorified Rice at Grandma's house every Thanksgiving and Christmas. Grandma and Betty Crocker® taught me to mix rice with crushed pineapple, whipped cream, and maraschino cherries ... but now that so many people in our family are vegan, I wanted to come up with a non-dairy, sans [neon] cherries version. I did it! The flavor is so spot-on, even Grandma would approve."*

1 Cup Short Grain White Rice, Uncooked
1 20-Ounce Can Crushed Pineapple, Well Drained
3/4 Cup Granulated Sugar or Evaporated Cane Juice, Divided

1 12.3-Ounce Package Firm Silken Tofu, Well Drained
2 Tablespoons Lemon Juice
1 Pint Strawberries, Sliced

Cook the white rice according to the package directions. While the rice is still hot, place it in a large mixing bowl and stir in the crushed pineapple and 1/2 cup of the sugar. Let the mixture rest at room temperature for one hour to cool. Cover and refrigerate until cold.

Place the silken tofu, the remaining 1/4 cup of sugar, and the lemon juice in a blender. Blend until completely smooth. Fold the blended tofu into the rice mixture, breaking apart any clumps of rice with a wooden spoon. Top with fresh sliced strawberries to serve.

Better Than Ice Cream

Yields 4 Servings

Recipe adapted from The Vegetarian Mother's Cookbook by Cathe Olson - This recipe is not only a taste of Cathe's most popular cookbook, but also of what we have to look forward to; she has a dairy-free/ vegan "ice cream" cookbook in the works. This simple blend is surprisingly rich and creamy, yet very nutritious and easy to whip up sans ice cream maker. The nuts add a good dose of luxury, but feel free to omit them if you have a nut allergy, or would like to stick with a virtually fat free version.

1/2 Cup Nuts (almonds, pecans, etc.) (optional)
1 Cup Frozen Banana Slices
1 Cup Frozen Diced Peaches or Berries

1/4 to 1/2 Cup Plain Milk Alternative of Choice
1/2 Teaspoon Vanilla Extract

Place the nuts (if using) in your food processor* and pulse until coarsely chopped. Add the bananas and berries or peaches. Pulse until the fruit is coarsely chopped. Add the milk alternative a little at a time through the top of the processor, along with the vanilla, and puree until creamy. This is best eaten right after it is made, but if you want to save it for later, freeze it in individual containers and leave at room temperature for about 10 minutes before eating.

* If you don't have a food processor, grind the nuts in your spice grinder (if using), and add them to your blender along with the remaining ingredients. You will need the full 1/2 cup of milk alternative (and possibly a touch more) to get things moving, or you may want to let the fruit defrost for just a few minutes before blending.

Simply Vanilla Frozen Yogurt

Yields 1 Pint

There are many complicated frozen yogurt recipes out there, but I like this basic version, which focuses on the yogurt aspect. I use coconut-based yogurt, which tends to be a bit sweeter and less tangy than soy yogurt, but feel free to adjust the sugar (or sweetener of choice) to your tastes. If using an ice cream maker, you may need to double this recipe if a pint is too little for your equipment's capacity.

2 cups Strained Plain or Vanilla Dairy-Free Yogurt*
6 Tablespoons Granulated Sugar, or More to Taste

1 Teaspoon Vanilla Extract
1 teaspoon Lemon Juice

In a medium-sized mixing bowl, combine all ingredients until the sugar has dissolved and the mixture is smooth. Freeze in your ice cream maker according to the manufacturer's instructions.

Without an Ice Cream Maker: Pour the mixture into an ungreased 8-inch square dish or a 9x13-inch dish for a quart-sized batch. Cover and freeze for 3 to 4 hours or until partially set, but not frozen solid. Blend the yogurt in your food processor, blender, or mixing bowl until smooth. Transfer the mixture to a container, cover, and freeze until firm, about 2 hours.

* To strain the yogurt, line a fine mesh strainer with a double layer of cheesecloth and place a bowl under the strainer. Put the yogurt atop the cheesecloth, fold the corners of the cheesecloth over to cover, and place the entire apparatus in your refrigerator. Allow it to sit overnight to strain. About 4 to 5 6-ounce containers (24 to 32 ounces) of dairy-free yogurt should yield the 2 cups you will need for this recipe.

Very Vanilla "Ice Cream"

Yields 1 Quart
Recipe created by Hannah Kaminsky, author of *My Sweet Vegan* - *If you don't have an ice cream maker, see the instructions for the Simply Vanilla Frozen Yogurt (p245).*

3 Cups Plain or Vanilla Soymilk
3/4 Cup Granulated Sugar
1/2 Cup Canola or Vegetable Oil

1/4 Cup Light Agave Nectar
1 Tablespoon Vanilla Paste or Extract
Pinch Salt

Take out your food processor or blender and begin by combining the soymilk and sugar. Let the machine run for a minute or two, until the sugar has dissolved. Stream in the oil very, very slowly as it continues to run, giving it time to emulsify properly. Add in the agave, vanilla, and salt, and simply pulse to combine. If it's still somewhat cold and completely smooth, you're free to start churning immediately. Otherwise, let the mixture chill in your refrigerator for an hour or two before freezing it in your ice cream maker according to the manufacturer's directions. Transfer the "ice cream" into a container and freeze for at least two hours before serving.

Luxurious Peanut Butter "Ice Cream"

Yields Roughly 1 Quart
Recipe adapted from the blog, Have Cake Will Travel (www.havecakewilltravel.com) by Celine Steen - *Celine demonstrates her versatility in the kitchen, and continued love for peanut butter, with this simple, yet incredibly rich, frozen dessert. As she notes, the coconut flavor in this "ice cream" is quite subdued, letting the peanut butter take center stage. But, if you prefer, you can substitute silken tofu or even soy yogurt for the coconut milk. If you don't have an ice cream maker, see the instructions for the Simply Vanilla Frozen Yogurt (p245).*

1-1/3 Cup Regular Coconut Milk (do not shake the can; grab as much cream as possible) (see intro)
1 Cup Plain Rice Milk
1 Cup Crunchy Salted Natural Peanut Butter

3/4 Cup Granulated Sugar or Firmly Packed Light Brown Sugar
2 Teaspoon Vanilla Extract

Blend all of the ingredients together in your food processor or blender. Place the mixture in a covered container, and allow it to sit in your refrigerator for at least 4 hours, or overnight. While the mixture is chilling, place the ice cream container of your ice cream maker in your freezer. Once chilled, place the mixture in your ice cream maker, and follow the manufacturer's instructions. If using any of the Optional Add-Ins below, toss (or drizzle) them in when the ice cream maker is almost (but not quite) done churning. When it is finished, place the ice cream container in the freezer for at least 30 minutes to allow it to set.

Optional Add-Ins (add during the last 5 minutes of preparation):
Chocolate Chips / Chunks
Chocolate Syrup
Brownie Pieces
Graham Cracker Pieces

Chocolate Fudge Pieces
More Peanut Butter to Make Swirls
Jelly of Choice to Make Swirls
Fruit Leather Pieces

Coconut Ginger "Ice Cream"

Yields 1 Quart

Recipe created by Hannah Kaminsky, author of *My Sweet Vegan - This frozen dessert is so creamy that you'd swear it's an ultra-premium ice cream made with dairy, yet the base is actually nothing but coconut! With just a hint of lemon and ginger to give it a bright, fresh taste, this is a tropical treat you simply won't be able to get enough of. If you don't have an ice cream maker, see the instructions for the Simply Vanilla Frozen Yogurt (p245).*

1 14-Ounce Can Coconut Milk
1 Tablespoon Cornstarch or Arrowroot Powder
1 15-Ounce Can Cream of Coconut

1/4 Cup Granulated Sugar
1/2 Teaspoon Lemon Juice
2 Teaspoons Fresh Ginger Root, Grated

Set aside 1/4 cup of the coconut milk and mix it with the cornstarch or arrowroot until the powder is completely dissolved. Combine the remaining coconut milk with the cream of coconut, sugar, lemon juice, and ginger in a saucepan and gently heat until it just begins to boil. Add in the mixture of coconut milk and arrowroot, whisking thoroughly so that there are no lumps. Continue cooking everything for 3 to 4 minutes longer until slightly thickened, and remove from the heat. Let it cool to room temperature (or refrigerate it for a few hours) before freezing it according to the manufacturer's directions for your ice cream maker.

After churning for the appropriate amount of time, you will want to transfer your ice cream into a medium sized container, cover and let it set up for at least 3 hours in the freezer. You could always eat it as is for a consistency similar to soft serve, but be warned - It melts very quickly in this state!

Pineapple Sherbet

Yields 1-1/2 Pints

Recipe created by Hannah Kaminsky, author of *My Sweet Vegan - This makes for one easy and refreshing summery treat! If you don't have an ice cream maker, see the instructions for the Simply Vanilla Frozen Yogurt (p245).*

1 Cup Pineapple Juice
1 Cup Plain Soymilk

1 Cup Plain Soy Creamer
2/3 Cup Granulated Sugar

Begin by combining the pineapple juice and soymilk, and let it sit for about 5 minutes to become better acquainted. Add in the soy creamer and sugar, stir well, and freeze the mixture in your ice cream maker according to the manufacturer's instructions. It should take approximately 25 to 30 minutes to achieve the ideal consistency.

The sherbet will still be fairly soft at this point and you're welcome to eat it as is, but I would suggest moving it all into a large tub and letting it harden further your freezer for a few hours.

Soy-Free Option: For a slight piña colada vibe, substitute the soymilk and soy creamer for 2 cups of light coconut milk, or 1 cup of regular coconut milk and 1 cup of plain milk alternative of your choosing.

Mint Stracciatella

Yields 1 Quart

My first attempt at creating a dairy-free mint chip "ice cream" actually turned out quite well, but the flavor wasn't quite perfect. Rather than wrestle with the subtle nuances myself, I turned the recipe over to the dairy-free (and vegan) dessert expert, Hannah, of My Sweet Vegan. Not only did she adjust the sugar and mint to just the right levels, but she also masterfully changed my chunky mint chip to a stracciatella. The wafer thin chocolate shards are actually very simple to create, and they offer a true melt-in-your-mouth chocolate experience. If you don't have an ice cream maker, see the instructions for the Simply Vanilla Frozen Yogurt (p245).

2 Medium/Smallish Avocados (about 6 ounces of avocado flesh)
1 14-Ounce Can Regular Coconut Milk
1 Cup Plain Soymilk or Other Milk Alternative of Choice
1/2 Cup Agave Nectar

6 Tablespoons Granulated Sugar
1 Teaspoon Lime or Lemon Juice
1-1/2 Teaspoons Peppermint Extract
1/2 Teaspoon Vanilla Extract
1/8 Teaspoon Salt
4 Ounces Bittersweet or Semi-Sweet Chocolate

Blend all of the ingredients, except for the chocolate, together in your food processor or blender. Place the mixture in a covered container, and allow it to sit in your refrigerator for at least 4 hours, or overnight. While the mixture is chilling, place the ice cream container of your ice cream maker in your freezer. Once chilled, place the mixture in your ice cream maker, and follow the manufacturer's instructions.

When the "ice cream" is nearing the end of its cycle, chop the chocolate. Place the chocolate in a microwave-safe bowl and microwave it on HIGH in 30 second intervals (just 2 to 3 should suffice), stirring vigorously between intervals, until the chocolate has just melted and is smooth. Be careful not to overheat the chocolate, as it can scorch easily. Let the chocolate cool for a minute or two. Transfer the ice cream to the tub you will be using to store it, and drizzle the melted chocolate over the top in a thin stream. Cover and freeze completely.

When you are ready for dessert, just mash the hardened chocolate on top to break it up and mix it into the "ice cream." Alternately, you can slowly drizzle the melted chocolate into the ice cream maker in a thin stream, once it nears the end of its cycle. Let it churn for just a minute to break up the chocolate and disperse it throughout the "ice cream."

Mint Chip Option: If stracciatella isn't your style, feel free to add 1/3 cup of mini chocolate chips to the ice cream maker near the end of its cycle.

Intense Chocolate Sorbet

Yields 1 Pint

Recipe created by Hannah Kaminsky, author of My Sweet Vegan - You may think that a concoction without any non-dairy milk or chocolate pieces would be a bit lacking in flavor or texture, but you will be surprised at how rich and luscious this simple sorbet is. Even more decadent than full-fledged chocolate ice cream, this is a frozen treat for true chocoholics only! For instructions without an ice cream maker, see the Simply Vanilla Frozen Yogurt recipe (p245).

2 Cups Warm Water, Divided
1 Cup Granulated Sugar
1 Cup Dutch-Processed Cocoa Powder

1 Teaspoon Vanilla Extract
1/2 Teaspoon Salt

Combine 1/4 cup of the water and the sugar in a medium saucepan over medium-high heat. Don't stir for the first couple of minutes, until the sugar dissolves and the mixture comes to a boil. Continue cooking, stirring occasionally, until the sugar becomes a golden caramel color after about 5 to 10 minutes. Add the remaining water carefully, standing back in case of splashing. The caramel will seize and sputter a bit, and don't worry if it appears to harden. Cook gently once again until the caramel is dissolved, immediately removing the pot from the heat once smooth. Thoroughly whisk in the cocoa powder, vanilla, and salt, making sure there are absolutely no lumps. Chill thoroughly before freezing in your ice cream maker per the manufacturer's instructions. Once churned, pack the sorbet into a container and freeze it solid before serving.

Basic Fruit Sorbet

Yields 4 Servings

Recipe adapted from the blog, The Urban House Wife (theurbanhousewife.blogspot.com), by Melisser Elliott - For fun, I did a brief ice cream survey on Go Dairy Free, requesting to know the favorite flavors of readers. To my great surprise, there were numerous sorbet responses. To appeal to this fruit-loving, dairy-free crowd, Melisser perfected her simple sorbet recipe for me to share within this guide. Thank you, Melisser! If you don't have an ice cream maker, see the instructions for the Simply Vanilla Frozen Yogurt (p245).

1 Cup Water
1/2 Cup Granulated Sugar
1/4 Cup Lemon Juice

2 Cups Fresh Fruit of Choice (for liquid fruits such as lemon, lime, and orange, use 1-1/2 cups of the fruit's juice)

Place the water and sugar in a small saucepan and heat over medium-low heat until the sugar dissolves. Turn off the heat, stir in the lemon juice, and set this mixture aside to cool. Puree or squeeze the fruits of your choice until you have 2 cups worth of puree or 1-1/2 cups of the juice. If using berries, strain the seeds, if desired. Add the liquid mixture to the fruit puree and stir until combined. Place the mixture in the refrigerator and allow it to chill for 1 hour or longer. Pour the mixture into your ice cream maker and follow the manufacturer's instructions.

Cinnamon Coconut Pops

Yields 5 to 6 Frozen Treats

This is a very versatile treat that will cater to a variety of flavors; see the options below for some ideas.

1 14-Ounce Can Regular or Light Coconut Milk*   1 Teaspoon Ground Cinnamon
1/3 Cup Agave Nectar or Sweetener of Choice

In a medium-sized bowl, whisk together all ingredients until the cinnamon is well dispersed or combine the ingredients in your blender and give it a quick bled. Pour the mixture into freezer pop molds or ice cube trays. Freeze for several hours, or until the pops are frozen solid. If you don't have freezer pop molds, fill 5-ounce paper cups with the mixture. Top the cups with foil and make a slit into the center of each and insert a wooden stick before freezing.

Carob or Cocoa Option: Omit the cinnamon. When making carob pops, I add 1/4 cup (4 tablespoons) carob powder and increase the agave by 1 tablespoon, but I would start with 2 tablespoons of carob or cocoa powder and add more 1 tablespoon at a time until it reaches your desired intensity.

Plain Old Vanilla Option: Omit the cinnamon but whisk in 1-1/2 to 2 teaspoons of pure vanilla extract.

Piña Colada Option: Blend in 1/2 cup of crushed (drained) pineapple and stir in 1/4 cup of shredded coconut (sweetened or unsweetened). You can optionally toast the coconut before adding it to enhance the coconut flavor.

Easiest "Ice Cream" Option: Freeze the mixture in half-filled ice cube trays for about 1 hour, or until "soft" frozen. Puree the cubes in your food processor or blender (begin by pulsing) until creamy. If frozen solid, then you may need to allow the cubes to defrost for 10 minutes or so before blending.

* I go for the full indulgence, using regular coconut milk for the richest consistency.

Magical Shell

Yields approximately 1 Cup

I loved this stuff as a kid, so when I discovered the magical solidifying properties of coconut oil, I knew it was time to recreate this old favorite at home.

6 Ounces Semi-sweet Chocolate Chips   1/4 Cup Grapeseed or Vegetable Oil
1/4 Cup Coconut Oil

Place the chocolate in a microwave-safe bowl and microwave it on HIGH in 30 second intervals (just 2 to 3 should suffice), stirring vigorously between intervals, until the chocolate has just melted and is smooth. Be careful not to overheat the chocolate, as it can scorch easily. Stir in the two oils until smooth and drizzle away! Store at room temperature or in the refrigerator, warming the sauce as needed.

Hot Fudge Sauce

Yields 1-1/4 Cups or 10 Servings

*Recipe adapted from T*he Ice Dream Cookbook *by Chef Rachel Albert-Matesz - According to Rachel, this sauce makes the perfect topping for almost any flavor of "ice cream." You can also layer it with "ice cream" for a rippled effect or serve the sauce over a fresh fruit salad. To keep the sweet taste without the added calories, Rachel uses a combination of agave or honey and stevia. If you don't have any stevia handy, you can sweeten to taste with the agave, honey, or your sweetener of choice.*

3/4 Cup Cold Regular or Light Coconut Milk or Plain Almond, Cashew, or Hazelnut Milk Alternative

2 Teaspoons Arrowroot Powder

1/4 Cup Honey or Agave Nectar, Plus 1 to 3 Tablespoons as needed

1/8 Teaspoon Salt

2 Ounces Unsweetened Baker's Chocolate, Coarsely Chopped or Broken into 1/2-Inch Pieces

1/2 Teaspoon Clear Stevia Liquid Extract

1 Teaspoon Vanilla Extract or Alcohol-Free Vanilla Flavoring

Combine the coconut milk or nut milk and arrowroot in a small saucepan. Whisk to dissolve. Add the honey or agave and salt. Bring the mixture to a boil over medium heat, stirring or whisking constantly, until the mixture thickens, about 3 to 5 minutes. Remove from the heat, and add the chocolate, stevia, and vanilla, stirring until the chocolate melts. If desired, adjust the sauce to taste with additional honey or agave. Let it stand for 10 minutes to cool slightly before servings. Refrigerate any unused sauce in a covered heatproof bowl, a few custard cups, or a wide mouth jar.

Gently warm the leftover sauce in a heatproof bowl in a 250ºF (120ºC) oven, or in a double boiler or saucepan over very low heat, stirring periodically. If too thick, add 1 to 2 tablespoons of additional coconut milk or milk alternative.

Almond Fudge Sauce Option: Add 1/2 teaspoon almond extract.

Peppermint Fudge Sauce Option: Add 1/4 to 1/2 teaspoon peppermint extract or natural peppermint flavoring or 1 tablespoon crème de menthe, with the vanilla.

Chocolate-Orange Fudge Sauce Option: Add 1-1/2 tablespoons minced or finely grated orange zest and/or 1-1/2 tablespoons orange liqueur, such as Grand Marnier, with the vanilla.

Mocha Fudge Sauce Option: Add 2 to 3 teaspoons instant coffee granules or espresso powder with the arrowroot powder.

Spiked Fudge Sauce Option: Add 1-1/2 tablespoons light or dark rum, brandy, or your favorite liqueur, with the vanilla.

Sweet and Silky Butterscotch Sauce

Yields 2 Cups

This super sweet sauce adds that extra touch of indulgence to "ice cream" or your favorite desserts.

1 Cup Light Brown Sugar, Firmly Packed
2/3 cup Agave Nectar or Corn Syrup
1/4 Cup Dairy-Free Margarine
1/3 Cup Water + 1/3 Cup Regular Coconut Milk or 2/3
    Cup Evaporated Milk Alternative*

1 Teaspoon Vanilla Extract
1/8 Teaspoon Baking Soda
Scant 1/8 Teaspoon Salt

Combine the sugar, agave or corn syrup, and margarine in a medium-sized saucepan over medium heat. Stir and cook until the sugar has dissolved and the mixture comes to a full rolling boil. Allow it to boil, without stirring, for exactly 1 minute. Remove the sauce from the heat and allow it to sit and cool while you prepare the other ingredients. In a glass measuring cup, combine the water and coconut milk or the evaporated milk alternative with the vanilla, baking soda, and salt. Gradually stir this liquid into the slightly cooled sauce until smooth and combined. Pour the sauce into a large glass jar, cover, and refrigerate. It will thicken as it chills. If it thickens too much for your liking, gently warm the jar in a pot of hot water on the stove.

To make evaporated milk alternative, add 1-1/3 cups of plain or unsweetened milk alternative of choice to a small saucepan over medium-low heat. Cook, stirring frequently, until the volume has reduced in half (2/3 cup).

Dulce de Coco

Yields approximately 1 Cup

Recipe created by Hannah Kaminsky, author of My Sweet Vegan – Hannah states, "I was on a mission, determined to bring dulce de leche back into my life. Sure, recipes for similar results do exist in various corners of the Internet, but all called for strange, hard to find ingredients. After finally realizing that I would need to take things into my own hands if I was ever to enjoy my most cherished sweet caramel topping again, I discovered that... It really wasn't so hard to make! Truly effortless, the greatest difficulty involved is having enough patience to stay in the kitchen as it cooks down, and then wait for it to fully cool before digging in. Trust me; your perseverance will be rewarded!"

1 14-Ounce Can Regular Coconut Milk
1 Cup Dark Brown Sugar, Firmly Packed

1/4 Teaspoon Salt
1/2 Teaspoon Vanilla Extract

Combine all ingredients except for the vanilla in a medium sauce pan over medium-high heat. Once the mixture comes to a boil, reduce the heat to medium-low, cover, and simmer for about 20 minutes. Remove the lid; turn the heat down to low and simmer for approximately 35 to 40 more minutes, stirring occasionally, until thickened. Stir in the vanilla and pour it into a glass jar for storage, allowing it to cool completely before covering.

Quick Caramelita Sauce
Yields 2/3 Cup
This simple caramel-like sauce is lighter in both taste and calories/fat than butter and cream-laden caramels as it uses dairy-free yogurt instead.

3/4 Cup Light Brown Sugar, Firmly Packed   Pinch Salt (optional)
1/4 Cup Plain Dairy-Free Yogurt   1/4 Teaspoon Vanilla Extract

Combine the brown sugar, yogurt, and salt in a small saucepan over medium-low heat. Whisk until the sugar dissolves. When it begins to bubble, allow it to cook and boil for about 4 minutes. Remove from the heat and let it cool for 10 minutes. Whisk in the vanilla extract. Store any leftovers in the refrigerator; the sauce should keep for a few days.

Perfect World Whipped Coconut Cream
Yields 1 Cup
Whenever I find a coconut milk that separates beautifully (in other words, it doesn't contain too many additives and stabilizers), I like to make this recipe. If your coconut milk is too homogenized, and doesn't exhibit a nice separation, then I recommend using the Cool Whipped Coconut Cream recipe (below) instead.

2 14-Ounce Cans Regular Coconut Milk, Chilled   1-1/2 Tablespoons Superfine or Powdered /
1/4 Teaspoon Vanilla Extract (optional)   Confectioner's Sugar

Place the can of coconut milk (unshaken) in the refrigerator to chill for several hours (or days if you like). Place a medium-sized metal bowl and whisk or beaters in the freezer for 10 minutes. Remove the coconut milk from the refrigerator and skim 1/2 cup of the thickest cream from the tops of each, so that you end up with 1 cup of coconut cream. Make sure to avoid the thin liquid from the bottom of the can (it can be used in another recipe as light coconut milk), or the cream will not become stiff when whipped. Place the metal bowl in a larger bowl filled with ice (optional), add the coconut cream to the metal bowl and beat with a hand mixer (you can whip with a whisk, but this will give your arm quite the workout), until thick and stiff. Whip in the vanilla extract, if using, and the sugar. Serve immediately or store covered in the refrigerator.

Cool Whipped Coconut Cream
Yields approximately 1 Cup
When the cream doesn't separate nicely in my cans of coconut milk, I turn to this recipe. This is a great make-ahead option, as it will thicken as it chills. This is a sweeter whipped cream, but you can reduce the sugar a bit if desired.

1 14-Ounce Can Regular Coconut Milk or Cream   1/4 Cup Rice or Soymilk Powder
1/4 to 1/3 Cup Superfine or Powdered /   1/2 Teaspoon Vanilla Extract
     Confectioner's Sugar   1/2 Teaspoon Lemon Juice (optional)

Place the can of coconut milk (unshaken) in the refrigerator to chill for several hours (or days if you like). Place a medium-sized metal bowl and whisk in the freezer for 10 minutes. Remove the coconut milk from the refrigerator and skim as much cream from the top as you can, leaving any watery portions for use in another recipe. Add the coconut cream to the metal bowl and beat with a hand mixer (you can whip with a whisk, but this will give your arm quite the workout), until thick and stiff. Gently whip in the remaining ingredients. If the mixture is too thin, allow it to chill in the refrigerator for several hours or overnight.

Some Store-Bought Recommendations:

There are many great brands on the market, but the following recommendations only include products that I purchase with some regularity or that a colleague highly recommended. For full lists of non-dairy, packaged foods and brands, see the product lists available on www.godairyfree.org.

Cherrybrook Kitchen® (www.cherrybrookkitchen.com, (978) 974-0200) ~ boxed cake mixes
If you can't find dairy-free cake mixes, then you just haven't stumbled across this company. Cherrybrook's mixes include cookies, cakes, frostings, and brownies, and they are made in a kitchen that is free from dairy, eggs, peanuts, and tree nuts. They also have a gluten-free mix line (still free from dairy, eggs, and nuts), and most of their products are free from soy. The boxes are adorably animated too, making them very fun to make with kids.

Coconut Bliss® (www.coconutbliss.com, (541) 345-0020) ~ frozen dessert
Luna and Larry really outdid themselves with this ultra-rich frozen dessert. In fact, I do not exaggerate when I say that it could easily rival premium ice cream. The ingredients are pure and natural, and they use a modest hand with the agave nectar, sweetening to the perfect taste, but not a bit more. I have fallen in love with the Cherry Amaretto flavor, but there are still so many flavors to trial.

Divvies™ (www.divvies.com, (914) 533-0333) ~ fresh baked cookies and cupcakes, and caramel corn
If you have a little one with food allergies, then Divvies is a company to know about. They ship party-friendly buckets of popcorn, cupcakes with frosting, and bakery fresh cookies, which are all prepared in their dairy-, egg-, and nut-free kitchen. While I haven't sampled their goodies myself, I hear nothing but rave reviews from the dairy-free little ones of colleagues.

Enjoy Life® (www.enjoylifefoods.com, (847) 260-0300) ~ cookies
You don't have to be gluten-free to love the soft little cookies from Enjoy Life. They are positively addictive and delicious in their own right. You can snack on them (they are even a bit virtuous), use them to prepare a pie crust, or crumble them atop pudding or "ice cream." Everyone I know who has tried these, loves them ... the whole free from gluten, dairy, soy, nuts, etc, is just a side benefit, really.

Gluten-Free Pantry (www.glutenfree.com, (800) 291-8386) ~ gluten-free dessert mixes
This is reportedly the best GFCF chocolate cake mix ever. But, if chocolate isn't your thing, Gluten Free Pantry does offer a wide range of gluten-free / dairy-free cake mixes.

HomeFree™ (formerly Gak's Snacks) (www.homefreetreats.com, 800) 552-7172) ~ baked cakes and cookies
If you haven't already heard of Gak's Snacks ... well, you're a little late, as the company name has now changed to HomeFree. Luckily, the organic goodies churning out of this dairy-, egg-, nut-, and wheat-free kitchen (not gluten-free) haven't changed, as they are so delicious. HomeFree ships full-sized coffeecakes (kid-friendly taste, and excellent for birthday parties) and a variety of bakery fresh cookies to customers throughout the U.S. I am a big fan of the jumbo cookies and the apple coffeecake.

Kinnikinnick (www.kinnikinnick.com, (780) 424-2900) ~ gluten-free goodies
I believe this is the third time I have mentioned this company (and to remind you, I am not actually gluten-free myself), but their K-Too cookies are awesome. They taste nearly identical to Oreos™, offering the same "milk"-dunking satisfaction.

Lagusta's Luscious Truffles (www.lagustasluscious.com, (845) 255-8VEG) ~ truffles
If you want to give a special gift to someone who can't consume dairy (including yourself of course), look no further than the handmade boxes of truffles from Lagusta's Luscious. You have to place your order early, as Lagusta tends to sell out quickly, which isn't surprising when you take a peak at her affordable prices and incredible quality. She uses just organic coconut milk, organic coconut butter, and organic and fair trade dark chocolate to create a variety of unique flavors.

Luigi's® Italian Ice (www.luigis.com, 800-486-9533) ~ frozen desserts
When Luigi's was mentioned, childhood memories came rushing back. I absolutely loved these fruity cups of Italian Ice when I was growing up. Definitely a good treat for kids.

Namaste Foods (www.namastefoods.com, (866) 258-949) ~ gluten-free dessert mixes
I thought I had died and gone to sugar-overload heaven when I prepared the Blondies Mix from Namaste. Keep in mind, I am not gluten-free, but this dessert was spectacular by all standards. Equally glowing reviews have come from my colleagues. Namaste has other tasty gluten-free dessert mixes too, but the Blondies knocked our socks off.

Newman's Own (www.newmansownorganics.com) ~ cookies
Newman O's are remarkably similar to Oreos™, but they are organic, and made without milk ingredients (all flavors upon last check), high fructose corn syrup, and hydrogenated oils. They are perfect for snacking or making pie crusts or parfaits, and beyond the basic chocolate sandwich crèmes you can find unique varieties such as Ginger-O's and a Wheat-Free (but not gluten-free) version.

Pamela's Products™ (www.pamelasproducts.com, (707) 462-6605) ~ gluten-free cookies and cake mixes
When one of the Go Dairy Free reviewers claims that a cookie is better than Chips Ahoy (without dairy or gluten no less), I have to take notice. Pamela's Simplebites Mini Cookies (chocolate chip, extreme chocolate, and ginger snapz) captured Amy's taste buds and therefore received this spot on my most recommended desserts list.

Rice Dream® (www.tastethedream, (800) 434-4246) ~ frozen desserts
This brand of frozen desserts has received mixed reviews among my family and friends; it seems to exude a love / hate reaction. Nonetheless, I find the Rice Dream Frozen Pies (individually packaged rice-based "ice cream" sandwiches with a chocolate or carob coating) to be completely addictive. In the summer, I often see them at the natural food store for just $.99 a piece, making them impossible to resist.

Sjaak's (www.sjaaks.com, (707) 775-2434) ~ boxed chocolates
Sjaak's is another one of those reliable companies that is certified organic and fair trade. They offer a very large and luxurious range of vegan / dairy-free chocolates, including bars, bites, boxed chocolates, and seasonal items, which I find handy for gift giving. They do follow rigorous cleaning procedures (since they do have a milk chocolate line too), but admit that trace milk may be possible, so contact them before purchasing if this is a concern.

Soyatoo!® (www.soyatoo.de, +49 6 593 99 670 – Germany) ~ whipped topping cream
Sold in a ready-to-spray canister, Soyatoo!® Soy Whip™ is the quick, dairy-free answer to that swirl of fluffy whipped topping to complete desserts. Like most alternatives, it garners conflicting reviews, though I definitely here more raves than rants about Soyatoo. They also have a rice-based version (soy-free), but at the time of writing this version was only available in Europe.

The Ginger People (www.gingerpeople.com, (800) 551-5284) ~ candies
I was so excited when I spotted candies from The Ginger People in my local store. Believe it or not, even candy labels need to be checked for milk ingredients, but I feel "safe" with this all-natural (and gluten-free) line of grown-up ginger chews and hard candies. Most of their products are potent, but perfect for ginger lovers. They also offer some ginger tonics, which are delicious and excellent for queasy mom-to-be stomachs.

Tofutti® (www.tofutti.com, (908) 272-2400) ~ frozen desserts
While tofu and "ice cream" don't sound like they belong in the same sentence, let alone in the same food, Tofutti Cuties® have become a mainstay in dairy-free frozen desserts. These simple ice cream sandwiches come in various flavors, and are the perfect treat to splurge on when the bells of the ice cream truck beckon. Sarah of No

Whey, Mama (nowheymama.blogspot.com) sends her milk allergic daughter to parties with a Tofutti Cutie in tow, so that she can partake in the sweet festivities, rather than feeling left out.

Turtle Mountain (www.turtlemountain.com, (866) 3TURTLE) – frozen desserts
Where would we be without Turtle Mountain? They have created more incredible dairy-free frozen desserts under their Purely Decadent® and So Delicious® labels than one could possibly taste-test in an entire year. My personal favorite is their Purely Decadent made with Coconut Milk "Ice Cream" line, which is rich, creamy, and also free from soy. Hannah loves the It's Soy Delicious® fruit-sweetened "Ice Cream" line, and Amy is wild for the Purely Decadent soy-based line, if for nothing else than their gluten-free cookie dough "ice cream." From chocolate covered "ice cream" sandwiches to luxurious pints in numerous flavors, Turtle Mountain is one of those companies that makes dairy-free easy.

Whole Soy & Co.® (www.wholesoyco.com, (415) 434-3020) ~ frozen yogurt
You didn't think dairy-free frozen yogurt existed, did you? Well it does, and it is in fact the most decadent soy-based vegan "ice cream" I have ever trialed, and with just 1 gram of fat per serving. No kidding. Of course, there is a catch ... this stuff can be difficult to locate, but ask for it at your local natural food store and they will surely order some in.

Section 6

More Recommended Resources

CHAPTER 27:
ONLINE READING & RESOURCES

It would take an entire book for me to tell you all of the wonderful websites and blogs I have discovered while surfing the Internet. To keep things manageable, the following includes a *short* list of sites that I highly recommend (trust me, there are more!). Type the underlined URL into your web browser to pay them a visit.

Strictly Dairy-Free

Avoiding Milk Protein (www.avoidingmilkprotein.com, website and blog) – This information portal for milk allergies was created and is maintained by milk-free mom, Karen Blue.

Go Dairy Free (www.godairyfree.org, website and blog) – Well of course I have to mention my own site. Trust me, it is packed full of more information than you could surf in a day. Product reviews, news, recipes, health information, etc., all lurk within. I update it with new information several times per week.

Got No Milk (blog: gotnomilk.wordpress.com) – This lactose intolerant blogger shares dairy-free recipes every week, and unlike the sweet tooth nature of the blogosphere, you will find many savory dishes and meal ideas on this blog, along with the occasional dessert, of course.

Must Follow Recipes (blog: mustfollowrecipes.blogspot.com) – Becky is a stay-at-home mom who shares sweet and savory dairy-free (and typically egg-free) recipes that she has created or trialed from other sources.

No Whey, Mama (blog: nowheymama.blogspot.com) –I don't know where I would be without Sarah, dairy-free mother extraordinaire. She shares stories, tips, and kid-friendly recipes. (*Sample Recipes on p230 and p240*)

Planet Lactose (blog: planetlactose.blogspot.com) – Steve Carper, creator of the Lactose Intolerance Clearinghouse (below), updates this blog several times per week with news on all things milk. If it has anything to do with the white stuff, Steve is on it.

Steve Carper's Lactose Intolerance Clearinghouse (website: www.stevecarper.com) – When I first began my website, this website was the only extensive resource I could find on living dairy-free. I still reference it often.

The Milk Documentary (website: www.milkdocumentary.com) – I try to steer clear of political and social issues in the dairy industry, but this documentary is a must watch for everyone.

The Non-Dairy Queen (blog: thenondairyqueen.blogspot.com) – Sarena keeps her blog for "the lactose challenged," but anyone looking for good dairy-free posts and recipes will definitely enjoy her writing. (*Sample Recipes on p154 and p184*)

The Parve Baker (blog: www.theparvebaker.com) – Rebecca Joseph keeps this neat and tidy blog with a goal to provide dairy-free recipes for home bakers that are worth the effort (and calories!) and don't rely heavily on dairy substitutes.

Vegan

Bittersweet (blog: bittersweetblog.wordpress.com) – Hannah Kaminsky, author of *My Sweet Vegan*, keeps this colorful "crafting" blog, which fuses her mouth-watering baking and vegan recipes with photography, knitting, and other creative ventures. (*Sample Recipes on p135, p159, and p235*)

Chocolate Covered Vegan (blog: howtogainweightonavegandiet.blogspot.com) – Katie kindly shares what she eats, offering easy ideas and recipes that can be whipped up in minutes.

Diet, Dessert and Dogs (blog: dietdessertndogs.wordpress.com) – Ricki's posts are always entertaining, filled with cute pictures of her dogs, and of course they almost always contain a great recipe. She is focused on a wheat-free diet that is also free from processed sugars. Yet, I can vouch that the results of her creations are delicious! (*Sample Recipe on p158*)

Domestic Affair (blog: domesticaffair.blogspot.com) – With over three years of posts, I consider jae a pioneer on the foodie blogging scene. Plus, I love the many all natural, soy-free recipes she shares. (Sample Recipe on p199)

Everyday Dish TV (videos: www.everydaydish.tv) – Julie Hasson created this site filled with cooking/baking demos and corresponding recipes. It is great to connect the recipes with visuals, as the creators of each recipe step you through the process in their own videos. (*Sample Recipes on p242 and p244*)

Fat Free Vegan (blog: blog.fatfreevegan.com) – This is one of the most popular food blogs on the Internet, period. It just happens to be vegan, dairy-free, and filled with incredible recipes and photos. (*Sample Recipes on p133 and p147*)

Gone Raw (website: www.goneraw.com) – Even if you aren't a raw foodist this website has many wonderful recipes to offer, from milk alternatives to "ice cream." All recipes are dairy-free, vegan, and of course, raw.

Have Cake Will Travel (blog: www.havecakewilltravel.com) – After receiving numerous requests for dairy-free bread machine recipes, I was elated to find Celine's blog. She churns out countless bread recipes, along with desserts, dinners, and anything she happens to create that day. (*Sample Recipes on p156, p175, and p246*)

Kitchen Ramblings of a Fairly Odd Tofu Mom (blog: tofu-n-sproutz.blogspot.com) – This tofu mom knows comfort food. Enjoy her down-home stories and recipes.

No Whey Jose (blog: www.nowheyjose.com) – Aspiring cookbook authors and vegan bakers, Josh Maines and Chelsea Kirk, dish up comfort food on their vegan blog. A recipes tab makes finding dishes easy.

Notes from the Vegan Feast Kitchen (blog: veganfeastkitchen.blogspot.com) – It is near impossible to match the inventiveness of Bryanna Clark Grogan. If you need an alternative to any food, Bryanna is your chef. Beyond her many cookbooks, she shares scores of well-tested recipes on her blog. (*Sample Recipe on p120*)

Post Punk Kitchen (website: www.postpunkkitchen.com) – If you are vegan, then you probably already know about the PPK, but it is a fantastic website for anyone seeking tested dairy-free recipes and a well-populated forum to ask special diet food questions.

The Healing Feast (website: www.thehealingfeast.com) – Aptly named, this site is a visual feast for the eyes, with a vivid look, delicious "raw" recipes, and enticing color photos, created and maintained by Janet L. Doane, the author of *Almond Essence*. (*Sample Recipes on p121 and p195*)

The Urban Housewife (blog: theurbanhousewife.blogspot.com) – Melisser's enjoyment of food and sweets shines through on her eclectic blog of recipes, reviews, and restaurant reports. In her "spare time" she runs Sugar Beat Sweets (www.sugarbeatsweets.com), a custom order baking business in San Francisco. (*Sample Recipes on p249*)

The Urban Vegan (blog: urbanvegan.blogspot.com) – This is my number one "idea" blog. There are many wonderful recipes, but beyond these, the Urban Vegan frequently details simple meal ideas.

The Vegan Chef (website: www.veganchef.com) - Beverly Lynn Bennett, co-author of two Complete Idiot's Guides (Vegan Living and Vegan Cooking), has stocked this website with hundreds of original recipes that are always vegan, and often raw, gluten-free, low-fat, and/or sugar-free. (*Sample Recipe on p121*)

The Vegan Diet (blog: thevegandiet.blogspot.com) – Jackie writes food-centric posts, each focusing on a single food, its virtues, and a handful of recipes that utilize it. The Vegan Diet helps me discover other websites and blogs and is great when I need recipes for a certain ingredient.

Vegan Dad (blog: vegandad.blogspot.com) – Yes, there are male food bloggers out there. Vegan Dad keeps his blog updated very regularly with easy recipes he prepares for his family.

Vegan Lunch Box (blog: veganlunchbox.blogspot.com) – Jennifer McCann, author of the cookbook Vegan Lunch Box, delights with simple, fun, kid-friendly recipes and food ideas. (*Sample Recipe on p244*)

Vegan Planet (blog: veganplanet.blogspot.com) – With 18 cookbooks under her belt (#19 is on the way), it is no wonder that Robin Robertson's blog has a good deal of natural appeal. Her blog has a nice clean feel, offering select recipes, tips, and ideas.

Vegan Visitor (blog: veganvisitor.wordpress.com) – It was love at first site when I discovered Vegan Visitor. This Canadian based blogger entices with beautiful photos and surprisingly easy recipes that she creates for her vegan in-laws and her own family. (*Sample Recipe on p205*)

Vegan Yum Yum (blog: www.veganyumyum.com) – Enticing recipes, beautiful step-by-step photos ... what more could you want in a blog? Lolo has been posting for a couple of years now, so there are many sweet and savory options to choose from.

VegFamily (online magazine: www.vegfamily.com) - This website covers essential topics for parents raising children who are vegan or dairy-free. Though already popular with the vegan community, it is an undiscovered gem for families with milk allergies. (*Sample Recipes on p200 and p228*)

VeggieGirl (blog: veggiegirlvegan.blogspot.com) – It is hard not to feel inspired by the energy with which Liz (aka Veggiegirl) bakes and writes for her blog. She provides an interesting cross-section of baked goodies (including gluten-free treats) and raw food recipes. (*Sample Recipes on p152, p153, and p237*)

VegWeb (website: www.vegweb.com) - VegWeb holds hundreds of reader submitted recipes, all dairy-free, and many with reviews. There is also a wealth of information through the network of external links they provide.

Vitalita (e-cookbooks: www.vitalita.com/cookbooks.html) – Over 150 recipes are available in the free e-cookbooks A Taste of Vitality and Desserts of Vitality. Health is the focus, so all of the recipes are vegan, and most are gluten-free and low-fat. While it is free to download the cookbooks, donations are appreciated.

Vive le Vegan (blog: vivelevegan.blogspot.com) – Dreena Burton just can't stay out of the kitchen, so she created this blog, which I would refer to as a creative outlet for her three cookbooks. She links to the recipes she created for the Canadian Food Network, provides sample recipes from her books, and offers tips for using the recipes in her cookbooks.

Gluten-Free / Casein-Free

Cindalou's Kitchen Blues (blog: cindalouskitchenblues.blogspot.com) – This evolving blog is rich with recipes that follow the Paleolithic diet principals, and are consequently gluten-free, dairy-free, and low in sugar.

Elana's Pantry (blog: www.elanaspantry.com) – Elana focuses on all natural cooking and baking, using low sugar ingredients and packing in as much nutrition as possible into each of the recipes she shares.

Gluten a Go Go (blog: glutenagogo.blogspot.com) - As one of the pioneering gluten-free bloggers, Sheltie Girl cooks and bakes gluten-free (and typically dairy-free) for her three toughest critics, her gluten-eating family. Living with celiac disease, she experiments quite a bit with alternative flours and sweeteners, and takes a healthy approach to both cooking and baking.

Gluten-Free for Good (blog: www.glutenfreeforgood.com) – Beyond just recipes, this blog has a strong emphasis on health. Post categories include such topics as gluten-free (and dairy-free) recipes, nutrition therapy, seasonal foods, and superfoods.

Karina's Kitchen (blog: glutenfreegoddess.blogspot.com) – This is another "wow" blog. It doesn't matter if you are following a special diet or not, Karina's recipes and photos are impossible to resist. Technically, her recipes cater to multiple food allergies, but since gluten-free is her focus, I have included her blog in this category. (*Sample Recipe on p210*)

TACA (website: gfcf-diet.talkaboutcuringautism.org) – Talk About Curing Autism has dedicated a large portion of their site to the GFCF diet, offering numerous resources and a plethora of information and tips.

The GFCF Diet (website: www.gfcfdiet.com) – Touting itself as the "official" GFCF diet support group website, I must admit that this is a good starting place for parents seeking information on dietary intervention or treatment for autism spectrum disorders and support groups.

The Gluten-Free Casein-Free Diet Experience (blog: gfcfexperience.blogspot.com) – Thomas Dzomba is the father of four children, one with autism. He writes about their experiences with the GFCF diet and with autism.

The Good Eatah (blog: thegoodeatah.blogspot.com) – After discovering a gluten and dairy intolerance, the Good Eatah began this blog to archive her GFCF recipes as she learns to cook and eat in a whole new way.

Multiple Food Allergies

Allergic Child (website: www.allergicchild.com) – This website provides a large amount of information for parents of children with food allergies. The content is focused on "safe" living with informational articles and tips. Nicole Smith (one of the founders of the site) is also an author of food allergy children's books.

Allergy Kids (website and blog: www.allergykids.com) – Action-oriented mom Robyn O'Brien started a line of allergy awareness products, maintains a food politics blog, supports food allergy research toward a cure, and speaks out in the media ... and her work can all be followed on the Allergy Kids website.

Allergy Moms (website and blog: www.allergymoms.com) – Gina Clowes created this news portal exclusively for food allergies. It houses blog posts, current news, and a regular e-newsletter on a wide range of topics, including new food allergy research, allergy related product/food recalls, kid and allergy-friendly recipes, and tips for dealing with food allergies in and out of the home. (*Sample Recipe on p196*)

Cooking Allergy Free (website: www.cookingallergyfree.com) – This site offers a recipe database and discussion forum for those living with food allergies. To get the most out of the site, you will need to register, but at last check it was free.

Food Allergy Initiative (research: www.foodallergyinitiative.org) – This non-profit organization raises funds to research a cure and improve the clinical treatment of food allergies.

Foods Matter (e-magazine: www.foodsmatter.com) – Foods Matter magazine is produced specifically for those who live with food allergies and intolerances. They provide a print magazine to customers in the UK, as well as an online version to customers in the US and the UK. Even if you opt to hold off on a subscription, their website is filled with an abundance of helpful information.

Kids with Food Allergies (website: www.kidswithfoodallergies.org) – KFA is a nonprofit online support group for parents of children with food allergies. With a quick and free registration you will have access to their support forums and recipe database on a read only basis. A small annual fee allows full access and use.

Please Don't Pass The Nuts (blog: allergicgirl.blogspot.com) – Sloane Miller (aka Allergic Girl) doesn't just have food allergies; she has dedicated her life to them. Sloane shows people how to still enjoy dining out with severe food allergies via her blog and her latest invention, Worry-Free Dinners™. She also consults school groups and food service organizations on food allergy management.

Test for Allergy (website: www.testforallergy.com) - Neocate®, the makers of infant formula, have provided this quick online allergy test to assess if your child may be suffering from an allergy. It is certainly not meant for diagnosis, but it is a handy little questionnaire to help identify when it may be time to consult a pediatrician.

The Allergic Kid (blog: allergickid.blogspot.com) – This food allergy mom turned blogger offers daily recipes, tips, and findings as she raises her child who has severe allergies to peanuts, eggs, beef, lamb, shellfish, and dairy.

The National Institute of Allergy and Infectious Diseases (NIAID) (website: www.niaid.nih.gov) - If you are interested in finding out about current and past government research in the areas of food allergies or autoimmune disease, then this is the site for you.

YummyAllergenFree (blog: yummyallergenfree.blogspot.com) – Charmaine's husband and three daughters all have severe food allergies. As you may have guessed, her blog possesses family-friendly allergen-free recipes, including many gluten-free options.

More Websites Worth Mentioning

Is that my Bureka? (blog: is-that-my-bureka.blogspot.com) – Bureka boy offers from-scratch recipes with very detailed step-by-step photos. You will find everything from full entrées to homemade pasta and pita pockets. Learning to prepare foods from scratch can be invaluable on a special diet, and luckily, most of his recipes are dairy-free friendly.

Love & Olive Oil (blog: www.loveandoliveoil.com) – There are a few dairy-containing recipes lurking within, but over 100 beautiful dairy-free recipes are just a click away thanks to the neat and tidy format created by Lindsay and Taylor.

Steamy Kitchen (blog: www.steamykitchen.com) – This modern Asian food blog is a site for hungry eyes. Jaden, the author and photographer, is a cooking instructor, and since her focus is Asian food, most of the recipes are dairy-free.

World's Healthiest Foods (website: www.whfoods.org) - This is my primary resource for nutrition related information. When I am seeking foods with certain vitamins or minerals or a way to incorporate some new-to-me vegetables into my diet, this is the first place I go.

Online Shopping

Some people live in major cities with easy access to natural food stores and specialty ingredients, while so many others must rely on a small rural market or mainstream grocers alone for all ingredient needs. For the latter group, I highly recommend you get cozy with online shopping for specialty products. Even though I live in a fairly sizable city, I do find myself purchasing several products online because they are often quite a bit cheaper. Below are some online grocers you may find useful.

Amazon Grocery (www.amazon.com) – Yes, Amazon sells food, and I am a regular customer. At the time of writing, all food had the same deal as their books, free shipping on grocery orders over $25. Food products sold directly from Amazon are typically sold at reasonable prices in bulk quantities, which is excellent for frequently used foods. You will find mostly non-perishable items for sale.

Online Vegan Grocers
The following online stores all sell hard-to-find dairy alternatives for cheese, whipped cream, cream, chocolate, etc., in addition to specialty baking and cooking ingredients, GFCF foods, and vegan vitamins and supplements:

U.S. Based
~   Cosmo's Vegan Shoppe (www.cosmosveganshoppe.com) – ships internationally
~   Ethical Planet (www.ethicalplanet.com) – only ships domestically
~   The Vegan Store from Pangea (www.veganstore.com) – ships internationally
~   The Vegetarian Express (www.thevegetarianexpress.com) – ships internationally
~   The Vegetarian Site (www.thevegetariansite.com) - ships internationally
~   Vegan Essentials (www.veganessentials.com) – ships internationally

Canada Based
~   Viva Granola (www.vivagranola.com) – only ships domestically

U.K. Based
~   Alternative Stores (www.alternativestores.com) - ships internationally
~   Veganstore (www.veganstore.co.uk) – ships internationally

Australia Based
~   The Cruelty-Free Shop (www.crueltyfreeshop.com.au) - only ships domestically

Online Food Allergy & Specialty Grocers

The following online stores also sell hard-to-find dairy alternatives for cheese, whipped cream, cream, milk, chocolate, etc., in addition to specialty baking and cooking ingredients, GFCF foods, and vitamins and supplements ... but they are not specifically vegan. Special diets are their niche, so they each have easy-to-find categories or searches for various "free-from" food allergy needs:

U.S. Based
~ Allergy Grocer (www.allergygrocer.com) - ships internationally
~ Glutenfree.com (www.glutenfree.com) – ships within the U.S. and Canada
~ Juniper Foods (www.juniperfoods.com) - only ships domestically
~ Navan Foods (www.navanfoods.com) - only ships domestically
~ ShopOrganic (www.shoporganic.com) - only ships domestically

U.K. Based
~ Dietary Needs Direct (www.dietaryneedsdirect.co.uk) - only ships domestically
~ Goodness Direct (www.goodnessdirect.co.uk) - only ships domestically
~ The Natural Grocery Store (www.naturalgrocery.co.uk) - only ships domestically
~ Wheat and Dairy-Free (www.wheatanddairyfree.com) - ships internationally

Also, many manufacturers sell/ship their products directly to consumers. I have included company websites throughout the guide as their products are mentioned, and you can find a company contact list (with websites and phone numbers) from www.godairyfree.org.

CHAPTER 28:
OFFLINE READING & RESOURCES

Like websites, there are so many special diet books and cookbooks on the market that it can be mind-boggling. Luckily, the Go Dairy Free team of reviewers (including myself) has had a chance to test-run dozens of them. The books listed below (with mini-summary) include only those that we have trialed and given two thumbs up to.

As you will note, the section for "Strictly Dairy-Free" is quite sparse. Vegan and food allergy cookbooks have eclipsed dairy-free cookbooks in recent years, merging the needs for milk-free with additional special diet requests. Even if you are "just dairy-free" I urge you to enjoy cookbooks that cater to multiple free-from needs, and consequently just happen to be dairy-free. There really are some gems among them.

Strictly Dairy-Free

Levana Cooks Dairy-Free! by Levana Kirschenbaum – Levana invites you to think like a chef, pairing elegant flavors to create rich and creamy sauces, while recognizing comfort food cravings with simple chocolate chip cookies and homemade lasagna. It should be noted that Levana does not shy away from dairy substitutes, nor does she depend on them. They are used where most appropriate in this neatly laid out cookbook complete with full color photos throughout. (*Sample Recipe on p190*)

Vegan

Ani's Raw Food Kitchen by Ani Phyo – I have dabbled in a few raw food cookbooks, but Ani's is the only one that has captured the attention of this avid baker. Unlike the odd complexity of most raw food recipes, Ani actually sticks with the simplicity theme, creating easy recipes that use few ingredients and are generally appealing. Though some raw foodists do use raw dairy in their recipes, Ani keeps it dairy-free and vegan.

Eat Drink & Be Vegan by Dreena Burton – Dreena puts a heavy emphasis on natural foods. She has a fondness for hearty ingredients such as spelt flour and coconut milk, she tosses in extra vegetables at every possible occasion, and she uses just the right amount of sweetener, no more. Yet, she is a master of flavor, and not one of her recipes has let me down to date. The book format is very neat and tidy, with just a handful of pictures thrown in. (*Sample Recipes on p173 and p206*)

Get it Ripe! by jae steele – As someone who loves the taste of "all-natural" foods, I have truly enjoyed the recipes in this cookbook. jae's focus isn't on alternatives for non-vegan recipes, but rather flavorful dishes and desserts that use whole food ingredients. Instead of store-bought dairy and meat substitutes, the ingredient lists call for grains (she typically avoids wheat, using spelt or other grains for most baked goods), natural sweeteners, vegetables, fruits, legumes, nuts, herbs and spices. (*Sample Recipe on p220*)

More Great Good Dairy-Free Desserts Naturally by Fran Costigan – Though the title merely claims dairy-free, this is actually a vegan dessert cookbook (no eggs or honey either). Fran keeps the indulgence factor in her recipes, which range from peanut butter mousse to a colossal chocolate cake, but she sneaks in some whole wheat flour and natural sweeteners whenever suitable. The book layout is a bit hard to follow, with a few pictures randomly thrown in, but the recipes are reliable.

My Sweet Vegan by Hannah Kaminsky – This gift-worthy cookbook offers a beautiful full color photo with every recipe. But beyond looks, the recipes in this dessert and baked goods cookbook really perform, challenging the myth that vegan and indulgence don't belong in the same sentence. In fact, I have come to rely on the Triple Threat Chocolate Cheesecake and Bananas Foster Cake for non-vegan entertaining and the Nut Case Cookies for my own personal cravings. (*Sample Recipe on p242*)

Nonna's Italian Kitchen by Bryanna Clark Grogan – Bryanna is the mother of vegan invention, constantly working to replicate and perfect traditional favorites sans dairy, eggs, and meat. While she has numerous titles under her belt, this is the one I am drawn to most for dairy-free expertise. Bryanna does an excellent job in recreating traditional Italian cuisine, while offering numerous recipes for creamy sauces, "butters," essential faux cheeses, and complete comfort meals. Egg-free consumers will also like the homemade fresh pasta recipes. Keep in mind that creating some of these authentic recipes can be a bit time-consuming. (*Sample Recipes on p172 and p216*)

The Ultimate Uncheese Cookbook by Jo Stepaniak – I actually gravitate toward Jo's Vegan Vittles cookbook (below) for its variety, but if you are seeking a cookbook that offers loads of dairy alternative recipes, then this is your book. Of course, you will find no shortage of "cheesy" sauces and sliceable "cheeses" within, but Jo goes beyond the basics with recipes for blintzes, fondue, pizza, quiche, cheesecakes, lasagna, etc. (*Sample Recipes on p122, p174, and p198*)

The Vegetarian Mother's Cookbook by Cathe Olson – I do not qualify as a vegetarian mother or mother-to-be, but this cookbook is a personal favorite. It contains an abundance of simple, flavorful, and healthy recipes (over 300 in fact) using a wide range of basic, all-natural ingredients. The layout is excellent, with several helpful sections including mothers' only needs, grain and bean cooking charts, notes on high calcium recipes, and more. This cookbook is not a one-size-fits-all for special diets, but most of the recipes are dairy-free and vegan, and there are many gluten-, soy-, egg-, and nut-free recipes throughout. (*Sample Recipes on p123, p134, and p245*)

Vegan Bites by Beverly Lynn Bennett – At the time of writing, I had only just begun exploring this cookbook, but so far the recipes have turned out excellent. Beverly caters to health-oriented single and two person households with recipes that yield 1 to 4 servings and have a quick and easy theme. The cookbook is a nice size, very attractively laid out, and the recipes are far from intimidating. In fact, I would venture to say that even though the recipes target whole food ingredients, they appear to be quite kid-friendly. I expect that this will quickly become one of my go-to cookbooks. (*Sample Recipe on p145*)

Vegan Cupcakes Take Over the World by Isa Chandra Moskowitz and Terry Hope Romero – This mini-sized cookbook is filled exclusively with cupcake and frosting recipes, but they are tasty and creative.

Vegan Fire & Spice by Robin Robertson – Robin is coming very close to obtaining 20 cookbooks under her belt, and with some shame I must admit that this is the first of her cookbooks I have trialed … but it certainly won't be the last. This cookbook is for those who are seeking flavor and a little international adventure, but still want recipes that are simple to create and don't require exotic ingredients. Each recipe is coded from mild to hot, but most can be easily adjusted to taste. The recipes are, for the most part, savory in nature, and the chapters are divided by geographical region. (*Sample Recipe on p200*)

Vegan Lunch Box by Jennifer McCann – I haven't viewed the "upgraded" version of this cookbook, but even the first edition was a fun compilation of easy, kid-friendly recipes and ideas to make even the most novice of cooks look like a creative genius to their little ones. Jennifer's recipes are not elaborate nor are they advanced, but rather they are simple, doable, and down-right tasty.

Veganomicon by Isa Chandra Moskowitz and Terry Hope Romero – This iconic cookbook was famous even before its release. Many vegans I know rely almost solely on this cookbook for their sustenance, referring to it as the vegan bible. Okay, that may be taking things a bit far, but from what I hear, the recipes within are generally tasty, and the cookbook takes an excellent instructional approach.

Vegan Vittles, Second Helpings by Jo Stepaniak – This cookbook is the vegan answer to home-style cooking. All of Jo's cookbooks are vegan, but I have always felt like she has a special place in her kitchen for dairy-free diners. She never fails to address creamy cravings with an abundance of simple yet creative recipes. However, this is my favorite of her cookbooks as it offers a big cross-section of flavors (beyond creamy and cheesy) while including some of the "necessity" recipes from the Ultimate Uncheese Cookbook.

Vegan with a Vengeance by Isa Chandra Moskowitz – Since Veganomicon was released, Isa's first cookbook has been enjoying a quiet resurgence … and some believe that it is still her best work. Vegan with a Vengeance possesses Isa's fun tone of storytelling and political remarks that have helped to make all of her cookbooks a good read, along with recipes that will ease any omnivore into vegan cooking.

Vice Cream by Jeff Rogers – This "cookbook" contains over 70 dairy-free "ice cream" recipes, but it is still on the petite side as far as cookbooks go. The recipes do tend to rely heavily on cashews for their creaminess, so I would not recommend it for the nut allergic. You will need an ice cream maker to fully enjoy these recipes.

Gluten-Free / Casein-Free

Gluten-Free 101 by Carol Fenster – Since the biggest GFCF challenge is baking, I highly recommend this cookbook, which is primarily focused on baking and desserts. The recipes are straight-forward, and though not completely dairy-free, most of the recipes are easily customized (as noted) with milk alternatives (soy, rice, etc.) and dairy-free margarine, without sacrifice to taste or performance. Note that this is not an egg-free cookbook, and you will need ingredients such as a range of gluten-free flours, xanthan gum, guar gum, and gelatin, which are all fairly standard to gluten-free baking.

Gluten-Free Girl by Shauna James Ahern – Shauna loves cheese, so I wasn't expecting to love her book, but this isn't really a cookbook. Rather it is a story that any adult living with a food allergy, intolerance, or autoimmune disease can relate to. At times her poetic writing style gets stuck on repeat, but overall it was a very pleasant and easy read that reminded me I am not alone in my struggles and discoveries. For fun, there are a few recipes randomly (yet strategically) placed throughout this book.

The Gluten-Free Vegan by Susan O'Brien – Finding recipes that are gluten-free, dairy-free, and egg-free is no easy feat. Susan addresses a definite missing link in the special diet cookbook world, and for that reason alone, I feel that her collection is invaluable. The recipes themselves are creative and fairly easy to prepare.

The Ice Dream Cookbook by Rachel Albert-Matesz – Unlike Vice Cream, Rachel whips up dairy-free "ice cream" recipes that focus on the luxuriousness of coconut milk and glycemic-friendly sweeteners, such as agave nectar and stevia. While one might assume an "ice cream" cookbook would be naturally gluten-free, Rachel goes above and beyond, offering gluten-free recipes for "ice cream" cookies, cakes, pies, and of course brownies for those sundae necessities. (*Sample Recipe on p251*)

Food Allergy

Allergen-Free Baking by Jill Robbins – Jill is the founder of HomeFree™ treats, a delicious line of food allergy-friendly cakes and cookies. In this cookbook Jill shares her secrets to fabulous wheat-, nut-, egg-, and dairy-free desserts. Some of the ingredients she uses may seem new-to-you, but the results are perfect, and Jill offers resources to obtain a starter pack of ingredients. This cookbook is not gluten-free. (*Sample Recipe on p230*)

Food Allergy Survival Guide by Vesanto Melina, Dina Aronson, and Jo Stepaniak - The authors of this guide cover "required material," such as explaining food allergies / sensitivities and food allergy testing, but they then move on to new ground that is seldom discussed in the surface world of food allergies, such as "creating and maintaining a healthy intestinal boundary" and "nutrition planning for adults and children." Some of the informational sections are an easy read, while others tackle a little biology. The latter half of this guide is a cookbook with over 100 recipes, all of which are free-from dairy, eggs, fish, gluten, peanuts, shellfish, soy, tree nuts, wheat, and yeast. Some of the recipes are repeats from Jo's other cookbooks, but some are originals from her and the other authors.

How to Manage Your Child's Life-Threatening Food Allergies by Linda Coss - It is essential for anyone who spends time with a food allergic child to understand how to create a safe environment and how to handle an emergency. Linda's book frankly and thoroughly addresses the subject, and is the best introduction to child food allergies that I have ever read. Linda addresses every detail from how to use an EpiPen® to grocery shopping and "play dates." Plus, to really send the message home, she includes stories and testimonials from dozens of parents.

Multi-Lingual Phrase Passport (from the Let's Eat Out! series) by Kim Koeller and Robert La France – I hesitate to recommend the main Let's Eat Out guide here, as it is primarily geared toward gluten-free dining, and contains some inaccuracies about dairy-free dining. However, this passport-sized mini-guide from the same series is excellent for food allergic travel to major countries. It is English-based with French, German, Spanish, and Italian translations for relevant words and phrases. The phrases address various situations (from conversing with waiters to describing symptoms to a doctor) and the food translations cover the "top eight" food allergens (milk, wheat, eggs, soy, fish, shellfish, peanuts, and tree nuts), plus gluten and corn.

Sophie-Safe Cooking by Emily Hendrix – This is an excellent starter cookbook for parents of children with multiple food allergies. All of the recipes are quite simple with tastes and portion sizes that are geared toward little ones. The entire cookbook uses ingredients you can find at virtually any grocery store, and is free of the top eight allergens (milk, eggs, peanuts, tree nuts, wheat, soy, fish, and shellfish). To replace the wheat, Emily relies heavily on oat flour, so gluten-free individuals should proceed with caution. (*Sample Recipe on p222*)

The Whole Foods Allergy Cookbook by Cybele Pascal – This is one of my go to cookbooks as it seamlessly merges gourmet with simple comfort food. I also like that there is no guessing or sifting through recipes. All are free from the top eight allergens: milk, eggs, peanuts, tree nuts, wheat, soy, fish, and shellfish. However, this is not a gluten-free cookbook; Cybele uses spelt flour and oats in many of the recipes. (*Sample Recipe on p202*)

What's to Eat? by Linda Coss – This is truly one of the best basic recipe collections I have come across in years, allergen-free or not. The book itself is meticulous. Concise recipes are neatly framed, one per page, no more, no less. All are dairy-, egg-, and nut-free, yet they do not rely on obscure ingredients. Linda utilizes everyday pantry items to create easy recipes that seldom require more than ten ingredients. (*Sample Recipes on p147, p192, and p219*)

What Else is to Eat? by Linda Coss – Aptly named, this cookbook is like a continuation of Linda's first cookbook. I had the opportunity to act as a recipe tester for this cookbook, and was once again pleased with the ease in preparation, use of common grocery store items, and reliable results.

More Cookbooks Worth Mentioning

Artisan Bread in 5 Minutes a Day by Jeff Hertzberg and Zoe Francois – This cookbook was recommended by a food allergy mom who manages her children's dairy, egg, and nut allergies. Since inexpensive, allergen-free, store-bought bread is becoming a scarce commodity, she found this cookbook to be a wonderful resource for simplifying the at-home bread making process. Most of the recipes suit her special diet needs, or can be easily converted. She uses rice milk in place of the milk and dairy-free margarine in place of the butter. Beyond the recipes themselves, she found the tips and techniques within this book to be invaluable.

Simply Natural Baby Food by Cathe Olson – This is a perfect gift for new moms who are interested in health and nutrition for baby, and who may want to dabble in preparing baby food at home. It is not focused on one single special diet, but rather it offers a variety of recipes for various dietary needs, from vegan to carnivorous. Most of the recipes are dairy-free and vegetarian, but a few contain milk-based products. This is a petite book, but seems to be packed with a good deal of information and recipes, without being overwhelming.

I'm Just Here for the Food by Alton Brown – My dairy-free foodie friend, Sarah, highly recommends this Alton Brown series as "good for understanding food science." She owns his 2002 cookbook, I'm Just Here for the Food: Food + Heat = Cooking. As a long time fan of Alton Brown's recipes from the Food Network online, I have added this one to my own wish list.

Children's Books

Abby the Alley Cat – Staying Safe from Dairy by Myronie McKee, Sam McKee, Adi Rom – This kid-approved book contains cute drawings and a positive, upbeat message that is well received by milk-allergic little ones. It also includes some allergy-related information for parents.

Cody the Allergic Cow by Nicole Smith – Nicole has written several children's books geared toward food allergies, but this is the milk version in her series. Cody is perfect for helping young children and their friends (aged 3 to 5) understand milk allergies.

The Very Non-Dairy Christmas by Stephanie Haag Foraker – Expect this Christmas classic to be on repeat request as the holidays approach in dairy-free households. Stephanie's Santa can't have dairy either, making little ones feel as if they aren't alone. The book is whimsically illustrated and provides a lot of informational dialogue that seems to be well accepted by young ears.

Health-Oriented Books

The China Study by Dr. T. Colin Campbell, Thomas M. Campbell II - This book is a true must read. These researchers embarked on a 20-year real world study of diet, weight loss, long-term health, and nutrition in rural China. Raised on a dairy farm and a former researcher on animal protein, Dr. Campbell's findings during the China Study were remarkable and unbiased to say the least.

The Okinawa Program by Bradley J. Willcox, D. Craig Willcox, Makoto Suzuki - The authors are three doctors who conducted a 25-year Okinawa Centenarian Study to see what made the longest living group tick. It is a fascinating insight into social, physical, and dietary aspects that promote a healthy life.

The Inflammation Syndrome by Jack Challem - This easy to follow book addresses a recent medical focus on internal inflammation, and its role in many chronic and life-threatening diseases. Mr. Challem explains the science and offers simple diet and lifestyle suggestions.

Healthy Women, Healthy Lives: A Guide to Preventing Disease, from the Landmark Nurses' Health Study (Harvard Medical School Book) - This enormous study out of Harvard Medical School followed 225,000 women throughout a 30-year study. The results have offered key insights into heart disease, breast and ovarian cancer, diabetes and other serious illnesses. This isn't an easy read, but it is an eye-opener that expands beyond nutrition, looking at various lifestyle factors and how they affect the health of women.

As we read more, I will continue to update www.godairyfree.org with more product and cookbook reviews, so feel free to check-in.

APPENDIX

Metric Conversions & Equivalents

LIQUID / DRY MEASURES

U.S.	Metric
1/4 Teaspoon	1.25 Milliliters
1/2 Teaspoon	2.5 Milliliters
1 Teaspoon	5 Milliliters
1 Tablespoon	15 Milliliters
1 Fluid Ounce	30 Milliliters
1/4 Cup	60 Milliliters
1/3 Cup	80 Milliliters
1/2 Cup	120 Milliliters
2/3 Cup	160 Milliliters
3/4 Cup	180 Milliliters
1 Cup (8 Fluid Ounces)	240 Milliliters
1 Pint (2 Cups)	480 Milliliters
1 Quart (4 Cups)	960 Milliliters
1 Ounce (by Weight)	28 Grams
4 Ounces (by Weight)	114 Grams
8 Ounces / 1/2 lb (by Weight)	227 Grams
16 Ounces / 1 lb (by Weight)	454 Grams

COOKING MEASUREMENT EQUIVALENTS

U.S.	Metric
1 Tablespoon	3 Teaspoons
1/8 Cup	2 Tablespoons
1/4 Cup	4 Tablespoons
1/3 Cup	5 Tablespoons + 1 Teaspoon
1/2 Cup	8 Tablespoons
1 Cup	16 Tablespoons
1 Gallon	4 Quarts
1 Quart	2 Pints
1 Pint	2 Cups

LENGTH

U.S.	Metric
1/8 Inch	3 Millimeters
1/4 Inch	6 Millimeters
1/2 Inch	12 Millimeters
1 Inch	2.5 Centimeters
1 foot (12 inches)	30 Centimeters

BAKING PANS

U.S.	Metric	Metric Volume
8x5-Inch (Loaf)	20x13 Centimeters	1.8 Liters
9x5-inch (Loaf)	23x13 Centimeters	2 Liters
8x8-Inch	20x20 Centimeters	2 Liters
7x11-Inch	18x27 Centimeters	1.5 Liters
8x12-Inch	20x30 Centimeters	3 Liters
9x13-Inch	23x33 Centimeters	3.5 Liters
8-Inch Round (Cake)	20x4 Centimeters	1.2 Liters
9-Inch Round (Cake)	23x4 Centimeters	1.5 Liters
9-Inch Round (Pie)	23x3 Centimeters	1 Liter

Additional References

CHAPTER 1 - What is Dairy?

~ "Milk Composition and Nutritional Value", Michel A. Wattiaux; Ch. 19 of Dairy Essentials Report; The Babcock Institute for International Dairy Research and Development.

~ "Milk & Milk Products", Clark Ford, Ph.D; Ch. 11 of Food and the Consumer, FSHN 101, Fall 2000; Department of Food Science and Human Nutrition, Iowa State University.

~ "Why It Takes 2,000 Gallons of Fresh Water to Produce One Gallon of Milk," by Mike Adams. The Natural News Network, June 2, 2008.

~ "Which Do You Choose?" A Campaign for Real Milk, The Weston A. Price Foundation.

~ "MDA's role in preventing antibiotic resistance" Minnesota Department of Agriculture.

~ "Milk & Milk Products", Ch.11, Clark Ford, Ph.D; Department of Food Science and Human Nutrition, Iowa State University.

~ "How USDA's Dairy Grading Program Works", US Department of Agriculture.

~ "Newer Knowledge of Milk and Other Fluid Dairy Products," rev. ed., National Dairy Council®: 1993.

~ "The Facts About Pasteurization and Homogenization of Dairy Products," by Jo Hartley. The Natural News Network, April 9, 2008.

~ "Milk Homogenization and Heart Disease," Mary G. Enig, PhD; Wise Traditions in Food, Farming and the Healing Arts, Weston A. Price Foundation, Summer 2003.

~ "An rBGH Overview"; Vermont's Voice (a consumer advocacy organization).

~ "Insulin-like growth factors 1 and 2 in bovine colostrum. Sequences and biological activities compared with those of a potent truncated form."; Biochem J. 1988 Apr 1;251(1):95-103.

~ "Modification of sweet acidophilus milk to improve utilization by lactose-intolerant persons," by McDonough FE, Hitchins AD, Wong NP, Wells P, Bodwell CE. American Journal of Clinical Nutrition 1987 Mar;45(3):570-4.

~ "What is a2 milk™?" The A2 Corporation.

~ "Evolutionary distance from human homologues reflects allergenicity of animal food proteins," by John Jenkins, Heimo Breiteneder, Clare Mills. The Journal of Allergy and Clinical Immunology, DOI: 10.1016/j.jaci.2007.08.019

~ "The natural history of IgE-mediated cow milk allergy," Justin M. Skripak, MD, Elizabeth C. Matsui, MD, MHS, Kim Mudd, RN, Robert A. Wood, MD. Journal of Allergy and Clinical Immunology, Volume 120, Issue 5, Pages 1172-1177, November 2007.

~ "Mare's Milk ...," Foods Matter, October 2007, p12. Report from issue 2608 of New Scientist magazine, 16 June 2007, page 58.

~ "Food Allergies and Camel Milk", Yosef Shabo, Reuben Barzel, Mark Margoulis, and Reuven Yagil; Immunology and Allergies, 796-798, Vol 7, December 2005.

~ "Ask Dr. Sears: Advantages of Goat's Milk" By Dr. William Sears, parenting.com.

CHAPTER 2 – The Many Faces of Non-Dairy Dieters

~ "Milk Allergy Can Persist After Infancy" Clinical and Experimental Allergy study, Dr. A. Carroccio and colleagues, of the University of Palermo; 1998;28:817-823.

~ "Milk Allergy – An Immune System's Response to Milk Proteins", by Judy Tidwell, about.com

~ "Lactose Intolerance"; NIDDK — National Digestive Diseases Information Clearinghouse; NIH Publication No. 06–2751, March 2006.

~ "Specific oral tolerance induction in children with very severe cow milk–induced reactions," Giorgio Longo, MD, Egidio Barbi, MD, Irene Berti, MD, Rosanna Meneghetti, MD, Angela Pittalis, MD, Luca Ronfani, MD, Alessandro Ventura, MD. The Journal of Allergy and Clinical Immunology, Volume 121, Issue 2, Pages 343-347, February 2008.

~ "Lactose Intolerance", Praveen, Roy MD; NIH Publication No. 98-2751, April 1994.

~ "Lactose Intolerance", British Nutrition Foundation, 2000

~ "Lactose Intolerance," Digestive Health, MayoClinic.com

~ "Lactose Maldigestion Fact Sheet," National Dairy Council®. "Overview of lactose maldigestion (lactase nonpersistence)," Inman-Felton AE. Journal of the American Dietetic Association. 1999; 98:481-9.

~ "Lactose Intolerance", Journal of the American Dietetic Association, May 2003.

~ "Physicochemical characteristics of commercial lactases relevant to their application in the alleviation of lactose intolerance," O'Connell S, Walsh G (2006). Appl. Biochem. Biotechnol. 134 (2): 179–91. doi:10.1385/ABAB:134:2:179. PMID 16943638.

~ "The Really BIG List of Lactose Percentages," Steve Carper's Lactose Intolerance Clearinghouse.

~ "The Acceptability of Milk and Milk Products in Populations with a High Prevalence of Lactose Intolerance," Nevin S. Scrimshaw and Edwina B. Murray: American Journal of Clinical Nutrition, 1988;48:1080-1159.

~ "Ingredients for Bakers," Samuel A. Matz. McAllen, TX: Pan-Tech International, 1987.

~ "Galactosemia," National Institute of Health, Genetics Home Reference, January 2008.

~ "How Many Adults Are Vegetarian? The Vegetarian Resource Group Asked in a 2006 National Poll," by Charles Stahler. Vegetarian Journal 2006 Issue 4

~ "Prevalence of Autism Spectrum Disorders — Autism and Developmental Disabilities Monitoring Network, Six Sites, United States, 2000." Morbidity and Mortality Weekly Report, February 9, 2007, Vol. 56, No. SS-1; pages 1-2.

~ "Parent Ratings of Behavioral Effects of Biomedical Interventions," Autism Research Institute, ARI Publ. 34/March 2005.

~ "Fact Sheet: CDC Autism Research," Centers for Disease Control and Prevention, March 4, 2006.

~ "Biomedical and Dietary Approaches", Autism Society of America, autism-society.org.

~ "Diet Changes Give Hyperactive Kids New Taste for Life in Norway," by Nina Larson, AFP and Yahoo! News, Feb. 24, 2008.

~ "Avoiding milk is associated with a reduced risk of insulin resistance and the metabolic syndrome: findings from the British Women's Heart and Health Study." by Lawlor DA, Ebrahim S, Timpson N, Davey Smith G.; Diabetic Medicine, 2005;22:808-11.

~ The Rate of Growth of the Dairy Cow. Extrauerine Growth in Weight," by Samuel Brody and Arthur C. Ragsdale. The Journal of General Physiology (From the Department of Dairy Husbandry, University of Missouri Agricultural Experiment Station, Columbia. February 24, 1921.

~ "Milk, Dairy Fat, Dietary Calcium, and Weight Gain." By Catherine S. Berkey, ScD; Helaine R. H. Rockett, MS, RD; Walter C. Willett, MD, DrPH; Graham A. Colditz, MD, DrPH; Archives of Pediatrics and Adolescent Medicine, 2005;159:543-550.

~ "Avoiding milk is associated with a reduced risk of insulin resistance and the metabolic syndrome: findings from the British Women's Heart and Health Study." By Lawlor DA, Ebrahim S, Timpson N, Davey Smith G.; Diabetic Medicine, 2005;22:808-11.

~ "Dairy products do not lead to alterations in body weight or fat mass in young women in a 1-y intervention" by Carolyn W Gunther, Pamela A Legowski, Roseann M Lyle, George P McCabe, Marianne S Eagan, Munro Peacock and Dorothy Teegarden; American Journal of Clinical Nutrition, Vol. 81, No. 4, 751-756, April 2005.

~ "More Milk Means More Weight Gain." By Rob Stein; Washington Post, Tuesday, June 7, 2005; Page A03.

~ "Milk, Dairy Fat, Dietary Calcium, and Weight Gain." By Catherine S. Berkey, ScD; Helaine R. H. Rockett, MS, RD; Walter C. Willett, MD, DrPH; Graham A. Colditz, MD, DrPH; Archives of Pediatrics and Adolescent Medicine, 2005;159:543-550.

~ "Cheese Industry Profile," by Malinda Geisler, content specialist, AgMRC, Iowa State University and revised February 2008 by Diane Huntrods, AgMRC, Iowa State University.

~ "U.S. Agriculture—Linking Consumers and Producers - What Do Americans Eat?", USDA Agriculture Fact Book, 1998.

~ "A low-fat, vegan diet improves glycemic control and cardiovascular risk factors in a randomized clinical trial in individuals with type 2 diabetes." Barnard ND, Cohen, J, Jenkins DJ, Turner-McGrievy G, Gloede L, Jaster B, Seidl K, Green AA, Talpers S.; Diabetes Care, August 2006 volume 29: pp 1777-1783

~ Diabetes Care, July 2006 (29, 7:1579-84, 2006); Women's Health Study, UCLA

~ "A low-fat, vegan diet improves glycemic control and cardiovascular risk factors in a randomized clinical trial in individuals with type 2 diabetes," Barnard ND, Cohen, J, Jenkins DJ, Turner-McGrievy G, Gloede L, Jaster B, Seidl K, Green AA, Talpers S. Diabetes Care, August 2006 volume 29: pp 1777-1783.

~ "Weight Gain as a Risk Factor for Clinical Diabetes Mellitus in Women" by Graham A. Colditz, Walter C. Willett, Andrea Rotnitzky, and JoAnn E. Manson; Annals of Internal Medicine, April 1995, Volume 122 Issue 7, 481-486.

~ "Physical activity and incidence of non-insulin-dependent diabetes mellitus in women"; Channing Laboratory, Department of Medicine, Harvard Medical School, Boston, Massachusetts; Lancet. 1991 Sep 28;338(8770):774-8.

~ "Vitamin D and Flavonoids Examined for Impact on Breast and Ovarian Cancers," American Association for Cancer Research, April 4, 2006.

~ "A Call for More Vitamin D Research," American Cancer Society, May 27, 2006

~ "Milk and the Cancer Connection" by Hans R. Larsen, MSc ChE; International Health News Issue 76, April 1998.

~ "Milk link to ovarian cancer risk", BBC News, 29 November, 2004.

~ "Hormones in Milk Are Linked to Cancer", by Alison Stewart; Consumer Health Journal, March 2004.

~ "A Prospective Study of Dietary Lactose and Ovarian Cancer", by Fairfield KM, Hunter DJ, Colditz GA, Fuchs CS, Cramer DW, Speizer FE, Willett WC, Hankinson SE; Department of Medicine, Brigham and Women's Hospital, Harvard Medical School, Boston, MA; Int J Cancer, 2004 Jun 10;110(2):271-7.

~ "Harvard Researchers Link Prostate Cancer and Dietary Calcium", CNN, April 4, 2000.

~ "Animal Foods, Protein, Calcium and Prostate Cancer Risk: The European Prospective Investigation into Cancer and Nutrition," Allen NE. Cancer Epidemiology Unit, University of Oxford, Oxford, UK, Br J Cancer. 2008 Apr 1.

~ "Vegan Diet 'Cuts Prostate Cancer Risk", BBC News, 8 June, 2000.

~ "Preventing Prostate Cancer", Bonnie Liebman, Nutrition Action Health Newsletter, July/August 2001.

~ "Dairy, calcium, and vitamin D intakes and prostate cancer risk in the National Health and Nutrition Examination Epidemiologic Follow-up Study cohort", American Journal of Clinical Nutrition, Vol. 81, No. 5, 1147-1154, May 2005.

~ "Does high Soymilk intake reduce prostate cancer incidence? The Adventist Health Study," Jacobsen BK, Knutsen SF, Fraser GE., Institute of Community Medicine, University of Tromso, Norway; Cancer Causes Control. 1998 Dec 9(6):553-7.

~ "Dairy products, calcium, and prostate cancer risk in the Physicians' Health Study", American Journal of Clinical Nutrition, Vol. 74, No. 4, 549-554, October 2001.

~ "Dairy Product, Saturated Fatty Acid, and Calcium Intake and Prostate Cancer in a Prospective Cohort of Japanese Men," by Norie Kurahashi, Manami Inoue, Motoki Iwasaki, Shizuka Sasazuki, and Shoichiro Tsugane for the Japan Public Health Center–Based Prospective Study. Cancer Epidemiol Biomarkers Prev. 2008 Apr;17(4):930-937.

~ "Long-term dietary habits affect soy isoflavone metabolism and accumulation in prostatic fluid in caucasian men", Hedlund TE, Maroni PD, Ferucci PG, Dayton R, Barnes S, Jones K, Moore R, Ogden LG, Wahala K, Sackett HM, Gray KJ; School of Medicine, Department of Pathology, The University of Colorado Cancer Center, Denver; J Nutr. 2005 Jun;135(6):1400-6.

~ "Acne and Milk, the Diet Myth, and Beyond" by F. William Danby, MD, FRCPC; Manchester, New Hampshire; Commentary

~ "Acne: How Food Can Cause It", Food Allergy Solutions Review; News, Ideas & Strategies to Improve Your Health; February 2004.

~ "High School Dietary Dairy Intake and Teenage Acne" by Clement A. Adebamowo, MD, ScD, Donna Spiegelman, ScD, F. William Danby, MD, Lindsay Frazier, MD, Walter C. Willett, MD, DrPH, and Michelle D. Holmes, MD, DrPH; Boston, MA; Hanover, NH; and Ibadan, Nigeria; Research Paper.

~ "Dissociation of the glycaemic and insulinaemic responses to whole and skimmed milk", Hoyt G, Hickey MS, Cordain L, Department of Health and Exercise Science, Fort Collins, CO; Br J Nutr. 2005 Feb;93(2):175-7.

~ "Implications for the role of diet in acne." Cordain L., Department of Health and Exercise Science, Colorado State University; Semin Cutan Med Surg. 2005 Jun;24(2):84-91.

~ "Is migraine food allergy? A double-blind controlled trial of oligoantigenic diet treatment." By authors Egger J, Carter CM, Wilson J, Turner MW, and Soothill JF; Lancet, 1983 Oct 15, 2:8355, 865-9.

~ "Oligoantigenic diet treatment of children with epilepsy and migraine." By Egger J, Carter CM, Soothill JF, and Wilson J of the Department of Neurology, Hospital for Sick Children, London; Journal of Pediatrics, 1989 Jan;114(1):51-8.

~ "Food allergies and migraine." By Grant EC; Lancet. 1979 May 5;1(8123):966-9.

~ "Scientists Identify Migraine Chromosome," Deutsche Welle, September 10, 2005.

~ "Diet & Migraine" by Leira R, Rodriguez R, Servicio de Neurologia, Hospital General de Galicia Clinico Universitario, Santiago de Compostela; Rev Neurol. 1996 May;24 (129):534-8.

~ "What is inflammatory bowel disease?", By V. Alin Botoman, M.D., and Gregory F. Bonner, M.D., Cleveland Clinic Florida, Ft. Lauderdale, Florida; Daniela A. Botoman, M.D., North Broward Hospital District Family Practice Program of the University of South Florida, Coral Springs, Florida; American Academy of Family Physicians, January 1, 1998

~ "Increased prevalence of lactose malabsorption in Crohn's disease patients at low risk for lactose malabsorption based on ethnic origin." By Mishkin B, Yalovsky M, Mishkin S. at the Royal Victoria Hospital, Faculty of Medicine, McGill University, Montreal, Quebec, Canada; American Journal of Gastroenterol; 1997 Jul;92(7):1148-53.

~ "Dietary Factors in Gastrointestinal Diseases", International Foundation for Functional Gastrointestinal Disorders, Inc. (IFFGD); Article by Jarol B. Knowles, M.D., M.P.H.; Spring 2004 issue of Digestive Health Matters

CHAPTER 3 – Building Strong Bones, Calcium and Beyond

~ "Serum retinol levels and the risk of fracture", Michaelsson K, Lithell H, Vessby B, Melhus H. New England Journal of Medicine. 2003;348:387-94. 5.

~ "Dietary Changes Favorably Affect Bone Remodeling in Older Adults"; Journal of the American Dietetic Association 1999;99:1228–1233.

~ "Calcium & Milk: What's Best for Your Bones?" Nutrition Source, Harvard School of Public Health.

~ "Tea drinking is associated with benefits on bone density in older women," Devine, A. The American Journal of Clinical Nutrition, October 2007; vol 86: 1243-1247.

~ "Potassium citrate prevents urine calcium excretion and bone resorption induced by a high sodium chloride diet," Sellmeyer DE, Schloetter DE, Schloetter M et al. J Clin Endo Metab 2002;87(5):2008-12 2002.

~ "Build Better Bones with Bananas," The World's Healthiest Foods, George Mateljan Foundation.

~ "Quality of Rivers of the United States, 1975 Water Year" -- Based on the National Stream Quality Accounting Network (NASQAN): U.S. Geological Survey Open-File Report; Briggs, J.C., and Ficke, J.F. 78-200, 436 p. (1977)

~ "Bioavailability of vitamin D," van den Berg H. Eur J Clin Nutr 1997;51:S76-9. [PubMed abstract]

~ "Dietary Reference Intakes: Calcium, Phosphorus, Magnesium, Vitamin D, and Fluoride." Institute of Medicine, Food and Nutrition Board. Washington, DC: National Academy Press, 1997.

~ "Effectiveness and safety of vitamin D," Cranney C, Horsely T, O'Donnell S, Weiler H, Ooi D, Atkinson S, et al. Evidence Report/Technology Assessment No. 158 prepared by the University of Ottawa Evidence-based Practice Center under Contract No. 290-02.0021. AHRQ Publication No. 07-E013. Rockville, MD: Agency for Healthcare Research and Quality, 2007. [PubMed abstract]

~ "Orange, Grapefruit Juice for Breakfast Builds Bones in Rats", by Kathleen Phillips Texas A&M University, News and Public Affairs, June 5, 2006.

~ "Calcium, vitamin D, milk consumption, and hip fractures: a prospective study among postmenopausal women" by Diane Feskanich, Walter C Willett and Graham A Colditz; American Journal of Clinical Nutrition, Vol. 77, No. 2, 504-511, February 2003

~ J.A.T. Pennington, Bowes and Church's Food Values of Portions Commonly Used; Philadelphia: J.B. Lippincott, 1998.

~ United States Department of Agriculture, Human Nutrition Information Service, Agriculture Handbook Number 8-11.

~ "Calcium," Weaver, C.M. & Heaney, R.P. In Shils, M. et al. Eds. Nutrition in Health and Disease, 9th Edition. Baltimore: Williams & Wilkins, 1999: pages 141-155.

~ USDA Nutrient Database for Standard Reference, Release 19 Web version, Agricultural Research Service, 2006.

CHAPTER 4 – Infant and Childhood Milk Allergies

~ "Allergy Risk Tied to Early Solid Foods," Fiocchi, A. Annals of Allergy, Asthma, and Immunology, July 2006; vol 97: pp.10-21. Alessandro Fiocchi, MD, University of Milan Medical School; chairman, ACAAI Adverse Reactions to Foods Committee. Amal Assa'ad, MD, associate director, division of allergy and immunology, Cincinnati Children's Hospital Medical Center, Cincinnati.

~ "Eight Signs Your Baby Has A Milk Allergy", 365gay.com.

~ "Timing of Solid Food Introduction in Relation to Eczema, Asthma, Allergic Rhinitis, and Food and Inhalant Sensitization at the Age of 6 Years," Results From the Prospective Birth Cohort Study LISA; Anne Zutavern, MDa,b, Inken Brockow, MD, MPHa,c, Beate Schaaf, MDd, Andrea von Berg, MDe, Ulrike Diez, MD, PhDf, Michael Borte, MD, PhDf,g, Ursula Kraemer, PhDh, Olf Herbarth, PhDi, Heidrun Behrendt, MD, PhDj, H-Erich Wichmann, MD, PhDa,k, Joachim Heinrich, PhDa LISA Study Group. PEDIATRICS Vol. 121 No. 1 January 2008, pp. e44-e52 (doi:10.1542/peds.2006-3553).

~ "Effects of Early Nutritional Interventions on the Development of Atopic Disease in Infants and Children: The Role of Maternal Dietary Restriction, Breastfeeding, Timing of Introduction of Complementary Foods, and Hydrolyzed Formulas," Frank R. Greer, MD, Scott H. Sicherer, MD, A. Wesley Burks, MD and the Committee on Nutrition and Section on Allergy and Immunology. PEDIATRICS Vol. 121 No. 1 January 2008, pp. 183-191 (doi:10.1542/peds.2007-3022).

~ "Breast is best, but watch out for the allergies" by Matt Kaplan; New Scientist magazine, 05 August 2006, page 14, 05 August 2006, Issue 2563.

CHAPTER 5 – Other Dairy-Free Concerns

~ "Soy Allergy", about.com, August 13, 2006.

~ "The Science of Soy: What Do We Really Know?" by Julia R. Barrett; Environmental Health Perspectives Volume 114, Number 6, June 2006

~ "Extra Virgin Coconut Oil—the 'Good' Saturated Fat." The Doctors' Prescription for Healthy Living / Volume 7, Number 2, p35-37.

~ "Protein in diet." Medline Plus Medical Encyclopedia. (September 2, 2003). U.S. National Library of Medicine and National Institute of Health.

~ "Protein in the Vegan Diet," by Reed Mangels, Ph.D., R.D. The Vegetarian Resource Group.

~ The Rate of Growth of the Dairy Cow. Extrauerine Growth in Weight," by Samuel Brody and Arthur C. Ragsdale. The Journal of General Physiology (From the Department of Dairy Husbandry, University of Missouri Agricultural Experiment Station, Columbia. February 24, 1921.

~ Nutrition facts from calorie-count.com, nutritiondata.com, and product specific labels

CHAPTER 6 - Restaurant Dining

~ "Want to Watch Calories When Dining Out?" National Restaurant Association, Table service Restaurant Trends, 2001.

~ "Let's Eat Out! – Your Passport to Living Gluten and Allergy Free" by Kim Koeller & Robert La France; R&R Publishing LLC, 2005.
~ "Food Allergies & Other Food Sensitivities"; A Publication of the Institute of Food Technologists; Expert Panel on Food Safety and Nutrition; FoodTechnology, 68-83, Vol.55, No.9, September 2001.

CHAPTER 8 – Decoding Food Labels
~ "Cow's milk casein, a hidden allergen in natural rubber latex gloves," Ylitalo L, Mäkinen-Kiljunen S, Turjanmaa K, Palosuo T, Reunala T. Department of Dermatology, Tampere University Hospital, Tampere, Finland. J Allergy Clin Immunol. 1999 Jul;104(1):177-80.
~ "Dairy or Nondairy? The Experts Speak." Steve Carper's Lactose Intolerance Clearinghouse.
~ "Facts on Wax: Are Vegetable and Fruit Waxes Kosher?," by Rabbi Dovid Heber, Star-K Kashrus Administrator, Star-K Kosher Certification.

Chapter 13 - Moving Beyond Butter
~ "Fats & Oils; Smoking Points," The New Professional Chef, 6th edition, 1996, by The Culinary Institute of America published by John Wiley & Sons.
~ "Smoke Points of Various Fats," by Michael Chu, Cooking For Engineers.

Recipe / Food Allergy Index

This index notes if a recipe is vegan or free from certain ingredients, or if there is an option in the recipe to make the recipe vegan or free from certain ingredients. This index is for basic informational purposes only. Always evaluate the ingredients to ensure that the recipe is safe for you and the ones you are making it for. For example, choose soy-free shortening (p141) and oil (p55) when preparing soy-free meals.

M = Margarine is the only "necessary" soy-containing ingredient (soy-free margarine can be hard to locate)
O = Oats are the only gluten-containing ingredient (certified gluten-free oats may be safe for some)
C = Coconut is the only potential tree nut ingredient (coconut is not always a problem for tree nut allergies)

Dairy Alternatives

Recipe	Page	Vegan	Egg-Free	Soy-Free	Gluten-Free	Wheat-Free	Nut-Free*	Peanut-Free
Homemade Soy Milk	98	X	X		X	X	X	X
Basic Almond Milk	99	X	X	X	X	X		X
Almond-Seed Milk	100	X	X	X	X	X		X
Cooked Rice Milk	101	X	X	X	X	X	X	X
Rice-Cashew Milk Option	101	X	X	X	X	X		X
"Raw" Rice Milk	102	X	X	X	X	X	X	X
Effortless Overnight Oat Milk	103	X	X	X	O	X	X	X
"Authentic" Oat Milk	103	X	X	X	O	X	X	X
Instant Hemp Milk	106	X	X	X	X	X	X	X
Instant Nut Milk	107	X	X	X	X	X		X
Seed Milk	107	X	X	X	X	X	X	X
Potato Milk	108	X	X	X	X	X	X	X
Sweet Cantaloupe Milk	108	X	X	X	X	X	X	X
Apple-Pear Puree	114	X	X	X	X	X	X	X
Prune (Dried Fruit) Puree	114	X	X	X	X	X	X	X
Corn Buttery Spread	115	X	X	X	X	X	C	X
Carrot Whip	115	X	X	X	X	X	X	X
Creamy Margarine Spread	116	X	X	X	X	X	X	X
Whipped Coconut Buttery Spread	116	X	X	X	X	X	X	X
Basic Olive Oil Spread	117	X	X	X	X	X	X	X
Homemade Coconut Butter	117	X	X	X	X	X	C	X
Dairy-Free Feta-ish	120	X	X		X	X	X	X
Bryanna's Quick Tofu "Feta"	120	X	X		X	X	X	X
Sliceable Swiss-Style Cheese	121	X	X	X	X	X		X
Sunflower Seed "Cheese"	121	X	X	X	X	X	X	X
Port Wine Uncheese [Spread]	122	X	X	X	X	X	X	X
Cashew Crème "Cheese"	122	X	X	X	X	X		X
Rich & Nutty Ricotta	122	X	X	X	X	X		X

Recipe	Page	Vegan	Egg-Free	Soy-Free	Gluten-Free	Wheat-Free	Nut-Free*	Peanut-Free
Tofu Ricotta	123	X	X		X	X	X	X
Tofu Cottage "Cheese"	123	X	X		X	X	X	X
Easy Parmesan Substitute	123	X	X	X	X	X	X	X
Definitely Not Parmesan	124	X	X	X	X	X	X	X
Old Reliable Evaporated Milk Alternative	126	X	X	X	X	X	X	X
Evaporated "Milk" from Powder	126	X	X	X	X	X	X	X
Sweetened Condensed Coconut Milk	127	X	X	X	X	X	X	X
Sweetened Condensed "Milk" from Powder	127	X	X		X	X	X	X
"Buttermilk" for Baking	130	X	X	X	X	X	X	X
Silken "Sour Cream"	131	X	X		X	X	X	X
Sour Cashew Crème	131	X	X	X	X	X		X
Susan's Soy Yogurt	133	X	X		X	X	X	X
Coconut Yogurt	133	X	X	X	X	X	C	X
Cathe's Cashew Yogurt	134	X	X	X	X	X		X
White Chocolate	135	X	X	X	X	X	X	X
Quick Chocolate Chunks	136	X	X	X	X	X	X	X
Peanut Butter "Chips"	136	X	X	X	X	X	C	

Breakfast to Brunch

Recipe	Page	Vegan	Egg-Free	Soy-Free	Gluten-Free	Wheat-Free	Nut-Free*	Peanut-Free
Oatmeal Blender Waffles	143	X	X	X	O	X	X	X
Home Baked Granola	144	X	X	X	O	X	X	X
Cream of Multi-Grain Cereal	144	X	X	X	X	X	X	X
Maple Pecan French Toast	145	X	X	X	X	X		X
Pillowy Whole-Grain Pancakes	145	X	X	X		X	X	X
Real Donuts	146	X	X	X			X	X
Breakfast Parfaits	146	X	X	X	X	X	X	X
Mini Crustless Tofu Quiches	147	X	X		X	X	X	X
Cinnamon Roll Biscuits	147	X	X	M			X	X
Light Apricot Scones	148	X	X	X			X	X
Cocoa-Nut Scones	148	X	X	M			C	X

Baking Bread

Recipe	Page	Vegan	Egg-Free	Soy-Free	Gluten-Free	Wheat-Free	Nut-Free*	Peanut-Free
Carrot or Zucchini-Pineapple Bread	150	X	X	X			X	X
Multi-Purpose Muffins	151	X	X	X			X	X

Recipe	Page	Vegan	Egg-Free	Soy-Free	Gluten-Free	Wheat-Free	Nut-Free*	Peanut-Free
Idea: Breakfast "Cupcakes"	151	X	X	X	X	X	X	X
S'Mores Muffins	152	X	X	X			X	X
Maple Wheat Bran Muffins	152	X	X	X			X	X
Perfectly Pear Muffins	153	X	X	X			X	X
Apple Cinnamon Muffin Option	153	X	X	X			X	X
Pumpkin Pecan Raisin Loaf	153	X	X	X				X
Breakfast-Worthy Banana Bread	154	X	X	X		X	X	X
Sinful Cinnamon Bread	154	X	X	X			X	X
Whole Wheat Bread	155	X	X	X			X	X
Perfect Peanut Butter Bread	156	X	X	X			X	X
Tender Squash Dinner Rolls	157	X	X	X			X	X
Savory Sheesy Scones	157	X	X				X	X
Cheesy Potato-Onion Bread	158	X	X	X		X	X	X
Pizza Rolls	159	X	X				X	X

Sips & Smoothies

Recipe	Page	Vegan	Egg-Free	Soy-Free	Gluten-Free	Wheat-Free	Nut-Free*	Peanut-Free
Idea: Smoothie Customization	161	X	X	X	X	X	X	X
True Blue Smoothie	162	X	X	X	X	X	X	X
Peachy Keen Almond Smoothie	162	X	X	X	X	X		X
Super C Smoothie	162	X	X	X	X	X	X	X
Mango Colada	163	X	X	X	X	X	C	X
Cheater's Instant Horchata	163	X	X	X	X	X	X	X
Mexican Chocolate Option	163	X	X	X	X	X	X	X
Chocolate Peanut Butter Shake	164	X	X	X	X	X	X	
Chocolate Almond Shake Option	164	X	X	X	X	X		X
Minty Chocolate (or Carob) Shake	164	X	X	X	X	X	X	X
Minty Chocolate Pudding Option	164	X	X	X	X	X	X	X
Almost Vanilla "Milk" Shake	164	X	X	X	X	X		X
Thick & Spicy Pumpkin Pie Shake	165	X	X	X	X	X	X	X
Coco-Nog	165	X	X	X	X	X		X
Chocolate "Milk"	166	X	X	X	X	X	X	X
Carob "Milk" Option	166	X	X	X	X	X	X	X
Strawberry "Milk"	166	X	X	X	X	X	X	X
Hot Double Chocolate	167	X	X	X	X	X	X	X
Spiced Cocoa Option	167	X	X	X	X	X	X	X
Mocha Option	167	X	X	X	X	X	X	X
Peppermint Cocoa Option	167	X	X	X	X	X	X	X
Carob Cocoa	167	X	X	X	X	X	X	X

Snacks & Apps

Recipe	Page	Vegan	Egg-Free	Soy-Free	Gluten-Free	Wheat-Free	Nut-Free*	Peanut-Free
Instant Pudding	169	X	X	X	X	X	X	X
Instant Creamy Mousse Option	169	X	X	X	X	X	C	X
Pizza Fondue	170	X	X		X	X	X	X
Five-Minute Nachos	170	X	X	X	X	X		X
Rich Eggplant Dip	171	X	X	X	X	X	X	X
Wine-n-Cheese Spread	171	X	X		X	X	X	X
Bryanna's Bagna Cauda	172	X	X	X	X	X	X	X
Hazelnut Bagna Cauda Option	172	X	X	X	X	X		X
Rawesome Nut Dip	173	X	X	X	X	X		X
Perfect Popcorn	174	X	X	X	X	X	X	X
Cheezy Popcorn	174	X	X	X	X	X	X	X
Caramel Popcorn	174	X	X	M	X	X	X	X
Cheezy Quackers	175	X	X	X		X	X	X
Chocolate Figs	175	X	X	X	X	X	X	X
Carob Fudgies	176	X	X	X	X	X	X	X
Trail Mix Carob Fudgies Option	176	X	X	X	X	X		X
Chewy No-Bake Granola Bars	176	X	X	X	O	X	X	X
Fruity Frozen Yogurt Pops	177	X	X	X	X	X	X	X
Your Basic Vanilla Pudding	177	X	X	X	X	X	X	X
Instant Rice Pudding Option	177	X	X	X	X	X	X	X
Banana Pudding Parfaits Option	177	X	X	X	X	X	X	X
Custardy Option	177			X	X	X	X	X
More Menu Ideas: Quick Snacks	178	X	X	X	X	X	X	X

Soup's On

Recipe	Page	Vegan	Egg-Free	Soy-Free	Gluten-Free	Wheat-Free	Nut-Free*	Peanut-Free
Roasted Eggplant & Tomato Soup	181	X	X	X	X	X	X	X
Condensed "Cream" of Mushroom Soup	182	X	X	X	X	X	X	X
"Cream" of Celery Soup Option	182	X	X	X	X	X	X	X
Light Vichyssoise	182	X	X	M	X	X	X	X
Lightly Curried Cruciferous Soup	183	X	X	X	X	X	X	X
Potato Corn Chowder	184	X	X	M			X	X
"Cream" of Asparagus Soup	184	X	X	X	X	X	X	X
"Cream" of Broccoli Soup Option	184	X	X	X	X	X	X	X
Peanut Buttery African Stew	185	X	X	X	X	X	X	

Recipe	Page	Vegan	Egg-Free	Soy-Free	Gluten-Free	Wheat-Free	Nut-Free*	Peanut-Free
Quick & Creamy Bean Soup	185	X	X	X	X	X	X	X
Spiced Autumn Soup	186	X	X	X	X	X	X	X
Cheesy Broccoli Soup	187	X	X	X	X	X		X
Menu Ideas: Old Stand-by Soups	187	X	X	X	X	X	X	X

Simple Sides & Salads

Recipe	Page	Vegan	Egg-Free	Soy-Free	Gluten-Free	Wheat-Free	Nut-Free*	Peanut-Free
Cheese-Free Scalloped Potatoes	189	X	X	M	X	X	X	X
Sweet Potato Apple Casserole	189	X	X	M	X	X	X	X
Baked Cauliflower Au Gratin	190	X	X		X	X	X	X
Almost Traditional Green Bean Casserole	190	X	X		X	X	X	X
Oven Roasted Potatoes	191	X	X	X	X	X	X	X
Spicy Sweet Oven Fries	191	X	X	X	X	X	X	X
Traditional Mashed Potatoes	192	X	X	M	X	X	X	X
Whipped Potatoes	192	X	X	X	X	X	X	X
Lively Lemon Stir-Fry	193	X	X	X	X	X	X	X
Cumin-Spiked Rice and Peas	193	X	X	X	X	X	X	X
Spanish Baked Barley	194	X	X	X		X	X	X
Creamy Wild Rice Salad	194	X	X	X	X	X	X	X
Greek Pasta Salad	195	X	X		X	X	X	X
Seed "Cheese" and Tomato Salad	195	X	X	X	X	X	X	X
Seven Minute Salsa Salad	196	X	X	X	X	X	X	X
Carrot Cake Salad	196	X	X	X	X	X	X	X

Full Meal Deal

Recipe	Page	Vegan	Egg-Free	Soy-Free	Gluten-Free	Wheat-Free	Nut-Free*	Peanut-Free
Elegant Eggplant Cannelloni	197	X	X	X	X	X		X
Lightly Herbed Pasta Alfredo	198	X	X	X	X	X	X	X
French Bread Pizza	198	X	X		X	X	X	X
Creamy Pesto-Inspired Pasta	199	X	X	X	X	X		X
Grilled "Cheese"	199	X	X	M	X	X	X	X
Koushari	200	X	X	X			X	X
Pasta alla Puttanesca	200	X	X	X	X	X	X	X
Very Veggie Lasagna	201	X	X	X	X	X	X	X
Lasagna with Eggplant, Portobello Mushrooms, and Fresh Tomatoes	202	X	X	X	X	X	X	X
Mushroom & Sage Stuffed Bell Peppers	203	X	X	X	X	X	X	X

Recipe	Page	Vegan	Egg-Free	Soy-Free	Gluten-Free	Wheat-Free	Nut-Free*	Peanut-Free
Portobello-Ricotta Ravioli	204	X	X				X	X
Grilled Vegetable Strudel	205	X	X	X			X	X
Roasted Red Pepper Puree	205	X	X	X	X	X	X	X
Thai Chick-un Pizza	206	X	X		X	X	X	
Pizza: No Rise Pizza Crust	207	X	X	X			X	X
Pizza: Gluten-Free Pizza Crust	207	X	X	X	X	X	X	X
Pizza: Wheat-Free Spelt Pizza Crust	208	X	X	X		X	X	X
Pizza: Cooking Free Pizza Sauce	208	X	X	X	X	X	X	X
Nutty Guacamole Enchiladas	209	X	X	X	X	X		X
Red Enchilada Sauce	209	X	X	X	X	X	X	X
Karina's Sweet Potato & Black Bean Enchiladas	210	X	X	X	X	X	X	X
Quickie Green Chile Sauce	210	X	X	X	X	X	X	X
Chinese Five Spice Noodles	211	X			X	X	X	X
Lentil Curry in a Hurry	211	X	X	X	X	X	C	X
Pineapple Teriyaki Bowl	212	X	X		X	X	X	X
Almond Buttery Stir Fry	212	X	X		X	X		X
Sesame Soba Noodles with Calcium-Rich Kale	213	X			X	X	X	X
Menu Ideas: Dairy-Free Meals	214	X	X	X	X	X	X	X

Feelin' Saucy

Recipe	Page	Vegan	Egg-Free	Soy-Free	Gluten-Free	Wheat-Free	Nut-Free*	Peanut-Free
Bryanna's Béchamel or White Sauce	216	X	X	X	X	X	X	X
Mellow Cheesy Sauce	217	X	X	M	X	X	X	X
Macaroni & "Cheese" Option	217	X	X	M	X	X	X	X
Orange Cheesy Sauce	217	X	X	X	X	X	X	X
Macaroni & "Cheese" Option	217	X	X	X	X	X	X	X
Powdered "Cheese" Mix	218	X	X	X	X	X	X	X
Fresh Organic Tomato-Basil Sauce	218	X	X	X	X	X	X	X
Elegant Pantry Marinara	219	X	X	X	X	X	X	X
Sunflower Pesto	219	X	X	X	X	X	X	X
Flavorful Taco Seasoning	220	X	X	X	X	X	X	X
Cashew Gravy	220	X			X	X		X
Tahini Magic Sauce	221	X	X	X	X	X	X	X
Creamy Peanut Sauce	221	X	X		X	X	C	
Spicy-Sweet Mustard Dressing	222	X	X	X	X	X	X	X
Japanese-Style Ginger Dressing	222	X	X		X	X	X	X
Taco Vinaigrette	222	X	X	X	X	X	X	X
5-Star Ranch Dressing or Dip	223	X	X	X	X	X	X	X

Recipe	Page	Vegan	Egg-Free	Soy-Free	Gluten-Free	Wheat-Free	Nut-Free*	Peanut-Free
Creamy Garlic Salad Dressing	223	X	X		X	X	X	X
Menu Ideas: Typically Dairy-Free Dressings	223	X	X	X	X	X	X	X

Sweet Stuff

Recipe	Page	Vegan	Egg-Free	Soy-Free	Gluten-Free	Wheat-Free	Nut-Free*	Peanut-Free
Lemon Streusel Squares	225	X	X	X			C	X
Bakery Style Chocolate Chip Cookies	226	X	X	M			X	X
Chocolate Chip Cookies	226	X	X	X			X	X
Coffee House Cookies	227	X	X	X			X	X
Soft and Chewy Oatmeal Cookies	227	X	X	M			X	X
Maple Spice Pumpkin Cookies	228	X	X	X			X	X
Super Yummy Ginger Cookies	228	X	X	X			C	X
Coconut Fudge Brownies	229			X	X	X	C	X
Peanut Butter Brownie Option	229			X	X	X	X	
Fudge Brownie Cookies	229	X	X	X			X	X
Raisindoras	230	X	X	X		X	X	X
O'Henry Bars	230	X	X	M	O	X	X	X
Pecan Pralines	231	X	X		X	X		X
Peanut Butter "Truffles"	231	X	X	X	X	X	X	
Bittersweet Truffles	232	X	X	X	X	X	C	X
Peanut Butter Chews	232	X	X	X	X	X	X	
Yellow Birthday Cake	233			M			X	X
Simply Wonderful White Cake	234	X	X	X			X	X
Chocolate Wacky Cake	234	X	X	X			X	X
Rice Crispy Cake	235	X	X	X	X	X	X	X
Very Vanilla Frosting	235	X	X	X	X	X	X	X
Banana Crumb Coffee Cake	236	X	X	X			X	X
Sweet Apple Snackin' Cake	237	X	X	X			X	X
Cookies & Cream Muffin-Cakes	237	X	X				X	X
Orange Chocolate Chunk Cupcakes	238	X	X	X			X	X
Chocolate Ganache Frosting	238	X	X	M	X	X	X	X
Whipped Icing	238	X	X	M	X	X	X	X
"Buttercream" Frosting	239	X	X	M	X	X	X	X
Decorator's Option	239	X	X	M	X	X	X	X
Soy-Free White Frosting Option	239	X	X	X	X	X	X	X
"Cream Cheese" Frosting Option	239	X	X		X	X	X	X
Chocolate "Buttercream" Option	239	X	X	M	X	X	X	X
Idea: Baking Box Cake Mixes	239	X	X	X	X	X	X	X

Recipe	Page	Vegan	Egg-Free	Soy-Free	Gluten-Free	Wheat-Free	Nut-Free*	Peanut-Free
Fudgy Chocolate Frosting	240	X	X	M	X	X	X	X
Peanut Butter Fudge Frosting	240	X	X	M	X	X	X	X
Cashew Chai Frosting	240	X	X	X	X	X		X
Key Lime Mousse Pie	241	X	X	X	X	X	C	X
Pumpkin "Cheesecake"	241	X	X		X	X	X	X
Cookie Pie Crust	241	X	X	M	X	X	X	X
Mini Icebox "Cheesecake"	242	X	X		X	X	X	X
Graham Cracker Crust	242	X	X	M	X	X	X	X
Chocolate Espresso Truffle Pie	242	X	X			X	X	X
Virtuous Chocolate Mousse	243	X	X		X	X	X	X
Buttahscotch Dessert Pudding	243	X	X		X	X	X	X
White Chocolate Mousse	243	X	X	X	X	X	X	X
Triple Chocolate Pudding	244	X	X	X	X	X	X	X
Glorified Rice	244	X	X		X	X	X	X
Better Than Ice Cream	245	X	X	X	X	X	X	X
Simply Vanilla Frozen Yogurt	245	X	X	X	X	X	X	X
Very Vanilla "Ice Cream"	246	X	X		X	X	X	X
Luxurious Peanut Butter "Ice Cream"	246	X	X	X	X	X	X	
Coconut Ginger "Ice Cream"	247	X	X	X	X	X	C	X
Pineapple Sherbet	247	X	X	X	X	X	X	X
Mint Stracciatella "Ice Cream"	248	X	X	X	X	X	C	X
Intense Chocolate Sorbet	249	X	X	X	X	X	X	X
Basic Fruit Sorbet	249	X	X	X	X	X	X	X
Cinnamon Coconut Pops	250	X	X	X	X	X	C	X
Carob or Cocoa Pops Option	250	X	X	X	X	X	C	X
Plain Old Vanilla Option	250	X	X	X	X	X	C	X
Piña Colada Option	250	X	X	X	X	X	C	X
Easiest "Ice Cream" Option	250	X	X	X	X	X	C	X
Magical Shell	250	X	X	X	X	X	C	X
Hot Fudge Sauce	251	X	X	X	X	X	C	X
Sweet and Silky Butterscotch Sauce	252	X	X	M	X	X	X	X
Dulce De Coco	252	X	X	X	X	X	C	X
Quick Caramelita Sauce	253	X	X	X	X	X	X	X
Perfect World Whipped Coconut Cream	253	X	X	X	X	X	C	X
Cool Whipped Coconut Cream	253	X	X	X	X	X	C	X

* Tree nut-free (made without (or an option to make without) almonds, cashews, pecans, walnuts, hazelnuts, etc.)

General Index